AF148552

Genetics of Prader-Willi Syndrome

Genetics of Prader-Willi Syndrome

Editors

Merlin G. Butler
David E. Godler

MDPI • Basel • Beijing • Wuhan • Barcelona • Belgrade • Manchester • Tokyo • Cluj • Tianjin

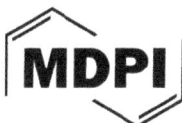

Editors

Merlin G. Butler
Departments of Psychiatry &
Behavioral Sciences and
Pediatrics, University of
Kansas Medical Center,
Kansas City, KS, USA

David E. Godler
Diagnosis and Development,
Murdoch Children's Research Institute,
Royal Children's Hospital,
Melbourne, VIC, Australia

Editorial Office
MDPI
St. Alban-Anlage 66
4052 Basel, Switzerland

This is a reprint of articles from the Special Issue published online in the open access journal *Genes* (ISSN 2073-4425) (available at: https://www.mdpi.com/journal/genes/special_issues/prader-willi_syndr).

For citation purposes, cite each article independently as indicated on the article page online and as indicated below:

LastName, A.A.; LastName, B.B.; LastName, C.C. Article Title. *Journal Name* **Year**, *Volume Number*, Page Range.

ISBN 978-3-0365-5025-1 (Hbk)
ISBN 978-3-0365-5026-8 (PDF)

© 2022 by the authors. Articles in this book are Open Access and distributed under the Creative Commons Attribution (CC BY) license, which allows users to download, copy and build upon published articles, as long as the author and publisher are properly credited, which ensures maximum dissemination and a wider impact of our publications.

The book as a whole is distributed by MDPI under the terms and conditions of the Creative Commons license CC BY-NC-ND.

Contents

About the Editors

Merlin G. Butler

Merlin G. Butler is a physician-scientist engaged in a clinical genetics practice and research programme for children and adults with an emphasis on neurodevelopmental disorders, congenital anomalies, cytogenetic defects, Prader–Willi syndrome, genetics of autism and morbid obesity, advanced genetic testing technology and pharmacogenetics with genotype–phenotype correlations, and the natural history and delineation of rare and uncommon genetic syndromes. He received his MD from the University of Nebraska and his PhD in medical genetics from Indiana University. He is an American Board of Medical Genetics-certified practitioner of Clinical Genetics and Clinical Cytogenetics and is a founding fellow of the American College of Medical Genetics and Genomics. He is a professor of psychiatry, behavioural sciences, and paediatrics; the director of the Division of Research and Genetics; and the medical director of KUMC Genetics Clinic at the University of Kansas Medical Center. He has published over 500 research articles in journals such as *Nature*, *New England Journal of Medicine*, *Lancet*, and *JAMA Network Open*, with 150 dedicated to Prader–Willi syndrome, and multiple book chapters and edited several journal issues and textbooks.

David E. Godler

David E. Godler is an associate professor at the University of Melbourne and a group leader of the Diagnosis and Development Laboratory at the Murdoch Children's Research Institute. He has a BSc (biomedical—honours) degree and PhD in genetics from Monash University. Dr Godler has performed postdoctoral research studies on epigenetic disorders associated with chromosomal abnormalities and developmental delays at the Murdoch Children's Research Institute, University of Melbourne and Victorian Clinical Genetics Services. His work centres on improved diagnoses, natural history studies, and outcome measures for clinical trials for rare diseases associated with intellectual disability and autism, including Angelman, Prader–Willi, Dup15q, and fragile X syndromes. His research also focuses on newborn screening for rare diseases and understanding underlying mechanisms responsible for epigenetic disorders associated with intellectual disability and autism. In recognition of his capability to deliver translational outcomes, in 2018, he was awarded the Clinical Researcher Career Development Fellowship funded by the Medical Research Future Fund to investigate the significance of low-level mosaicism to intellectual disability in paediatric disorders. He has published over 50 research articles, reviews in such quality journals as Genetics in *Medicine*, *Clinical Chemistry*, *Neurology*, *JAMA Neurology*, *JAMA Network Open*, and *Molecular Autism*, and has edited several journal issues.

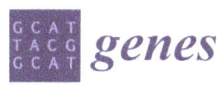

genes

Editorial

Special Issue: Genetics of Prader–Willi Syndrome

David E. Godler [1,2] and Merlin G. Butler [3,*]

[1] Royal Children's Hospital, Murdoch Children's Research Institute, Parkville 3052, Australia;
     david.godler@mcri.edu.au
[2] Department of Paediatrics, University of Melbourne, Parkville 3052, Australia
[3] Departments of Psychiatry & Behavioral Sciences and Pediatrics, University of Kansas Medical Center,
     Kansas City, KS 66160, USA
* Correspondence: mbutler4@kumc.edu; Tel.: +1-913-588-1800; Fax: +1-913-588-1305

Citation: Godler, D.E.; Butler, M.G. Special Issue: Genetics of Prader–Willi Syndrome. *Genes* **2021**, *12*, 1429. https://doi.org/10.3390/genes12091429

Received: 7 September 2021
Accepted: 10 September 2021
Published: 16 September 2021

Publisher's Note: MDPI stays neutral with regard to jurisdictional claims in published maps and institutional affiliations.

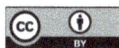

Copyright: © 2021 by the authors. Licensee MDPI, Basel, Switzerland. This article is an open access article distributed under the terms and conditions of the Creative Commons Attribution (CC BY) license (https://creativecommons.org/licenses/by/4.0/).

This Special Issue includes 15 peer-reviewed articles for publication by experts in Prader–Willi syndrome (PWS) and their reflective area of interest impacting this rare disorder. These articles were divided subjectively into three groups: (1) Genetics, three articles; (2) Clinical, 10 articles; (3) Other, two articles. They yield new information to improve our understanding of PWS and treatment approaches for those affected by this rare disorder. This Special Issue, captured in book form, includes the latest research reported by experts in the field of genetics, clinical observations, and disease natural history studies, as well as characterization and treatment approaches in PWS. This should be of great interest for families, care givers, health care providers, students of and experts in PWS, clinicians, research scientists and clinical and behavioral health providers, educators, and geneticists.

The Special Issue begins with a single case study of appetite control in PWS with experience reported over 12 years by Griggs [1] with the use of an Indian extract for management of hyperphagia in a case report format and illustration. This report introduces and emphasizes the importance of clinical trials and therapeutic options under development to treat the cardinal features of this condition, that is, hyperphagia and subsequent marked obesity, if uncontrolled. A second article in this Special Issue reported by Manzardo et al. [2] included a questionnaire survey of venous thrombosis in PWS, as attention to blood clots has emerged in clinical studies, and they are now recognized in individuals with PWS and should be monitored accordingly. Blood clots are significant risk factors for injury and death in PWS. Along the theme of thrombosis and blood clots in PWS, Butler et al. [3] reported on age distribution, comorbidities, and reported risk factors for blood clots and showed an increased occurrence of thrombotic events across all age cohorts with PWS, stressing the importance of surveillance for thrombosis.

Advances in database and diagnostic technologies have offered new opportunities to collect and integrate data from a broad range of sources at earlier ages to advance understanding of PWS. This awareness has led to the development of a global PWS registry, with participants from 37 countries completing over 23,000 surveys. Bohonowych et al. [4] reported that the emphasis of this registry was to improve understanding of natural history and to support medical product development for PWS. Furthermore, early diagnosis of PWS may reduce obesity and associated comorbidities. This concept was emphasized by Kimonis et al. [5] who reported that early diagnosis of PWS did delay the onset of obesity or children becoming overweight. Early diagnosis can lead to early treatment with growth and other hormones and approaches to further reduce the risk of obesity- associated comorbidities as an outcome. Holland et al. [6] further defined mental and behavioral disturbances that occur in genetically determined neurodevelopmental syndromes such as PWS and generated a model that brings together diagnostic–psychologic developmental approaches with the aim of matching specific behaviors and their neural mechanisms focused on PWS.

A PWS-like phenotype, caused by a rare atypical 15q11.2 microdeletion, was reported in a patient by Tan et al. [7] using whole exome sequencing; this was compared with others in the literature with similar atypical deletions. Their data further supports the notion that paternal *SNORD116* snoRNA plays a key role in cardinal PWS phenotypes. In an effort to describe food- and non-food-related behaviors of children with PWS between ages 3 to 18 years in the home and school settings, Gantz et al. [8] undertook a study utilizing questionnaire forms to better characterize and appreciate these behaviors in those with this rare disorder. Their research may help inform strategies to reduce behavioral problems and improve outcomes. On treatment and intervention of scoliosis in PWS, van Bosse and Butler [9] described clinical and surgical experiences in scoliosis, kyphosis, and kyphoscoliosis, which are commonly seen in children and adolescents with this disorder. They also described a higher prevalence rate for spinal deformities. The study suggested that a better understanding of the risk involved in surgically treating children with PWS is of clinical importance.

A potential role of activating the ATP sensitive potassium (KATP) channel in the treatment of hyperphagia and obesity was introduced and summarized by Cowen and Bhatnagar [10]. They reported on the role of potassium channel activation and the mechanistic involvement of the regulation of appetite in humans, and a better understanding of the breath and impact of this process remains a viable target for treatment in PWS. Furthermore, growth trajectories in PWS were described in a cohort of males and females, and their genetic subtypes were examined by Shepherd et al. [11]. Their cohort of 125 individuals with PWS showed that height was similar for males in both deletion and non-deletion subtypes. However, weight and BMI were estimated to be higher in the deletion subtype, with the size of difference increasing with advanced age. Peng et al. [12] also reported on the gut microbiota profiles in children with PWS, in which these data are sparse. They found that overall gut bacterial diversity was not different from those with PWS compared with controls, but specific bacterial genera and fungal community were different. The variation was not attributed to differences in dietary intake, or the impact of genetic subtypes seen in PWS. They propose that further longitudinal studies are needed to characterize the gut microbiota profile in PWS and its role. Rubin et al. [13] then reported on a 24-week physical activity intervention program in PWS and found increases in bone mineral content without changes in bone markers in the youth with PWS via this intervention. They found that the youth with PWS had increased spine bone mineral content following physical activity interventions; however, bone remodeling markers remained unaltered. Montes et al. [14] reported on genetic subtype–phenotype analysis in PWS while individuals were on growth hormone treatment and examined their psychiatric behavior. They found that skin picking was more frequent in those with the chromosome 15q11-q13 deletion compared to non-deletion (maternal disomy 15), while anxiety was more common in those with maternal disomy compared to the deletion. An increased frequency of anxiety was noted in the maternal disomy group when treated with the growth hormone when compared to the deletion group. Lastly, Forster et al. [15] reported on pharmacogenetic testing of cytochrome P450 drug metabolizing enzymes and medication management in a case series of patients with PWS and found differences in the frequency of specific P450 genes encoding liver enzymes metabolizing specific classes of drugs. A potential limitation of this study is the small number of subjects presenting for care with a skewed genetic subtype patterns (i.e., more patients with maternal disomy found than anticipated), but if replicated, the findings might have an impact on the response of drugs selected for medical care and treatment. Further studies are needed with a larger cohort of individuals with PWS to confirm these observations. The study also suggested that pharmacogenetic testing together with PWS genetic subtyping may inform clinicians of selection of psychotropic medications and dosing parameters for those at risk of adverse events or decreased therapeutic response in those with this rare genetic obesity related disorder.

There are now over 3500 published articles on PWS since its first description in 1956, and there is a growing need to gain a better understanding of cause, diagnosis, and treatment related to specific clinical presentations, genetic findings, and pathophysiology.

The contents of this Special Issue should stimulate clinical-based and basic research with the development of therapeutic approaches to treat hyperphagia, obesity, and the behavioral problems common in those affected with this disorder.

Funding: Next Generation Clinical Researchers Program—Career Development Fellowship, funded by the Medical Research Future Fund (MRF1141334 to D.E.G.).

Conflicts of Interest: The authors declare no conflict of interest.

References

1. Griggs, J. Single-Case Study of Appetite Control in Prader-Willi Syndrome, over 12-Years by the Indian Extract Caralluma fimbriata. *Genes* **2019**, *10*, 447. [CrossRef] [PubMed]
2. Manzardo, A.M.; Heinemann, J.; McManus, B.; Loker, C.; Loker, J.; Butler, M.G. Venous Thromboembolism in Prader–Willi Syndrome: A Questionnaire Survey. *Genes* **2019**, *10*, 550. [CrossRef] [PubMed]
3. Butler, M.G.; Oyetunji, A.; Manzardo, A.M. Age Distribution, Comorbidities and Risk Factors for Thrombosis in Prader–Willi Syndrome. *Genes* **2020**, *11*, 67. [CrossRef] [PubMed]
4. Bohonowych, J.; Miller, J.; McCandless, S.E.; Strong, T.V. The Global Prader–Willi Syndrome Registry: Development, Launch, and Early Demographics. *Genes* **2019**, *10*, 713. [CrossRef] [PubMed]
5. Kimonis, V.E.; Tamura, R.; Gold, J.-A.; Patel, N.; Surampalli, A.; Manazir, J.; Miller, J.L.; Roof, E.; Dykens, E.; Butler, M.G.; et al. Early Diagnosis in Prader–Willi Syndrome Reduces Obesity and Associated Co-Morbidities. *Genes* **2019**, *10*, 898. [CrossRef] [PubMed]
6. Holland, A.J.; Aman, L.C.S.; Whittington, J.E. Defining Mental and Behavioural Disorders in Genetically Determined Neurodevelopmental Syndromes with Particular Reference to Prader-Willi Syndrome. *Genes* **2019**, *10*, 1025. [CrossRef] [PubMed]
7. Tan, Q.; Potter, K.J.; Burnett, L.C.; Orsso, C.E.; Inman, M.; Ryman, D.C.; Haqq, A.M. Prader–Willi-Like Phenotype Caused by an Atypical 15q11.2 Microdeletion. *Genes* **2020**, *11*, 128. [CrossRef] [PubMed]
8. Gantz, M.G.; Andrews, S.M.; Wheeler, A.C. Food and Non-Food-Related Behavior across Settings in Children with Prader–Willi Syndrome. *Genes* **2020**, *11*, 204. [CrossRef] [PubMed]
9. Van Bosse, H.J.P.; Butler, M.G. Clinical Observations and Treatment Approaches for Scoliosis in Prader–Willi Syndrome. *Genes* **2020**, *11*, 260. [CrossRef] [PubMed]
10. Cowen, N.; Bhatnagar, A. The Potential Role of Activating the ATP-Sensitive Potassium Channel in the Treatment of Hyperphagic Obesity. *Genes* **2020**, *11*, 450. [CrossRef] [PubMed]
11. Shepherd, D.A.; Vos, N.; Reid, S.M.; Godler, D.E.; Guzys, A.; Moreno-Betancur, M.; Amor, D.J. Growth Trajectories in Genetic Subtypes of Prader–Willi Syndrome. *Genes* **2020**, *11*, 736. [CrossRef] [PubMed]
12. Peng, Y.; Tan, Q.; Afhami, S.; Deehan, E.C.; Liang, S.; Gantz, M.; Triador, L.; Madsen, K.L.; Walter, J.; Tun, H.M.; et al. The Gut Microbiota Profile in Children with Prader–Willi Syndrome. *Genes* **2020**, *11*, 904. [CrossRef] [PubMed]
13. Rubin, D.A.; Wilson, K.S.; Orsso, C.E.; Gertz, E.R.; Haqq, A.M.; Castner, D.M.; Dumont-Driscoll, M. A 24-Week Physical Activity Intervention Increases Bone Mineral Content without Changes in Bone Markers in Youth with PWS. *Genes* **2020**, *11*, 984. [CrossRef] [PubMed]
14. Montes, A.S.; Osann, K.E.; Gold, J.A.; Tamura, R.N.; Driscoll, D.J.; Butler, M.G.; Kimonis, V.E. Genetic Subtype-Phenotype Analysis of Growth Hormone Treatment on Psychiatric Behavior in Prader-Willi Syndrome. *Genes* **2020**, *11*, 1250. [CrossRef] [PubMed]
15. Forster, J.; Duis, J.; Butler, M.G. Pharmacogenetic Testing of Cytochrome P450 Drug Metabolizing Enzymes in a Case Series of Patients with Prader-Willi Syndrome. *Genes* **2021**, *12*, 152. [CrossRef] [PubMed]

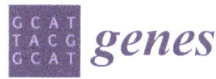

Case Report

Single-Case Study of Appetite Control in Prader-Willi Syndrome, Over 12-Years by the Indian Extract *Caralluma fimbriata*

Joanne Griggs

Institute of Health and Sports, College of Health and Biomedicine, Victoria University, P.O. Box 14428, Melbourne, VIC 8001, Australia; joanne.griggs@vu.edu.au; Tel.: +61-399-192-203

Received: 16 May 2019; Accepted: 5 June 2019; Published: 12 June 2019

Abstract: This paper reports on the successful management of hyperphagia (exaggerated hunger) in a 14yr-old female with Prader–Willi syndrome (PWS). This child was diagnosed with PWS, (maternal uniparental disomy) at 18 months due to developmental delay, hypertonia, weight gain and extreme eating behaviour. Treatment of a supplement for appetite suppression commenced at 2 years of age. This single-case records ingestion of an Indian cactus succulent *Caralluma fimbriata* extract (CFE) over 12 years, resulting in anecdotal satiety, free access to food and management of weight within normal range. CFE was administered in a drink daily and dose was slowly escalated by observation for appetite suppression. Rigorous testing determined blood count, vitamins, key minerals, HbA1c, IGF-1 and function of the liver and thyroid all within normal range. The report suggests a strategy for early intervention against hyperphagia and obesity in PWS. This case was the instigator of the successful Australian PWS/CFE pilot and though anecdotal, the adolescent continues to ingest CFE followed by paediatricians at the Royal Children's Hospital Melbourne, Victoria, Australia. Future clinical trials are worth considering, to determine an appropriate dose for individuals with PWS.

Keywords: Prader-Willi syndrome; appetite treatment; *Caralluma fimbriata* extract; single-case

1. Introduction

Prader-Willi syndrome (PWS) establishes a disrupted appetite with complex physical, behavioural and intellectual issues at a prevalence of 1:15,000–1:30,000 [1,2]. The predominant difficulty in PWS is an exaggerated appetite and a complex physiology which causes obesity. The hypothalamic dysfunction in PWS may be similar to early onset obesity or hypothalamic obesity [3,4] however, in PWS the disturbed neuroendocrine physiology is due to simultaneous non-functioning genes of the paternal chromosome in the critical region 15q11.2–q13. In PWS the characteristic appetite phenotype is established over three main phases [5] through: (1) 'failure to thrive' (newborn); (2a) increased weight gain with minimal adjustment in caloric intake; (2b) increased interest in food and caloric intake with a switch to hyperphagia at the median of 54 months and (3) the propensity to excessive eating (mean age 8 years). Typically, hyperphagia includes an impaired satiety [6,7]. Similar to obesity reported due to mutations in the PCSK1 gene [8], PWS establishes hypogonadotropic, hypogonadism and growth deficits. However, in PWS the obsessional eating behaviours determines the PWS phenotype to be life-threatening. Hypothalamic disruptions, the extent of which are unknown, interact with physiological deficits including growth hormone deficiency. Hypotonicity also exacerbates obesity propensity by making exercise and energy balance difficult. As in non-syndromic polygenic obesity, low caloric intake is important; however, in PWS this is constant and life-long. A range of interventions are necessary to correlate with each phase; however, to date there is no prescribed intervention or treatment for the switch to hyperphagia. Research into appetite supplements is limited [9,10] and management guidelines suggest interventions of diet, exercise and supervised access to food.

This is difficult due to individualized anxiety and obsessional behaviours. Typically the most utilized intervention is life-long familial limit setting and external food surveillance, which for many includes locked environments [11,12].

Caralluma fimbriata extract (CFE)—the intervention—is well known in Ayurvedic medicine. This shrub grows wild throughout India, Pakistan and Afghanistan [13] and has been ingested for centuries amongst populations as a natural appetite suppressant or as a vegetable substitute in times of famine [13,14]. It is reported that genetic deletion of small nucleolar RNA (SnoRNA) including the snord116 and snord115 contribute to the hyperphagia in PWS [15–17]. One of the most important recognized disruptions is within the hypothalamic pathways, which are disturbed due to disrupted SnoRNA115/HBII-52 transcription known to interact with transcription of the serotonin (5Hydroxytryptamine; 5-HT) 5-HT2c receptor. This receptor is involved in anorexigenic signalling within hypothalamic appetite pathways of the central nervous system (CNS). Previously we reported that an extract of *Caralluma fimbriata* (CFE) used as the intervention in this case study was involved in enhancing 5-HT2c receptor activity in a PWS animal model [18]. This activity conforms to a model of increased satiety.

This single-case reports on continued management of PWS hyperphagic behaviours for a 14 year-old female (M) who has exhibited appetite at the highest eating code level: 5 [5]. Unusually, chronic administration of the natural supplement, CFE—a powdered cactus succulent extract—has been successful in maintaining reduced interest in food and a normal weight, over a period of 12 years in individuals.

2. Case Study

This single female case-study was one of twins (2004). M's gestation was quiet compared to her brother and the birth was at 37 weeks by a double breach caesarean to a polyhydramnios mother of 42years-old. Both twins recorded a high Apgar score of 8/10, though M was administered oxygen straight after delivery. At 2 h M had multiple tonic-clonic seizures, was hypothermic, hypoglycaemic, had divergent gaze, hyperflexia and clonus. She was transferred to intensive care. A magnetic resonance imaging (MRI) determined the newborn had extra axial space in the brain. M was administered phenobarbital for seizures and was nasogastric tube fed due to "failure to thrive". The other twin was jaundiced, placed in special care and was discharged at 5 days. M was transferred to special care at 2 weeks and was discharged at 5 weeks still nasogastric tube fed. Even though the core features of PWS were apparent, including small size, hypotonicity (low muscle tone) and an inability to suck or swallow [19,20], chromosome analysis was only conducted to rule out common disorders. An electroencephalogram (EEG) scan showed abnormal spike wave activity and awkward postures were noted. The diagnosis was recorded at discharge as encephalopathy and suspected Cerebral Palsy, until further investigations. After discharge the parents stopped both the seizure medication and tube feeding at 8 weeks and M was fed by formula in an adapted bottle. No further tonic-clonic seizures were seen however, absence seizures continued till 10 years.

The parents devised an intervention program from 4 months [21] and M's feeding became normalized at 9 months, weight gain was seen at 12 months, however unusually—for encephalopathy—weight was recorded on the 90-percentile whilst height remained on the 3rd-percentile on the general public early weight/height for age guidelines. Hunger was noticed and celebrated; due to past difficulties at 14 months, however, M continued to eat past the amount of her twin brother. Observed behaviours included exaggerated crying, tantrums and reddening of the face. The facial reddening was perhaps due to unexplained seizures. As the parents were unaware of PWS, they utilized the exaggerated hunger to help M ambulate. For example, food was placed on a coffee-table and shifted around to help M weight-bare and walk. M would follow food with the table's assistance. When left to her own devices with food nearby, M would continue to eat and would not stop of her own accord (video recordings on request).

Diagnosis of PWS was made at 18 months due to M's weight gain and eating behaviour. The genetic female molecular karyotype showed one long continuous stretch of homozygosity (17.5 Mb) along chromosome 15, suggestive of maternal uniparental disomy (UPD). Other typical identifying features included small hands and feet, dysmorphic facial features, light skin pigmentation and severe developmental delay. Non appetite related issues experienced by M were vision impairment, deteriorating teeth, scoliosis, early puberty, repetitive questioning, skin picking until 12 years and anxiety.

3. Treatment Methodology

At 29 months of age CFE was sourced by the parents. Careful dosage of the product Slimaluma was considered by direct communication with the manufacturers. CFE was given for breakfast daily, in tropical juice (to cover the organic taste) at half a capsule (250 mg). The treatment dose was raised by 250 mg increments as necessitated by signals of reduced satiation. The commercially recommended adult dose is 1000 mg/d to be taken at 2×500mg doses. In M's case the full dose was taken at once and after 12 years (Table 1) is 2000 mg/d. Further increases may no longer be available.

Table 1. Age and anthropometric measurements in single-case with Prader-Willi syndrome (PWS) ingesting *Caralluma fimbriata* extract (CFE) . Anthropometric measurements behavioural indications of hyperphagia and additional intervention/exercise, in a single case of a female with PWS ingesting CFE over 12 years. The case begins as a newborn and ceases at 14 years and 4 months of age. Weight in Kg—kilograms, height in cm—centimetres, nil—represents no intervention, dose in mg—milligrams, per d—day.

Age Yr/Month	Weight Kg	Height Cm	Dose Mg/d	Food/Hyperphagia	Indication	Other Intervention
Birth	2.35	Unsure	nil	Failure to thrive	Unable to suck	Tube fed, phentobarbatal
2.3 months	3.7	55	nil	Feeding slowly	Take out nasogastric tube	Feeding extremely slowly; adapted bottle
8 months	6.5	65	nil	Normalised appetite	Bottle fed	Feeding slowly with adapted bottle
12 months	8.2	68	nil	Normalised appetite	Bottle fed and soft food	Adapted bottle exercise program
18 months	12	72	nil	Increased hunger	Obese and ambulating after food	Diet 100% home exercise program
20 months	12.9	78	nil	Eating constantly	Obese, always hungry ambulating after food	DIAGNOSIS
2 years	12.5	82.5	nil	Hyperphagia	Obesity, tantrums around food and always hungry	Diet 60% home exercise program
2 years, 4 months	12	85	250	Satiated	Saying no to dinner and leaving food on plate	Diet 60% home exercise program
4 years, 11months	19	104	500	Access to food with supervision	Saying no to dinner and minimal asking for food.	Diet 60% home exercise program
6 years, 6 months	23	112	NIL for 6 days	Ceased CFE hyperphagia returned after 1.5 days	Tantrums around food after 1.5 days. Licking empty plate	Diet 60% ballet once weekly
6 years, 6 months	23	112	500	Hunger persisted 1 day	Confirmation of satiety and interested in other activities	Diet 60% ballet once weekly
7 years, 1 month	23.5	114	750	Non-restricted with supervision	Both hunger and satiety	Diet 60% ballet once weekly
7 years, 9 months	25	119	1000	Non-restricted with supervision	Saying no to dinner and minimal hunger.	Diet 60% ballet once weekly
8 years, 8 months	29	124	1000	Non-restricted with supervision	Interested in food	Diet 60%, routine no exercise
9 years, 7 months	30	126	1250	Non-restricted with supervision	Forgetting to eat food provided	Diet 60%, routine no exercise
10 years, 1 months	34	128	1250	Non-restricted with supervision	Minimal communication of hunger.	Diet 60%, routine no exercise
11 years, 8 months	37	129	1250	Non-restricted with supervision	Minimal communication of hunger and throws out school treats.	Diet 60%, routine ballet once weekly

Table 1. *Cont.*

Age Yr/Month	Weight Kg	Height Cm	Dose Mg/d	Food/Hyperphagia	Indication	Other Intervention
12 years, 5 months	38	134	1500	Non-restricted with supervision	Minimal communication of hunger. Makes own lunch.	Diet 60%, routine swimming weekly
13 years, 1 month	39	136	1750	Non-restricted; attempting no supervision	Communication of both hunger, "I'm hungry", and satiation "I'm full".	Diet 60%, routine swimming weekly
14 years, 4 months	43	141	2000	Non-restricted environment.no supervision	Communication hunger and takes self out of difficult situations.	Diet 60%, self-managed swimming weekly

4. Results

During the earliest years of the intervention the child volunteered that "she felt full", and "was not hungry", instead wanting to draw (video if requested). This was a significant adjustment in comparison to recorded previous appetite behaviours, which were utilized as an instigator for movement. From 2–4 years, satiety eventually reduced in increments noticed by an increased asking for food. Each time this was observed the dose was increased by 250 mg/d. Within a day of increased administration, decreased hunger was noted. The dose therefore followed a simple pattern: expressed hunger, adjustment of dose and observed satiety. This process continued over 12 years with the most recent 250 mg/d increase raising the dose to 2000 mg/d in 2018. Each time with the amount settled upon there has been sustained successful appetite behaviour and freedom around food. All foods have been allowed within the diet however, M has been educated on the nutritional and caloric values of foods. It was noticed that M naturally initiates drinking a daily allowance of water (1 L/d).

Other medications administered were fluoxetine (LOVAN 20 mg, 9–14 years) for anxiety and Growth Hormone Therapy. Though there is clear evidence to support Growth Hormone (GH) use in PWS, it had been deemed that M was allergic to GH as after administration of a low dose of GH at two timelines, M showed signs of an allergic reaction including fluid retention and dark, puffy eyes. There is no known link to the intervention.

In 2010, M ceased taking the CFE extract for 6 days. Obvious changes to behaviour were recorded, including, crying and tantrums due to food. These remonstrations were far stronger than that observed by the parents when deciding to increase the dose. After 6 days the parents resumed administering CFE and continued with a routine of a broad diet with restricted daily caloric intake to 60%. The indicators of distress or hunger ceased within days and satiety resumed with M forgetting to eat after three days of CFE intervention (videos of before and after available).

Interestingly, certain of M's behaviours are not attenuated by CFE. These behaviours may be due to anxiety and not hyperphagia, as they occur when M reports no hunger. These behaviours are: Skin picking; asking and telling; feeding babies and animals and wanting to know the routine of the day. These behaviours are moved-on easily during CFE administration.

Over the 12 years of administration there have been no adverse effects. The parents suggest administration of savory salted foods increases focus after ingestion. Thirst for water may be an unusual effect of CFE. Over the 12 years gastric emptying had not been an issue. In 2011 after 4 years and 6 months administration of CFE, M was administered blood tests to determine any undue toxicity or adverse effect due to CFE administration. The measures noted in Table 2, including kidney, thyroid and liver function, blood count, IGF and HbA1C—measure of hyperglycaemia, were all within normal range. Endocrine tests for central adrenal insufficiency (CAI) also recorded levels within normal range. After 12 years, comprehensive blood tests determined M's blood serum to be all within normal range (Table 2) apart from the lowering of triglycerides.

Table 2. Blood serum measures after 12 years of treatment *Caralluma fimbriata* extract (CFE) intervention. Blood serum measures after 12 years of treatment CFE ingestion, in a single-case of a 14-year-old female with Prader-Willi syndrome (PWS). IFCC - International Federation of Clinical Chemists; NGSP - National Glycohemoglobin Standardization Program; Hct – haematocrit; RCC – red cell count; MCV – mean corpuscular volume; MCH – haemoglobin devided by the number or red cells; RDW – red blood cell width and distribution; EDTA as an anticoagulant, INR—international normalized ratio and APTT—activated partial thromboplastin.

Specimen Type/Time 13:52	Serum Value	Reference Range
25-OH Vitamin D	65	50–160 nmol/L
Vitamin A	1.2	0.9–2.5 µmol/L
Vitamin E	21	13–24 µmol/L
Calcium	2.27	2.10–2.60 nmol/L
Magnesium	0.70	0.70–1.20 nmol/L
Phosphate	1.45	1.10–1.80 nmol/L
Cholesterol	3.7	3.1–5.4 nmol/L
Triglyceride	0.8 (L)	0.9–2.0 mmol/L
Vitamin E/Lipid ratio	4.8	0.9–7.1 umol/mmol
Active Vitamin B12(Holotranscobalamin)	49.7	19–128 pmol/L
Ferritin	36	9–136 µg/L
Specimen type	**Whole Blood EDTA**	
HbA1c (IFCC)	31	26–39 mmol/mol
HbA1c (NGSP)	5.0	4.5–5.7%
Red Cell Folate	2925	1800–3700 µmol/L
Haemoglobin	122	120–160 g/L
Hct	0.36	0.36–0.46
RCC	4.00	$4.0–5.2 \times 10^{-12}$/L
MCV	90	78–97 fL
MCH	30.4	25–33 pg
RDW	12.5	11.0–14.0%
Platelets	197	$150–400 \times 10^{-9}$/L
White Cell Count	7.3	$4.5–13.5 \times 10^{-9}$/L
Neutrophils	4.22	$1.8–8.0 \times 10^{-9}$/L
Lymphocytes	2.59	$1.2–5.2 \times 10^{-9}$/L
Monocytes	0.42	$0.1–1.0 \times 10^{-9}$/L
Eosinophils	0.07	$0.0–0.5 \times 10^{-9}$/L
Basophils	0.02	$0.0–0.1 \times 10^{-9}$/L
Specimen	**Serum plasma**	
Zinc	9.5	9.2–15.4 µmol/L
Selenium	1.0	0.6–1.9 µmol/L
Thyroid stimulating hormone	2.96	0.50–4.50 mIU/L
Specimen	**Blood plasma**	
INR	1.1	0.8–1.2 ratio
APTT	34	27–44 s
Fibrinogen	2.4	1.5–4.3 g/L
Liver Function test	**Serum**	
Total Bilirubin	2	0–15 unmol/L
Unconjugated Bilirubin	2	0–10 unmol/L
Bilirubin	0	0–5 unmol/L
Neutrophils	26	10–30 IU/L
Lymphocytes	117	100–350 IU/L
Monocytes	<10	0–40 IU/L
Eosinophils	72	57–80 g/L
Basophils	44	33–47 g/L
Urea, Creatinine & Electrolytes		
Sodium	140	135–145 mmol/L
Potassium	4.2	3.5–5.0 mmol/L
Chloride	102	98–110 mmol/L
Urea	5.4	2.1–6.5 mmol/L
Creatinine	34	30–80 µmol/L

Weight reduced at the time of administration of CFE and had been stabilized to conform within a normal range. M's diet remained at a 60% ratio (of someone the same weight), though food with lower sugar was preferable. Lipids seemed necessary within the diet to maintain homeostasis and salt maintained alertness. Exercise was preferred, though due to GH allergy, M's muscle tone did not increase. Even so, M was active and energetic.

5. Discussion

This study establishes a case for management of hyperphagia by daily CFE administration in PWS. Over a 12-year-period hyperphagic behaviours have been contained without adverse effects in one child/adolescent with PWS. The prediction of obesity [22] has also been halted by this family's management of dietary routine, exercise, supervision and CFE supplementation. The reduction of food has been accepted with continual adjustment in dose of CFE. Further, the adolescent's weight has continued to decline over time. An important discussion point within this case-study is that continued maintenance of weight reduction could need a dose escalation past 2000 mg/d. The parents have chosen to longer increase the dose. Dose escalation has been gradual and though CFE is well tolerated, it is inevitable that the dose may continue to escalate until BMI and adolescent growth stop progressing. At this time, it has been confirmed that M's growth is close to its ceiling, therefore the set dose may not be a problem. Though CFE has been deemed safe by multiple safety assessments [23] dose may be a limitation to this intervention's capacity. Dose studies are necessary for a dose-weight ratio to be established. In the past Victoria University has piloted a successful study of CFE treatment in children and adolescents with PWS (n = 16), over a four-week period [10] —instigated by this anecdotal evidence. Future study will need to include adults with established hyperphagia; obesity and measures of glycaemic control would be preferable. Thirst may also be an important measure as M's instinct to drink is unusual for individuals with PWS.

Another point to consider is that the management of hyperphagic behaviours in PWS are quite taxing on families. In M's case her behaviours were similarly taxing during the 6 days without CFE in 2010, where vehement hunger was expressed. It is not clear if the hyperphagic distress experienced by M over the short experimental cessation of CFE was her natural hyperphagia or a stronger hyperphagia due to the years of satiety. Unfortunately, this connotes, anecdotally that there is no residual effect of CFE over time.

6. Conclusions

In conclusion, this single-case determined that an extract of the Indian cactus succulent *Caralluma fimbriata* eased hyperphagic over a 12-year-period. When the treatment was stopped for 6 days, excessive hunger returned. Therefore, anecdotally CFE administration appears to create abstinence from food within free access, leading to a routine natural cycle of appetite homeostasis, including both hunger and satiety. Unfortunately, CFE does not create a residual effect and dose-weight ratios must be defined to reduce confusion around dose adjustments to attenuate appetite behaviours. Even though this family aimed for independence without supervision for their daughter, dose escalation and phenotypical difficulties may have hindered this goal. This single-case study suggests that CFE increases satiety and maintains weight overtime, within parameters of caloric restriction without adverse effects or compromising blood serum measures.

Funding: This research received no external funding.

Acknowledgments: The author acknowledges Michael Mathai and Victoria University for their support and Gencor Pacific for its funding of VU's preliminary studies of this PWS intervention.

Conflicts of Interest: The author declares no conflict of interest. However, it is noted that the author of this single-case is also the parent of M.

References

1. Tuysuz, B.; Kartal, N.; Erener-Ercan, T.; Guclu-Geyik, F.; Vural, M.; Perk, Y.; Erginel-Unaltuna, N. Prevalence of Prader–Willi syndrome among infants with hypotonia. *J. Pediatr.* **2014**, *164*, 1064–1067. [CrossRef] [PubMed]

2. Whittington, J.; Holland, A. Neurobehavioral phenotype in Prader-Willi syndrome. *Am. J. Med. Genet. Part. C* **2010**, *154*, 438–447. [CrossRef] [PubMed]

3. Haliloglu, B.; Bereket, A. Central Control of Energy Metabolism and Hypothalamic Obesity Pediatric Obesity. *Springer* **2018**, *30*, 27–42.

4. Lee, J.M.; Shin, J.; Kim, S.; Gee, H.Y.; Lee, J.S.; Cha, D.H.; Uçar, A. Rapid-onset obesity with hypoventilation, hypothalamic, autonomic dysregulation, and neuroendocrine tumors (ROHHADNET) Syndrome: A systematic review. *BioMed. Res. Int.* **2018**. [CrossRef] [PubMed]

5. Goldstone, A.; Holland, A.; Butler, J.; Whittington, J. Appetite hormones and the transition to hyperphagia in children with Prader-Willi syndrome. *Int. J. Obes.* **2012**, *36*, 1564. [CrossRef] [PubMed]

6. Benelam, B. Satiation, satiety and their effects on eating behaviour. *Nutr. Bull.* **2009**, *34*, 126–173. [CrossRef]

7. Holland, A. The Paradox of Prader Willi syndrome: A genetic model of starvation. *J. Int. Disabil. Res.* **2008**, *52*, 811. [CrossRef]

8. Ramos-Molina, B.; Molina-Vega, M.; Fernández-García, J.; Creemers, J. Hyperphagia and obesity in Prader-Willi syndrome: PCSK1 deficiency and beyond? *Genes* **2018**, *9*, 288. [CrossRef]

9. Griggs, J.L.; Sinnayah, P.; Mathai, M.L. Prader–Willi syndrome: From genetics to behaviour, with special focus on appetite treatments. *Neurosci. Biobehav. Rev.* **2015**, *59*, 155–172. [CrossRef]

10. Griggs, J.L.; Su, X.Q.; Mathai, M.L. Caralluma fimbriata supplementation improves the appetite behavior of children and adolescents with Prader-Willi syndrome. *N. Am. J. Med. Sci.* **2015**, *7*, 509.

11. Butler, M.G. Management of obesity in Prader-Willi syndrome. *Nat. Rev. Endocrinol.* **2006**, *2*, 592–593. [CrossRef] [PubMed]

12. Miller, J.L.; Lynn, C.H.; Shuster, J.; Driscoll, D.J. A reduced-energy intake, well-balanced diet improves weight control in children with Prader-Willi syndrome. *J. Hum. Nutr. Diet.* **2013**, *26*, 2–9. [CrossRef] [PubMed]

13. Kuriyan, R.; Raj, T.; Srinivas, S.K.; Vaz, M.; Rajendran, R.; Kurpad, A.V. Effect of caralluma fimbriata extract on appetite, food intake and anthropometry in adult Indian men and women. *Appetite* **2007**, *48*, 338–344. [CrossRef] [PubMed]

14. Kamalakkannan, S.; Rajendran, R.; Venkatesh, R.V.; Clayton, P.; Akbarsha, M.A. Antiobesogenic and antiatherosclerotic properties of caralluma fimbriata extract. *J. Nutr. Metab.* **2010**, 285301.

15. Bortolin-Cavaillé, M.-L.; Cavaillé, J. The SNORD115 (H/MBII-52) and SNORD116 (H/MBII-85) gene clusters at the imprinted Prader-Willi locus generate canonical box C/D snoRNAs. *Nucleic Acids Res.* **2012**, *40*, 6800–6807. [CrossRef]

16. Falaleeva, M.; Surface, J.; Shen, M.; de la Grange, P.; Stamm, S. SNORD116 and SNORD115 change expression of multiple genes and modify each other's activity. *Gene* **2015**, *572*, 266–273. [CrossRef]

17. Polex-Wolf, J.; Lam, B.Y.; Larder, R.; Tadross, J.; Rimmington, D.; Bosch, F.; Rainbow, K. Hypothalamic loss of Snord116 recapitulates the hyperphagia of Prader-Willi syndrome. *J. Clin. Investig.* **2018**, *128*. [CrossRef]

18. Griggs, J.L.; Mathai, M.L.; Sinnayah, P. Caralluma fimbriata extract activity involves the 5-HT2c receptor in PWS Snord116 deletion mouse model. *Brain Behav.* **2018**, *8*, e01102. [CrossRef]

19. Holm, V.A.; Cassidy, S.B.; Butler, M.G.; Hanchett, J.M.; Greenswag, L.R.; Whitman, B.Y.; Greenberg, F. Prader-Willi syndrome: Consensus diagnostic criteria. *Pediatrics* **1993**, *91*, 398–402.

20. Whittington, J.E.; Holland, A.J.; Webb, T.; Butler, J.; Clarke, D.; Boer, H. Relationship between clinical and genetic diagnosis of Prader-Willi syndrome. *J. Med. Genet.* **2002**, *34*, 926–932. [CrossRef]

21. Griggs, J. *Miracle in Potential*; Braidwood Press: Melbourne, Australia, 2010.

22. Holson, L.; Zarcone, J.; Brooks, W.M.; Butler, M.; Thompson, T.; Ahluwalia, J.S.; Nollen, N.L.; Savage, C.R. Neural mechanisms underlying hyperphagia in Prader-Willi syndrome. *Obesity* **2006**, *14*, 1028–1037. [CrossRef] [PubMed]

23. Odendaal, A.Y.; Deshmukh, N.S.; Marx, T.K.; Schauss, A.G.; Endres, J.R.; Clewell, A.E. Safety assessment of a hydroethanolic extract of caralluma fimbriata. *Int. J. Toxicol.* **2013**, *32*, 385–394. [CrossRef] [PubMed]

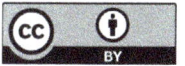 © 2019 by the author. Licensee MDPI, Basel, Switzerland. This article is an open access article distributed under the terms and conditions of the Creative Commons Attribution (CC BY) license (http://creativecommons.org/licenses/by/4.0/).

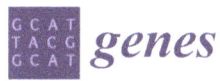

Article

Venous Thromboembolism in Prader–Willi Syndrome: A Questionnaire Survey

Ann M. Manzardo [1], Janalee Heinemann [2], Barbara McManus [2], Carolyn Loker [2], James Loker [3] and Merlin G. Butler [1,*]

[1] Departments of Psychiatry & Behavioral Sciences and Pediatrics, University of Kansas Medical Center, Kansas City, KS 66160, USA
[2] Prader-Willi Syndrome Association (USA), Sarasota, FL 34238, USA
[3] Department of Pediatrics, Bronson Hospital, Western Michigan University, Kalamazoo, MI 49008, USA
* Correspondence: mbutler4@kumc.edu; Tel.: +1-913-588-1800; Fax: +1-913-588-1305

Received: 5 June 2019; Accepted: 16 July 2019; Published: 19 July 2019

Abstract: Prader–Willi Syndrome Association (USA) monitors the ongoing health and welfare of individuals with Prader–Willi syndrome (PWS) through active communication with members by membership surveys and data registries. Thromboembolism and blood clots have emerged in clinical studies as significant risk factors for injury and death in PWS. A 66-item questionnaire was developed by a panel of PWS medical and scientific experts, with input from Prader–Willi Syndrome Association (USA) leadership, so as to probe their membership on the frequency, risk, and protective factors for venous thromboembolism, pulmonary embolism, and related findings. The characteristics of those with and without a reported history of blood clots and related health factors were tabulated and analyzed. Responses were obtained for 1067 individuals with PWS (554 females and 513 males), and 38 (23 females and 15 males) had a history of blood clots. The individuals with clots did not differ by gender, but were significantly older 32.8 ± 15 years vs 20.4 ± 13 years, and were more likely to have a reported history of obesity (76%), edema (59%), hypertension (24%), vasculitis (33%), and family history of blood clots (33%) than those without clots. Growth hormone treatment was more common in individuals without clots. The risk factors for thromboembolism in PWS overlap those commonly observed for the general population.

Keywords: Prader–Willi syndrome; thromboembolism; risk factors; vasculitis; blood clots

1. Introduction

Prader–Willi syndrome (PWS) is a complex neurodevelopmental genetic disorder as a result of errors in genomic imprinting. Characteristics include infantile hypotonia; hypogonadism and hypogenitalism; poor suck reflex with feeding difficulties during infancy; developmental delay with mental deficiency; growth and other hormone deficiencies with small hands and feet; short stature; a particular facial pattern and behavioral problems including skin picking, obsessive compulsions, and hyperphagia leading to obesity, if not externally controlled [1–4]. PWS is considered the most common genetic cause of marked obesity in humans, with an estimated 350,000 to 400,000 people worldwide, and more than 15,000 individuals in the USA [5]. The incidence is between 1 in 10,000–20,000. A paternally derived chromosome 15q11-q13 deletion is seen in about 60% of individuals, and maternal disomy 15 (both chromosome 15s inherited from the mother) is seen in about 35% of cases, while the remaining individuals have a defect of the chromosome 15 imprinting center controlling the imprinted genes or other chromosome 15 abnormalities (translocations or inversions) [6].

Recent reviews in causes of death and survival trends in Prader–Willi syndrome have increased our awareness of the mortality and risk factors contributing to death, specifically blood clots and pulmonary embolism [7,8]. Pulmonary embolism (PE) is the fourth most common reported cause of death in PWS, reported in over 400 deceased patients studied from the PWSA (USA) registry database, and blood clots as a cause of death have also been reported in clinical trials [7,9]. PE is also a recognized cause of death in obese individuals, as well as in our society. Beckman et al. [10,11]. further estimated that more than 300,000 Americans have had an episode of deep venous thrombosis (DVT) or pulmonary embolism, and it is now recognized as a growing public health concern associated with considerable morbidity and mortality. It affects all races, ethnicities, age groups, and both genders. Other known risk factors include an advanced age, surgery, and immobility. Learning more about the burden and causes of venous thromboembolism (VTE), and better surveillance by the public and medical community with advanced research, has the potential to prevent or at least reduce morbidity and death. This knowledge could also apply to obesity-related genetic disorders such as PWS, possibly at a young age. For example, a newborn female with PWS has been reported in the literature, with neonatal cerebral venous thrombosis [12].

Previous studies have shown that choking, swallowing difficulties, excessive eating, and obesity, if not externally controlled, can occur in early childhood, and gastric necrosis in adults, leading to death in PWS [2,13]. Furthermore, factors reported recently that contribute to mortality in PWS include increased weight, heart problems, sleep apnea and other respiratory complications, diabetes, osteoporosis, high pain tolerance, severe skin picking, and the duration of growth hormone use [8,14]. Hence, obesity and its subsequent consequences are primary contributors to mortality in PWS.

We developed a large nationwide survey to entertain questions about the natural history and factors related to thromboembolism and blood clots as a cause of death in PWS.

2. Materials and Methods

A health-related questionnaire was developed so as to assess the occurrence of vascular issues, blood clots, deep vein thrombosis, and/or pulmonary embolism in PWS, and to characterize the contributing factors based on the frequency of known risk factors from PWS and the general population. The survey material was compiled by a team of researchers and health care providers experienced in PWS in consultation, along with PWSA (USA) leadership. The resulting 66-item health-related questionnaire was posted at the PWSA (USA) website for access by more than 3000 parents or caregivers in the database registry, and was offered as a voluntary survey (see Questionnaire Form, (Figure 1)). Participation was also solicited from the PWSA (USA) membership through an email link, or, in some cases, as a hard copy sent to families if requested by regular mail. The caregivers of children and adults with PWS (living or deceased) were asked to fill out the survey, even without a history of clots, so as to help learn more about the contributing factors or aspects related to blood clots. The dates of that the survey occurred were between January 2015 to April 2016, with 1067 respondents participating in the study.

The questionnaire included standard demographic information (e.g., age, gender, weight, height, and PWS genetic subtype) and medical history, such as obesity status, presence or absence of metabolic syndrome, diabetes, edema, kidney problems, hypertension, vasculitis, and growth hormone treatment. Information on blood clots included the onset, location, duration, and severity, with or without a positive family history, vasculitis, or known blood clotting disorders such as Factor V Leiden, prothrombin (Factor II), methylene tetrahydrofolate reductase (MTHFR), Protein S, or Protein C deficiencies, and their treatment. Information about the PWS genetic subtypes and methylation status was requested, as well as PWS deletion subtypes.

Respondents were probed regarding experiences over the lifetime of their charge, with current biometrics of age, height, and weight; or the last data available if the individual was deceased. Individual responses to the questionnaire were initially screened for errors by the PWSA (USA) staff, who resolved inconsistencies and confirmed answers with respondents prior to analysis. If a history of blood clots or bleeding disorders were noted on the questionnaire form, a medical expert (e.g., physician knowledgeable about PWS and specialized in cardiovascular disease (co-author, J.L.)) and/or PWSA (USA; staff member (co-authors, B.M. or C.L.)) made contact with the respondent to clarify any questions and responses prior to data inclusion and analysis. The final de-identified dataset was examined, as well as the descriptive statistics, frequencies, and means generated using SAS statistical software version 9.2 (SAS Institute Inc. Cary, North Carolina, USA). Primary statistical analyses included an analysis of variance (ANOVA) for the continuous data and the chi-squared test for categorical measures.

Today's Date: _____ / _____ / _____

1. Name of person with PWS_____
2. Sex: Male___ Female____
3. Date of Birth: _____ / _____ / _____
4. Current height: inches _____
5. Current weight: pounds _____
6. Was genetic testing done for PWS (circle)? Y N UNKNOWN
7. Was the individual found to be methylation positive for PWS (circle)? Y N UNKNOWN
8. What PWS subtype was identified (circle)?
   a. Deletion
   b. Maternal disomy 15 (UPD)
   c. Imprinting defect (ID)
   d. PWS subtype not determined
9. If the individual is deletion subtype then are they,
   a. Deletion type 1
   b. Deletion type 2
   c. Atypical deletion
   d. Deletion type Unknown/Unspecified
10. Was the person with PWS ever on growth hormone? Y N UNKNOWN
11. Is the person a severe skin picker? Y N UNKNOWN
12. Is the person with PWS a smoker or former smoker? Y N UNKNOWN

Does/did the person with PWS have any of the following conditions?

13. Metabolic syndrome? Y N UNKNOWN
14. Diabetes mellitus? Y N UNKNOWN
15. Renal (kidney) disease? Y N UNKNOWN
16. A history of lower leg swelling (edema)? Y N UNKNOWN
17. Hypertension (high blood pressure)? Y N UNKNOWN
18. Vasculitis (inflammation of the blood vessels)? Y N UNKNOWN
19. Atrial fibrillation (heart rhythm problem)? Y N UNKNOWN
20. Heart failure? Y N UNKNOWN
21. Atherosclerosis (coronary artery disease)? Y N UNKNOWN
22. Antiphospholipid Antibody Syndrome (an autoimmune clotting disorder)? Y N UNKNOWN
23. Any Bone Marrow Disorders? Y N UNKNOWN
24. Thrombocythemia (high platelet count)? Y N UNKNOWN
25. Thrombotic Thrombocytopenic Purpura and Disseminated Intravascular Coagulation (rare blood clotting disorders)? Y N UNKNOWN
26. Was the person ever diagnosed or treated for cancer? Y N UNKNOWN

Family history of close blood relatives (parent, sibling and children) to the individual with PWS

27. Is there a family history of blood clots? Y N UNKNOWN
28. Is there family history of any of the following specific clotting/blood disorders:
   a. Factor 5 Leiden deficiency? Y N UNKNOWN
   b. Prothrombin (factor 2) deficiency? Y N UNKNOWN
   c. Methylene tetrahydrofolate reductase (MTHFR) deficiency? Y N UNKNOWN
   d. Protein S deficiency? Y N UNKNOWN
   e. Protein C deficiency? Y N UNKNOWN

Was the individual with PWS EVER taking the following medications?

29. Aspirin therapy to prevent clotting? Y N UNKNOWN
30. Blood thinners (Coumadin, Lovenox, Heparin, Plavix, etc.)? Y N UNKNOWN
31. For Females: Medicines that may contain estrogen such as birth control pills or hormone therapy? Y N UNKNOWN
32. For Males: testosterone? Y N UNKNOWN
33. Low (hypo) thyroid treatment? Y N UNKNOWN
34. High (hyper) thyroid treatment? Y N UNKNOWN
35. Adrenal gland treatment such as cortisol medication? Y N UNKNOWN
36. Has the person with PWS ever had DVT/clots/thrombosis? Y N UNKNOWN

IF #36 is No then skip to question 56.

37. At what age(s) did the DVT/clots/thrombosis occur?_____
38. At what age was the most severe episode? _____
39. Was this severe episode fatal? Y N UNKNOWN
40. What was the type of severe episode (circle)? DVT, Thrombosis, Embolism or a smaller surface vein clot?
41. Was the occurrence associated with a recent injury or surgical procedure? Y N UNKNOWN
42. Was the person with PWS diabetic at the time of the episode? Y N UNKNOWN
43. Was the person with PWS on growth hormone at the time of the episode? Y N UNKNOWN
44. Was the person with PWS taking any other hormones at the time of the episode? Y N UNKNOWN
45. If #44 is yes, then what hormones?_____
46. Was the clot in the lung or legs, UNKNOWN, other_____
47. Was hospitalization required? Y N UNKNOWN
48. Were blood tests (D-dimer) to look for clots abnormal? Y N UNKNOWN
49. Did the individual with PWS complain of pain with the clot? Y N UNKNOWN
50. On a scale of 0 (no pain) to 5 (severe pain) rate the pain (circle): 0 1 2 3 4 5 UNKNOWN
51. Have the clot or clots resolved? Y N UNKNOWN
52. Has the clot re-occurred? Y N UNKNOWN

If the clot was in the LEG,

53. Was there leg swelling at time of clot? Y N UNKNOWN
54. Was there brownish or reddish discoloration on the lower legs at the time of the clot? Y N UNKNOWN
55. Were compression stockings used? Y N UNKNOWN

Person filling out this form

56. Name _____
57. Relationship to person with PWS_____
58. Address_____
59. Email_____
60. Phone Number_____
61. May PWSA (USA) call or email you if any additional answers are needed? Yes No

Figure 1. Vascular Blood Clots, Deep Vain Thrombosis and/or Thrombosis in Prader-Willi Syndrome Questionnaire.

3. Results

A total of 1067 respondents completed the survey describing outcomes for n = 554 females and n = 513 males with PWS (Table 1). The described PWS subjects had a current mean age of 21.0 ± 14 years with a range of 0 to 63 years, with 502 (47%) being less than 18 years of age. Eight hundred and seventy-five of the 1067 (82%) respondents reported a PWS genetic subtype, with 527 (60%) reporting the typical 15q11-q13 deletion, 325 (37%) reporting maternal disomy 15, and 23 (3%) reporting an imprinting defect similar to the reported frequencies of the genetic subtypes recently described by Butler et al. [6] in a PWS cohort (n = 510 subjects) using advanced genetic testing (e.g., high-resolution chromosomal microarrays) in the largest analysis of PWS genetic subtype frequencies to date.

Table 1. Sample characteristics for n = 1067 total on Prader–Willi syndrome (PWS).

Variables	Overall (n = 1067)	Clots (n = 38)	No Clots (n = 1013)	χ^2; F	p–Value
Female sex	554 (52%)	23 (62%)	531 (52%)		
Male sex	513 (48%)	15 (41%)	498 (49%)	1.3	0.26
Reported PWS Subtype	**875 (82%)**	**20 (54%)**	**855 (84%)**		
Deletion Subtype	527 (60%)	12 (60%)	515 (60%)		
UPD15 Subtype	325 (37%)	8 (40%)	317 (37%)		
ID Subtype	23 (3%)	0	23 (3%)	0.58	0.75
Age	21.0 ± 14 years Range: 0–63	32.8 ± 15 years Range: 0–59	20.4 ± 13 years Range: 0–61	31.92	**<0.0001**
BMI	28.9 ± 12 Range: 3.6–104	41.3 ± 18 Range: 13–80	28.2 ± 12 Range: 4–104	42.27	**<0.0001**
Height	57.1 ± 10 inches Range: 17–77	58.8 ± 10 inches Range: 21–68	57.0 ± 10 inches Range: 17–77	0.96	0.33
Weight	144 ± 78 lb Range: 5–500	217 ± 104 lb Range: 8–490	140 ± 75 lb Range: 5–492	35.75	**<0.0001**

The sample characteristics are presented for the total sample (overall), those with a reported thromboembolism (clots), and without a reported thromboembolism (no clots). Thromboembolisms included all of the reported deep or small vein thrombosis events, pulmonary embolism, or other reported embolism. Chi-square test or analysis of variance (ANOVA) were used to test for differences between individuals with and without blood clots by gender, PWS subtype, age, weight, height, and body mass (BMI). A total of n = 502 (47%) were <18 years of age.

A thrombosis was reported for 38 (3%) PWS cases surveyed, involving 23 females (61%; 4% of females) and 15 males (39%; 3% of males). Of these cases, 33 (87%) events occurred in adults greater than 17 years of age (approximately 6% of adult respondents). The frequency of the blood clots did not differ by gender or PWS genetic subtype, and their occurrence was associated with a significantly greater age, weight, and body mass index (BMI; Table 2). The type of event was identified in 32 cases as a DVT (n = 8; 21%), thrombosis (n = 7; 18%), embolism (n = 4; 11%), PE (n = 6; 16%), smaller vein clot (n = 6; 16%), and one reported ventricular hemorrhage. Fourteen subjects had blood clots in the leg, five in the lung, and two in the brain, and the source of the blood clot was unknown in 17 subjects. The blood clot resolved in 23 individuals (64%) and recurred in seven (19%) subjects. The blood clot was fatal in four individuals, or 11% of the 38 subjects. Twenty-seven (75%) individuals required hospitalization, and eight had a prior injury or blood clot following a prior surgical procedure. Severe pain was reported in 22 (61%) individuals with PWS, and venous stasis, including leg swelling, reported in 23 (77%) individuals, with discoloration reported in 17 (57%). Medical conditions or treatments at the time of the blood clot formation included obesity in 22 (63%) subjects, 8 (23%) who had diabetes, and 5 (14%) who received growth hormone treatment.

A summary of the significant risk factors for thromboembolism in PWS is provided in Table 2. These predictors included established relationships with obesity, metabolic syndrome, and renal and cardiopulmonary dysfunction. The odds ratio for a reported clot was greatest when co-occurring with vasculitis (odds ratio (OR) = 36.9; 95% confidence interval (CI) 15.5 to 87.6), which is often associated with skin picking in PWS (OR = 1.9; 95% CI 1.0 to 3.7). Vasculitis was followed by edema (OR = 15.5; 95% CI 7.4 to 32.6) and kidney failure (OR = 14.9; 95% CI 5.3 to 41.9), heart failure (OR = 9.9, 95% CI 3.9 to 24.9), metabolic syndrome (OR = 5.6; 95% CI 1.8 to 17.4), obesity (OR = 5.4; 95% CI 2.1 to

14.1), and atrial fibrillation (OR = 5.4; 95% CI 1.8 to 16.6). Other predictors included behavioral factors (skin picking and smoking) and prior drug treatment with aspirin and blood thinners with a lower frequency. Of interest, previous treatment with growth hormone was associated with significantly reduced risk of thrombosis (OR = 0.2; 95% CI 0.1 to 0.39).

Table 2. Frequency and analysis of risk factors for thromboembolism in Prader–Willi syndrome.

Variable	Clots, N (%)	No Clots, N (%)	χ^2	p–Value
Medical Findings and History				
Obesity *	32 (86%)	539 (54%)	15.2	<0.0001
Edema *	28 (74%)	151 (15%)	86.6	<0.0001
Skin Picking *	19 (51%)	354 (35%)	4.0	0.045
Vasculitis *	13 (48%)	22 (2.5%)	150.0	<0.0001
Metabolic syndrome	5 (36%)	56 (9%)	11.3	<0.0008
Hypertension	12 (32%)	121 (12%)	12.9	<0.0003
Diabetes	7 (20%)	117 (12%)	1.92	0.16
Heart Failure	7 (19%)	23 (2.3%)	35.1	<0.0001
Kidney function	6 (17%)	14 (1.3%)	44.6	<0.0001
Smoker *	5 (13%)	36 (4%)	9.0	<0.0028
Atrial fibrillation *	4 (12%)	23 (2.4%)	10.9	<0.001
Cancer	4 (10.5%)	8 (0.79%)	30.6	<0.0005 (Exact)
Atherosclerosis	2 (6.3%)	2 (0.21%)	28.1	<0.0055 (Exact)
Antiphospholipid antibody syndrome *	1 (4.5%)	2 (0.22%)	12.8	0.004 (Exact)
Thrombocythemia *	1 (4.3%)	7 (0.8%)	3.3	0.18 (Exact)
Bone marrow disorder *	1 (3.1%)	5 (0.53%)	3.4	0.17 (Exact)
Family History				
Clotting *	9 (24.3%)	137 (14.4%)	2.8	0.09
Factor V deficiency *	2 (8%)	16 (2%)	4.7	0.03
MTHFR deficiency *	1 (5%)	10 (1%)	1.9	0.16
Factor II deficiency *	0	4		NA
Protein S deficiency *	0	5		NA
Protein C deficiency *	0	5		NA
Prior Treatments				
Growth hormone (ever)	14 (37%)	751 (75%)	26.4	<0.0001
Blood Thinners	25 (67%)	19 (2%)	370	<0.0001
Hypothyroidism	8 (24%)	183 (18%)	0.53	0.46
Aspirin	8 (22%)	30 (3%)	36.6	<0.0001
Hyperthyroidism	2 (6%)	6 (0.6%)	11.3	0.028 (Exact)
Adrenal Insufficiency	1 (3%)	40 (4%)	0.09	0.75

Summary of the characteristics and differences between the subjects with a reported thromboembolism (clots) and without a reported thromboembolism (no clots). Thromboembolisms included all of the reported deep or small vein thrombosis events, pulmonary emboli, or other reported emboli. Sample n = 1067; n = 38 individuals with blood clots: reported frequency of variable by clotting history and statistical analyses using a chi-squared test. * Represent factors that could contribute to the development of blood clots in an individual.

A total of 502 respondents were in the pediatric age group, with a collective mean age of 9.3 ± 5 years and a range of 0–17 years. Of these reports, thrombosis occurred in five (1%) children. The average age for the children with blood clots was 5.6 years, with a range of 0 to 14 years. Three of these children had the 15q11-q13 deletion, and three had a prior history of growth hormone treatment. All five children experiencing thrombosis possessed precipitating risk factors. One child had obesity with metabolic syndrome; two children had a history of skin picking, and one child had edema. One child had a genetic risk factor as a result of a positive family history of blood clots, and developed heart failure with thrombocytopenia.

4. Discussion

Blood clots, venous thromboembolism, and/or pulmonary embolism have recently emerged as major medical complications and as contributors to morbidity and mortality in PWS. A health-related questionnaire focused around blood clots was developed by medical experts and researchers in the study of PWS, and administered as a national survey to advance the understanding of and to characterize the frequency of blood clots and related risk factors in this rare obesity-related genetic disorder. Information on the presence or absence of growth hormone treatment, medication use, co-morbid health conditions, and relevant lifestyle factors were also collected. Each event was individually verified and characterized according to age and severity, and whether severe episodes were fatal.

A summary of the conclusions reached from the above data and from the information provided by each respondent showed that the occurrence of blood clots was predominantly seen in adults at rates of 3% to 4%, higher than the <1% rate reported for the general United States population by the U.S. Center for Disease Control (Beckman et al. [10]). Clot formation in the non-PWS population is known to follow an established male prevalence, which is attributed to gender differences in the hormone levels influential in clot formation. Our failure to identify similar gender differences in PWS cases may be related to disorder-specific neuroendocrine disruption, with associated hypogonadism and sexual immaturity that is characteristic of PWS. The frequency of PWS genetic subtypes (15q11-q13 deletion, maternal disomy 15, and imprinting center defects) provided in the survey was similar to the frequencies of the molecular classes reported by Butler et al. [6], supporting the validity of this voluntarily blood clot-related questionnaire via on-line access or by regular mail over a 15-month period. In addition, our study reports the largest number of individuals with PWS (N = 875) and known genetic subtypes, confirming the established frequencies of PWS molecular classes. PWS genetic subtypes did not appear to influence the probability of a reported thrombosis.

The risk factors identified in our analyses included excessive weight, metabolic syndrome and cardiovascular illness, as seen in the general population. The relative strength of association with vasculitis, edema, and kidney and heart failure support a progressive disease profile, potentially arising as secondary complications of exogenous obesity complicated by other neuroendocrine disruptions seen in PWS. Vasculitis is a critical risk factor interrelated with both the physiologic and behavioral features associated with PWS, which may be amenable to intervention and strict oversight to reduce skin picking, proactively address skin lesions, and mitigate infections, which may substantially reduce risks. Blood clots in children with PWS were not related to obesity, and appeared to reflect the medical and surgical complications or genetic risk factors related to the family history.

Growth hormone treatment was associated with a reduced risk of thrombosis in PWS, and may be due to a lower frequency of obese-related or comorbid illnesses, known to contribute to blood clotting events in the general population, and impacted positively by the treatment. The precise contributions of growth hormone treatment to the risk of thrombosis cannot be definitively established from these data, as growth hormone treatment is also a marker for more proactive medical management and vigilant behavioral monitoring in order to prevent the development of obesity not probed in our survey. Furthermore, the access and widespread availability of growth hormone treatment for PWS did not begin until approximately the year 2000, leading to significant differences between adult and child cohorts, impacting on the overall health and wellness in PWS. These cohort-related disparities in medical management, monitoring, and oversite necessitate confirmatory follow-up studies. This dataset and the survey results provide a baseline to monitor future data related to co-morbidities, natural history, survival trends, and causes of death in PWS.

Author Contributions: Conceptualization and precise methodology for the study including development and implementation of the survey incorporated contributions from M.G.B., J.L., J.H., and A.M.M.; M.G.B. was involved with funding acquisition. The investigation required project administration and data collection over several months by PWSA (USA) officials, J.H., B.M., and C.L. Data curation and validation were carried out by J.L., C.L., and B.M.; formal analysis was carried out by A.M.M. for writing the original draft preparation, with reviewing and editing done by all of the authors.

Funding: This research was funded by Zafgen, Inc (Boston, MA, USA) and the National Institute of Child Health and Human Development (NICHD), grant number HD02528.

Acknowledgments: We thank Charlotte Iannaci for assistance in the preparation of the manuscript. We thank all the PWS families and their efforts in completing the questionnaire form and for answering our questions.

Conflicts of Interest: The authors declare no conflict of interest.

References

1. Butler, M.G. Prader-Willi syndrome: Current understanding of cause and diagnosis. *Am. J. Med. Genet.* **1990**, *35*, 319–332. [CrossRef] [PubMed]

2. Butler, M.G.; Lee, P.D.K.; Whitman, B.Y. *Management of Prader-Willi Syndrome*, 3rd ed.; Springer: New York, NY, USA, 2003; pp. 1–550.

3. Cassidy, S.B.; Driscoll, D.J. Prader-Willi syndrome. *Eur. J. Hum. Genet.* **2009**, *17*, 3–13. [CrossRef] [PubMed]

4. Cassidy, S.B.; Schwartz, S.; Miller, J.L.; Driscoll, D.J. Prader-Willi syndrome. *Genet. Med.* **2012**, *14*, 10–26. [CrossRef]

5. Butler, M.G.; Thompson, T. Prader-Willi Syndrome: Clinical and Genetic Findings. *Endocrinologist* **2000**, *10*, 3S–16S. [CrossRef]

6. Butler, M.G.; Hartin, S.N.; Hossain, W.A.; Manzardo, A.M.; Kimonis, V.; Dykens, E.; Gold, J.A.; Kim, S.J.; Weisensel, N.; Tamura, R.; et al. Molecular genetic classification in Prader-Willi syndrome: A multisite cohort study. *J. Med. Genet.* **2019**, *56*, 149–153. [CrossRef] [PubMed]

7. Butler, M.G.; Manzardo, A.M.; Heinemann, J.; Loker, C.; Loker, J. Causes of death in Prader-Willi syndrome: Prader-Willi Syndrome Association (USA) 40-year mortality survey. *Genet. Med.* **2017**, *19*, 635–642. [CrossRef] [PubMed]

8. Manzardo, A.M.; Loker, J.; Heinemann, J.; Loker, C.; Butler, M.G. Survival trends from the Prader-Willi Syndrome Association (USA) 40-year mortality survey. *Genet. Med.* **2018**, *20*, 24–30. [CrossRef] [PubMed]

9. McCandless, S.E.; Yanovski, J.A.; Miller, J.; Fu, C.; Bird, L.M.; Salehi, P.; Chan, C.L.; Stafford, D.; Abuzzahab, M.J.; Viskochil, D.; et al. Effects of MetAP2 inhibition on hyperphagia and body weight in Prader-Willi syndrome: A randomized, double-blind, placebo-controlled trial. *Diabetes Obes. Metab.* **2017**, *19*, 1751–1761. [CrossRef] [PubMed]

10. Beckman, M.G.; Hooper, W.C.; Critchley, S.E.; Ortel, T.L. Venous thromboembolism: A public health concern. *Am. J. Prev. Med.* **2010**, *38*, S495–S501. [CrossRef] [PubMed]

11. Beckman, M.G.; Grosse, S.D.; Kenney, K.M.; Grant, A.M.; Atrash, H.K. Developing public health surveillance for deep vein thrombosis and pulmonary embolism. *Am. J. Prev. Med.* **2011**, *41*, S428–S434. [CrossRef] [PubMed]

12. Beretta, L.; Hauschild, M.; Jeannet, P.Y.; Addor, M.C.; Maeder, P.; Truttmann, A.C. Atypical presentation of Prader-Willi syndrome with cerebral venous thrombosis: Association or fortuity? *Neuropediatrics* **2007**, *38*, 204–206. [CrossRef] [PubMed]

13. Stevenson, D.A.; Heinemann, J.; Angulo, M.; Butler, M.G.; Loker, J.; Rupe, N.; Kendell, P.; Cassidy, S.B.; Scheimann, A. Gastric rupture and necrosis in Prader-Willi syndrome. *J. Pediatr. Gastroenterol. Nutr.* **2007**, *45*, 272–274. [CrossRef] [PubMed]

14. Proffitt, J.; Osann, K.; McManus, B.; Kimonis, V.E.; Heinemann, J.; Butler, M.G.; Stevenson, D.A.; Gold, J.A. Contributing factors of mortality in Prader-Willi syndrome. *Am. J. Med. Genet. A* **2019**, *179*, 196–205. [CrossRef] [PubMed]

 © 2019 by the authors. Licensee MDPI, Basel, Switzerland. This article is an open access article distributed under the terms and conditions of the Creative Commons Attribution (CC BY) license (http://creativecommons.org/licenses/by/4.0/).

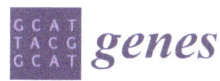

Article

The Global Prader–Willi Syndrome Registry: Development, Launch, and Early Demographics

Jessica Bohonowych [1], Jennifer Miller [2], Shawn E. McCandless [3] and Theresa V. Strong [1,*]

[1] Foundation for Prader–Willi Research, Walnut, CA 91789, USA; jessica.bohonowych@fpwr.org
[2] Department of Pediatrics, University of Florida School of Medicine, Gainesville, FL 32611, USA; millejl@peds.ufl.edu
[3] Section of Genetics and Metabolism, Department of Pediatrics, University of Colorado School of Medicine and Children's Hospital Colorado, Aurora, CO, USA; shawn.mccandless@ucdenver.edu
*   Correspondence: theresa.strong@fpwr.org

Received: 31 July 2019; Accepted: 9 September 2019; Published: 14 September 2019

Abstract: Advances in technologies offer new opportunities to collect and integrate data from a broad range of sources to advance the understanding of rare diseases and support the development of new treatments. Prader–Willi syndrome (PWS) is a rare, complex neurodevelopmental disorder, which has a variable and incompletely understood natural history. PWS is characterized by early failure to thrive, followed by the onset of excessive appetite (hyperphagia). Additional characteristics include multiple endocrine abnormalities, hypotonia, hypogonadism, sleep disturbances, a challenging neurobehavioral phenotype, and cognitive disability. The Foundation for Prader–Willi Research's Global PWS Registry is one of more than twenty-five registries developed to date through the National Organization of Rare Disorders (NORD) IAMRARE Registry Program. The Registry consists of surveys covering general medical history, system-specific clinical complications, diet, medication and supplement use, as well as behavior, mental health, and social information. Information is primarily parent/caregiver entered. The platform is flexible and allows addition of new surveys, including updatable and longitudinal surveys. Launched in 2015, the PWS Registry has enrolled 1696 participants from 37 countries, with 23,550 surveys completed. This resource can improve the understanding of PWS natural history and support medical product development for PWS.

Keywords: Prader–Willi syndrome; registry; natural history

---

1. Introduction

Prader–Willi syndrome (PWS) is a rare genetic disorder with a birth incidence of 1/10,000 to 1/30,000, and an estimated prevalence of approximately 10,000 to 20,000 living individuals in the United States [1–3]. It affects males and females equally, as well as all races and ethnicities [3]. PWS is caused by the absence of paternally-expressed, imprinted genes on chromosome 15q11–13. Loss of activity can occur by one of three major genetic mechanisms: Microdeletion of the paternally inherited chromosome (60%–70% of cases, further divided into type I and type II, 7 megabases (Mb) and 5 Mb in size, respectively); maternal uniparental disomy (UPD) subsequent to trisomic rescue (30%–40% of cases); or mutation/epimutation of the Prader–Willi syndrome/Angelman syndrome (PWS/AS) imprinting center (~3% of cases) [1–3]. Consensus clinical diagnostic criteria for PWS were reported in 1993 [4], but the phenotype is variable, and a definitive molecular diagnostic test for PWS is available, which accurately detects >99% of cases [3]. The PWS region of chromosome 15 is unusually complex and includes protein coding genes as well as long noncoding RNAs and embedded, short noncoding RNAs [5]. The exact contribution of each of the genes in the region to the overall phenotype has not been definitely determined and, to date, the molecular mechanisms underlying the PWS phenotype are

Genes **2019**, *10*, 713; doi:10.3390/genes10090713   www.mdpi.com/journal/genes

not fully understood. However, PWS is thought to be primarily a disorder of hypothalamic function, impacting multiple systems throughout the body [1,3,6].

PWS is associated with a constellation of symptoms that significantly negatively impact quality of life for affected individuals and their families. The initial clinical course of PWS is characterized by hypotonia in infants, with decreased movement, lethargy, feeding difficulties, and failure to thrive. A defining feature of PWS is the change in appetite over time, with the onset of hyperphagia (an unrelenting, pathologically excessive appetite) sometime after early childhood [3,7]. Whereas infants with PWS do not show normal signs of hunger and often require feeding via nasogastric tubes or other assistive means, feeding improves in young children and subsequently progresses to hyperphagia during childhood. Adolescents and adults with PWS will become morbidly obese if strict environmental controls restricting food intake are not implemented. Additional abnormalities associated with PWS include growth hormone deficiency, hypogonadotropic hypogonadism, sleep disorders, reduced pain sensitivity, poor bone health, decreased gastrointestinal motility, and scoliosis. Aspects such as central adrenal insufficiency, seizures, hypothyroidism, and hypoglycemia occur at frequencies higher than the normal population, but are not present in all individuals [1,3,6].

In addition to somatic symptoms, intellectual disability (ID) and neuropsychiatric issues are present to some degree in all individuals with PWS [3,8,9]. Individuals with PWS typically exhibit a characteristic behavioral phenotype that includes cognitive rigidity, heightened anxiety, severe temper outbursts, obsessive-compulsive behaviors, and self-injurious behaviors. Adolescents and adults are at risk of mental illness and autistic symptomatology is common, particularly in those with PWS by UPD. Hyperphagia-driven behaviors include food-seeking behavior, hoarding or foraging for food, eating of inappropriate food items (e.g., raw or discarded food), stealing food or money to buy food, and intense psychological stress and behavioral disturbances associated with food denial. Behavioral issues and an inability to control food intake represent the major impediments to independent living for individuals with PWS, and opportunities for community engagement, employment, independent living, and social activities are highly constrained by these issues.

There is a wide range of phenotypic variability in PWS, some of which is not attributable to the different genetic subtypes. With respect to major classes of genetic subtypes (deletion vs. UPD vs. imprinting mutations), overall there is more phenotypic variability within subtypes than across subtypes, including for features such as hyperphagia, scoliosis, sleep disruption, pain insensitivity, growth hormone deficiency and other endocrine dysfunctions, self-injurious behavior (skin picking), and obesity. Notable exceptions are autism spectrum disorder and psychosis, both of which are significantly more common in the UPD subtype compared to deletion, while major depressive disorder is more common in the deletion subtype [10,11].

Current treatments for PWS are limited and, to date, focus on the treatment of endocrine abnormalities with hormone replacement therapy [12,13]. Growth hormone (GH) is FDA-approved for treating children with PWS and is increasingly prescribed in infants and adults [14]. GH is effective in normalizing growth and improving body composition in PWS but has no effect on hyperphagia. To date, no FDA-approved drugs have proven effective in controlling appetite and food-related behavior in PWS. Thus, parent education, restricted diet, and environmental control are the only options for avoiding morbid obesity in PWS. However, a number of potential drugs and devices are currently in preclinical and clinical development and may provide new therapeutic options for those with PWS in coming years [15–23]. While the number of therapeutic avenues being pursued is encouraging, a better understanding of natural history, as well as a robust database of potential participants for clinical studies, can facilitate the development and evaluation of novel therapeutics for PWS.

The US National Institutes of Health (NIH)-funded PWS Rare Disease Consortium studied approximately 350 individuals with PWS over an eight-year period (2006–2014) [24], providing valuable insights into the natural history of PWS. However, many critical gaps remain. Long-term longitudinal description of disease manifestations, onset and progression of characteristic behaviors, as well the aging process in PWS individuals are incompletely defined. Gaps also exist in understanding the co-morbidities of PWS; the relationship between genotype and phenotype; the impact of genetic variants and environmental considerations on the clinical course of disease; and treatment outcomes across a broad population of individuals with PWS. Finally, as care changes and novel therapies become available, a flexible platform for gathering data on current real-world experiences and outcomes in the PWS population is needed.

The Global Prader–Willi Syndrome Registry (www.pwsregistry.org) was launched in 2015 by the Foundation for Prader–Willi Research (FPWR) in collaboration with leading clinicians to accelerate research and support the development of treatments for PWS. The Registry aims to document the natural history of PWS; understand the full spectrum of PWS features across the entire population; identify unmet medical needs, rare complications, and understudied areas; facilitate partnerships with stakeholders; expedite completion of clinical trials; guide the development of standards of care; and allow participants to centrally store their PWS medical data.

2. Materials and Methods

Registry Architecture and Security: The Global PWS Registry is web-based and is hosted on the National Organization for Rare Disorders (NORD) "IAMRARE" Registry Platform. NORD's Registry platform was developed with input from experts at the NIH, patient advocacy groups, and the US Food and Drug Administration (FDA). The Global PWS Registry is compliant with US Health Information Privacy Laws, FDA regulations on electronic records, and the security requirements of the European Union General Data Protection Regulation (GDPR). Registry data is only accessed by registry study personnel. De-identified data can be shared with researchers and other stakeholders as per the Registry protocol. All protocols, surveys, and recruitment materials are reviewed and approved by a central Institutional Review Board (IRB).

Registry Governance: The Global PWS Registry is governed by the Global PWS Registry Advisory Board. The members of the Advisory Board represent stakeholders in the PWS and rare disease communities including PWS patient groups, parents, caregivers, clinicians, and experts in Registry development and governance. The Advisory Board is tasked with (1) reviewing requests for de-identified data by researchers, clinicians, and other stakeholders; (2) reviewing requests from sponsors to send out IRB-approved recruitment materials to participants that meet study inclusion/exclusion criteria; and (3) reviewing proposals to run research projects through the Registry, particularly those that may include development of new surveys.

Survey Development: Survey development was a collaborative effort, led by the Registry investigators. The development team included input from various stakeholders with expertise in PWS including clinicians, academic researchers, parents, and other caregivers. The process was informed by resources including publications on best practices in Registry development [25], communications with other disease registries, and recommendations from the NORD IAMRARE Team. Surveys were beta tested with a small cohort of PWS families that provided feedback on any questions where the language was confusing or too technical. Beta testers also provided input on improving or expanding answer options for questions, which was incorporated into the final surveys.

Data Curation: Registry administrators continually review new participant accounts and remove duplicate accounts, or accounts created in error as determined by duplicate names and/or email addresses. Accounts with invalid contact information are also removed. On an ongoing basis, data points within the registry are curated for date of birth, diagnosis, and relationship of the respondent or person managing the account, to the person with PWS. Any errors that are identified are corrected by Registry administrators. Curation is done through communicating with respondents directly when their contact preferences grant permission, and also through comparing and validating common data elements across surveys within the Registry. An example of this includes comparing the date of birth on the account, with the date of birth on an uploaded medical record within the account. Data for this publication was accessed on 30 May 2019, and includes all completed responses for each question. Some questions were not completed by all respondents, thus the number of responses per question varies.

3. Results

3.1. Registry Design and Initial Recruitment

The Global PWS Registry is open to parents, guardians, caregivers, and to individuals with PWS. More than 90% of Registry accounts are managed by parents, guardians, or legal authorized representatives. However, there is a subset of accounts that are managed by self-reporting individuals with PWS.

The Global PWS Registry launched in April 2015 with 35 surveys (Table 1). The surveys are designed to capture the full spectrum and natural history of PWS, including birth history and diagnosis, a comprehensive battery of specific medical systems, as well as demographics, well-being, and quality of life. The initial 35 surveys are all updatable and serve as a comprehensive record over time, wherein participants return on an annual basis to add new information. In addition to these updatable surveys, the Registry platform also supports longitudinal surveys which repeatedly capture the same information at time point intervals.

Table 1. Surveys included in the Global Prader–Willi syndrome (PWS) Registry launch, and the number of submissions per survey. The initial launch of the PWS Registry included 35 surveys. Surveys have been completed by varying numbers of participants.

Survey Name	# of Participants
Getting Started	1207
Contact Information	1074
Participant Demographics	969
Research Trials	959
Diagnosis	952
Pregnancy History	861
Birth History	821
Biological Family History	810
General Medical History	787
Neurological History	767
Vision History	756
Developmental Milestones	708
Psychological and Mental Health	682
Speech, Occupational, and Physical Therapy	654
Sleep History	613
Pulmonary History	609
Gastrointestinal History	605
Sexual and Reproductive History	603
Dental History	584
Education and Employment	582
Endocrinological History	573
Dermatological History	570
Orthopedic History	565
Ear, Nose, and Throat Health History	560
Sociodemographic and Socioeconomic	555
Well–Being	548
Nutritional Phase and Diet	547
Medications–Endocrinology	545
Supplements A–M	526
Medications–Cardiology, GI, and Others	520
Supplements N-Z and Others	511
Medications–Psychiatric A–M	509
Medications–Psychiatric N–Z and Others	502
Hippotherapy, Psycotherapy, and Behavioral Therapies	488
Behavior	428
TOTAL	**23,550**

3.2. Enrollment and Survey Completion

The Global PWS Registry currently has 1696 participants who have completed the consent process (Table 2). Survey completion rates vary, with 21% of participants having completed all 35 of the initial surveys. Thirty-five percent (35%) of participants have completed between five to 34 surveys, and 17% have completed one to five surveys. There is also a group of 27% of participants that have consented, but not yet submitted any surveys. This all translates to a total of 23,550 survey submissions (Table 1). The "Getting Started" survey, which is the first survey of the Registry, has the most submissions at 1207. The surveys with the least number of submissions include the six surveys related to medications and supplements, as well as the two surveys covering "Behavior" and "Hippotherapy, Psychotherapy, and Behavioral Therapies".

Table 2. Survey completion percentages. The number of surveys completed by each participant ranges from 0 surveys to all 35 surveys.

# of Surveys Completed	# of Participants	% of Participants
0 surveys	463	27%
1–5 surveys	280	17%
6–10 surveys	208	12%
11–20 surveys	179	11%
21–34 surveys	209	12%
All surveys	357	21%
Total	**1696**	**100%**

3.3. Geographical Distribution of Registry Participants

In total, 37 countries are represented within the Global PWS Registry (Table 3). Participants are predominantly from the United States and U.S. Territories, making up over 75% of Registry participants. Canada has the second highest representation at 8.9%. Australia, the United Kingdom, and New Zealand each make up between 1% to 3% of the Registry. The remaining countries each constitute less than 1% of the Registry.

Table 3. Distribution of participants within the Global PWS Registry by country.

Country	# of Participants	% of Participants
United States	842	78.8%
Canada	90	8.4%
Australia	29	2.7%
United Kingdom	22	2.1%
New Zealand	12	1.1%
Mexico	7	0.7%
Spain	7	0.7%
France	5	0.5%
Germany	4	0.4%
Ireland	4	0.4%
South Africa	4	0.4%
Belgium	3	0.3%
Brazil	3	0.3%
India	3	0.3%
United States Minor Outlying Islands	3	0.3%
Austria	2	0.2%
China	2	0.2%
Colombia	2	0.2%
Finland	2	0.2%
Greece	2	0.2%
Israel	2	0.2%
Sweden	2	0.2%

Table 3. *Cont.*

Country	# of Participants	% of Participants
Bangladesh	1	0.1%
Bermuda	1	0.1%
Bulgaria	1	0.1%
Croatia	1	0.1%
Denmark	1	0.1%
Hong Kong	1	0.1%
Italy	1	0.1%
Lebanon	1	0.1%
Malaysia	1	0.1%
Netherlands	1	0.1%
Norway	1	0.1%
Poland	1	0.1%
Portugal	1	0.1%
Puerto Rico	1	0.1%
Singapore	1	0.1%
Taiwan, Province Of China	1	0.1%
United Arab Emirates	1	0.1%
TOTAL	**1069**	**100%**

Within the United States, there are Registry participants from all 50 states, as well as from the District of Columbia, and Puerto Rico (Table 4). The four states with the highest percentage of Registry participants are California (7.6%), Texas (6.8%), New York (5.7%), and Florida (5.1%). There are eight states that each have between 3% to 5% of US Registry participants, 19 states each with 1% to 3%, and the remaining states, districts, and territories each have less than 1%. Within Canada, eight of the 10 provinces are represented with over 40% of Canadian participants residing in Ontario (Table 5). The next highest percentages are British Columbia (17.4%), Alberta (15.1%), and Quebec (14%).

Table 4. Distribution of US participants within the Global PWS Registry by state. Participants within the Registry represent all 50 states within the United States. Of participants that live in the United States, California, Texas, New York, and Florida have the highest reported number of participants.

US State	# of Participants	% of US Participants
Alabama	14	1.7%
Alaska	7	0.8%
Arizona	22	2.7%
Arkansas	6	0.7%
California	63	7.6%
Colorado	19	2.3%
Connecticut	14	1.7%
Delaware	1	0.1%
District of Columbia	1	0.1%
Florida	42	5.1%
Georgia	31	3.7%
Hawaii	4	0.5%
Idaho	4	0.5%
Illinois	31	3.7%
Indiana	22	2.7%
Iowa	9	1.1%
Kansas	12	1.5%
Kentucky	7	0.8%
Louisiana	9	1.1%
Maine	3	0.4%
Maryland	11	1.3%

Table 4. *Cont.*

US State	# of Participants	% of US Participants
Massachusetts	24	2.9%
Michigan	27	3.3%
Minnesota	19	2.3%
Mississippi	3	0.4%
Missouri	17	2.1%
Montana	5	0.6%
Nebraska	7	0.8%
Nevada	4	0.5%
New Hampshire	4	0.5%
New Jersey	23	2.8%
New Mexico	7	0.8%
New York	47	5.7%
North Carolina	25	3.0%
North Dakota	1	0.1%
Ohio	39	4.7%
Oklahoma	7	0.8%
Oregon	8	1.0%
Pennsylvania	34	4.1%
Puerto Rico	1	0.1%
Rhode Island	5	0.6%
South Carolina	9	1.1%
South Dakota	2	0.2%
Tennessee	17	2.1%
Texas	56	6.8%
Utah	17	2.1%
Vermont	1	0.1%
Virginia	23	2.8%
Washington	30	3.6%
West Virginia	4	0.5%
Wisconsin	29	3.5%
Wyoming	0	0.0%
TOTAL	**827**	**100%**

Table 5. Distribution of Canadian participants within the Global PWS Registry by province. Participants within the Registry represent eight of the Canadian provinces. Participants from Ontario make up the largest group of Canadian participants. Shown are the responses from those specifying a province; four Canadian participants did not answer this question.

Canadian Province	# of Participants	% of Participants
Alberta	13	15.1%
British Columbia	15	17.4%
Manitoba	2	2.3%
New Brunswick	2	2.3%
Newfoundland & Labrador	1	1.2%
Ontario	37	43.0%
Quebec	12	14.0%
Saskatchewan	4	4.7%
TOTAL	**86**	**100%**

3.4. Race, Ethnicity, Age and Gender Demographics

Of those reporting race and ethnicity, the majority of Registry participants (person with PWS) are Caucasian (85.1%) and non-Hispanic or Latino (82%) (Tables 6 and 7). The age of participants at the time of enrollment is predominantly under the age of 15 years old (68%) (Figure 1). The two- to five-year old and six- to 10-year old age groups makeup the highest percentages, at 18% and 20%, respectively. These percentages demonstrate that the majority of participants within the Global PWS Registry are minors, and that there is an underrepresentation of young adults and adults with PWS. As expected, the gender distribution of participants is relatively equal at 51% male and 49% female (Figure 2).

Participants within the Registry represent 35 countries throughout the world. Participants from the United States make up the majority of the Registry. Shown are the responses from those specifying their country of origin; 627 participants did not answer this question.

Table 6. Race of participants within the Global PWS Registry.

Race	# of Participants	% of Participants
Caucasian	796	85.1%
Multi–Ethnic	66	7.1%
Asian	28	3.0%
Black or African American	14	1.5%
Other	17	1.8%
Native Hawaiian or Other Pacific Islander	3	0.3%
Prefer not to Answer	6	0.6%
American Indian or Alaska Native	4	0.4%
Don't know	1	0.1%
TOTAL	**935**	**100%**

Table 7. Ethnicity of participants within the Global PWS Registry.

Ethnicity	# of Participants	% of Participants
Non–Hispanic or Latino	629	82.0%
Hispanic or Latino	73	9.5%
Ashkenazi Jewish	19	2.5%
Unknown	30	3.9%
Prefer not to answer	16	2.1%
TOTAL	**767**	**100%**

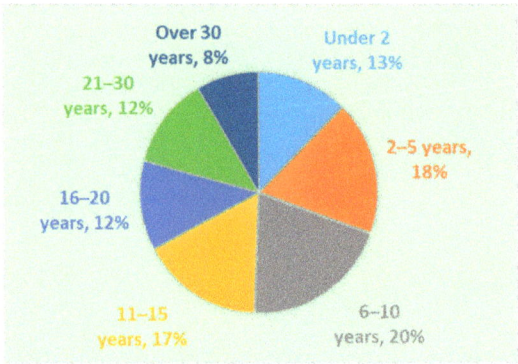

Figure 1. Age of Registry participants at time of enrollment. Registry participants range in age from newborn infants to adults. The majority of registry participants are under 15 years of age.

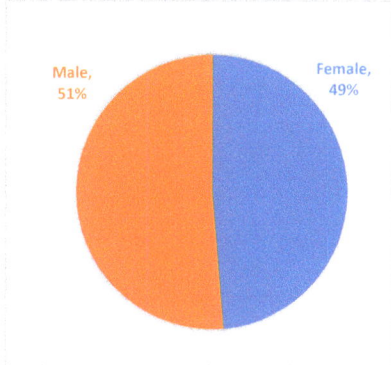

Figure 2. Gender of Registry participants.

3.5. PWS Genetic Subtype

Of participants within the Registry who have a reported genetic subtype, 49.3% reported having PWS due to a paternal deletion and 35.6% reported having uniparental disomy (UPD) (Figure 3). Approximately 3.3% of participants reported having an imprinting defect. A small percentage of Registry respondents (1.7%) indicated that the participant fell into an "other" category. Open ended responses to a follow up question for "other" showed that these individuals include participants with PWS due translocations, atypical microdeletions, or "acquired PWS" (e.g., PWS-like symptoms subsequent to a hypothalamic tumor). In addition, a small number of participants (n = 2) in the Global PWS Registry have a diagnosis of Schaaf-Yang syndrome [26], a PWS-related disorder caused by truncating mutations in the *MAGEL2* gene, which resides in the PWS-region of chromosome 15. Genetic subtype is unknown for 10.1% of participants. These participants may have been diagnosed with PWS based on a clinical diagnosis only (more common in older participants), or they may have received a molecular diagnosis of PWS based on DNA methylation analysis only, without additional testing to discern genetic subtype.

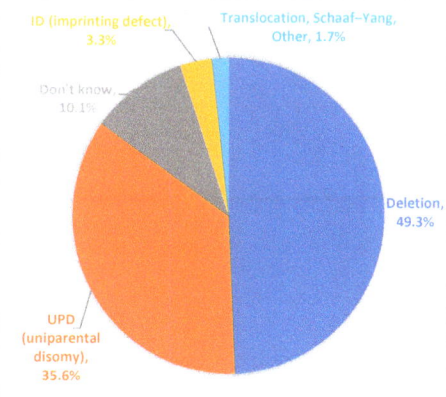

Figure 3. PWS genetic subtype of Registry participants. PWS by deletion is the predominant genetic subtype of participants within the Registry. PWS by uniparental disomy (UPD) is the second most common diagnosis. PWS by imprinting defect, translocation, and micro-deletions are also represented within the Registry. Approximately 10% of Registry participants do not know their PWS genetic subtype.

Of those reporting genetic subtype, maternal age at conception was also reported for 593 participants (352 PWS with PWS due to deletion and 241 with PWS due to UPD). The mean maternal age for PWS participants with the UPD genetic subtype was significantly older than for those with PWS due to deletion (34.8 years, SD 5.6 for UPD compared to 29.2 years, SD 5.3 for deletion; $p < 0.0001$), consistent with advanced maternal age and trisomy 15 rescue as the genetic mechanism underlying the UPD subtype [1].

3.6. Community Engagement

The initial recruitment for the Registry involved a multipronged approach including social media, newsletters, and e-mails in cooperation with PWS advocacy groups, presentations at PWS family conferences and fundraisers, brochures at PWS clinics, and informational webinars. A number of helpful resources have been created to guide families through the registration and informed about the consent process. These include a "getting started video", a "getting started PDF", a private Facebook group, webinars, brochures, FAQ documents, and direct engagement at family conferences. As the Registry has developed, additional outreach to PWS group homes, clinics, physicians, and international patient groups has occurred. An important aspect of Registry communication is the return of results to the PWS community. Through the Registry platform, participants are immediately able to view graphs of de-identified aggregate data for any surveys they have completed. In addition, at regular intervals, infographics addressing aspects of PWS are developed from Registry data and shared with the community through social media and email (Figure 4).

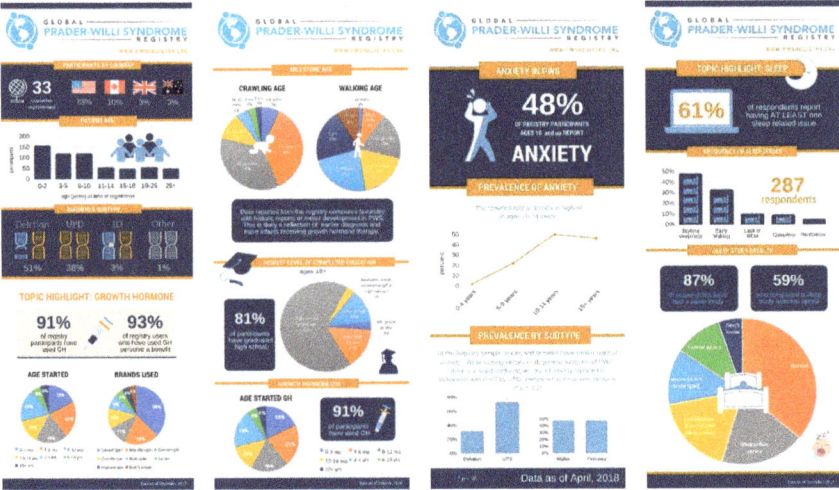

Figure 4. Infographics of Registry data shared with the PWS community. De-identified aggregate data is exported from the Registry, analyzed, and represented in infographics, and shared through social media, print newsletters, and other communications. Each infographic is designed to highlight a specific topic area of interest to PWS families, clinicians, and other stakeholders within the PWS community. Infographics and accompanying descriptions are available at https://www.fpwr.org/blog.

4. Discussion

Since it was launched in 2015, the Global PWS Registry has steadily grown in enrollment and now includes an estimated 5% to 10% of the US PWS population, with individuals from 37 countries represented in all. The IAMRARE platform provides the flexibility of both updatable as well as longitudinal surveys. These formats provide a means to capture the medical history of onset and severity of PWS symptoms throughout a participant's life, as well as to track changes over shorter periods of time for aspects of the PWS phenotype such as behavior, anxiety, or sleep. NORD continues to make improvements and enhancements to the IAMRARE platform to support survey development, data analysis, and the development of sub-studies focusing on specific groups or phenotypes. Additional long-term goals include integrating other data sources, including real-world data. The richness of the data collected to date within the PWS Registry is already supporting the development of novel therapeutics for PWS and facilitating partnerships with academic clinicians and pharmaceutical industry stakeholders. However, several challenges remain, most notably recruiting a population to the Registry that better reflects the demographics and entire spectrum of PWS (age, nationality, race and ethnicity, socio-economic status, PWS experience).

Although age estimates for the general PWS population are difficult to establish, the age distribution currently represented in the Registry is likely younger than the actual PWS population. Mortality rates are higher in PWS than the general population across all ages [27]. With only 13% of current Registry participants over the age of 25, there is a large population of adults that is not represented in the Registry. Challenges for enrolling and completing surveys for adults with PWS include navigating guardianship/consent for adults not living at home and/or for adults whose parents are deceased, assembling a long-accumulated history of medical records, lack of knowledge about the database, and engaging an older parent population that may be less comfortable with a web-based format. However, this adult PWS population group represents a critical segment of the Registry in gaining an understanding of the natural history of PWS. Moreover, there are early reports of premature aging in the PWS population [28]. This is a poorly understood area and the Registry can help identify health issues in adults with PWS, as well as direct priorities for clinical care in adults with PWS.

The Registry has enrolled a significant portion of the US PWS population, as well as participants from numerous other countries. However, more than 87% of the Registry is from the US and Canada, and additional work is needed to establish a participant population that more accurately reflects the global PWS population. The main hurdle in addressing this challenge is that the Registry is currently only available in English. There are plans to eventually offer the Registry in additional languages. This will entail medically-certified translations of all of the questions and informed consents. It will also require software enhancements to the IAMRARE platform to provide the site in multiple languages and to support appropriate data coding so that answers from multiple language versions of the same questionnaire can be queried together. Although challenging, the ability to offer the Registry in multiple languages will facilitate comparison of health care, treatment standards, and quality of life across countries.

With respect to population profile, currently, minorities make up a very small percentage of Registry participants. For example, 1.5% and 3% of Registry participants identify as African American and Asian, respectively. According to the 2010 US Census, those minority populations comprise 12.6% and 4.8% of US residents. Considering that the incidence of PWS is not associated with race or ethnicity, and that US participants comprise almost 80% of the Registry, these percentages highlight the underrepresentation of non-whites within the Global PWS Registry and suggest that the current Registry population is not fully representative of the ethnic and racial diversity of the expected PWS population. Offering the registry in multiple languages, as described above, may allow a more diverse US population to enter the Registry as well. Developing additional recruitment strategies to improve representation that more accurately reflects the racial and ethnic diversity in the US is also a priority. Collaborating with patient groups, clinics, and group homes to understand how to better reach these underrepresented demographic groups, as well as any hurdles/challenges to their participation in the Registry, is critical. Working with these stakeholders will also help broaden the phenotypic spectrum of individuals with PWS (i.e., individuals who are doing very well, as well as those who are more severely impacted). All of these demographics are critical to understanding the full spectrum of the disorder.

Outside of improving demographic representation within the Registry, additional concerns around this research tool include the potential limitations of parent/caregiver-reported data, and the challenge of completing all surveys for each participant with annual updates. Although the clinical accuracy of parent/caregiver-reported data may have limitations, the IAMRARE platform allows clinical notes and records to be uploaded to support or supplement the parent/caregiver-reported information. Encouraging parents/caregivers to upload diagnostic reports to allow reported genetic subtype to be confirmed, for example, is a current priority. In addition, engaging with the PWS community and demonstrating the value of the Registry is critical to increasing survey completion and having participants regularly update their profiles.

Return of results to the community is a critical component of retaining active participation in the Registry. Infographics highlighting data from topics of interest are shared through newsletters and social media, and the input of the community on topics of interest is encouraged. Data has also been presented at several family conferences. Launching new surveys, and special projects or sub-studies with researchers, also brings people back into the Registry.

With growing participation, the Global PWS Registry is poised to continue leveraging de-identified data through collaborations with researchers, industry, and other partners to advance the understanding of PWS, direct efforts in basic and clinical research, and support the development of novel therapies for this challenging disorder.

Author Contributions: Conceptualization and development, J.B., J.M. and T.V.S.; methodology, J.B., J.M., S.E.M. and T.V.S.; analysis, J.B., J.M., S.E.M. and T.V.S.; data curation, J.B.; writing—original draft preparation, J.B. and T.V.S.; writing—review and editing, J.B., J.M., S.E.M. and T.V.S.

Funding: This research was funded by the Foundation for Prader–Willi Research

Acknowledgments: The authors gratefully acknowledge the families who participate in the Global PWS Registry, as well as the input of many PWS experts in the development of Registry surveys, including Harold von Bosse for Orthopedics, James Strong for Neurology, and. Tony Holland for general registry discussion. We thank Lauren Schwartz-Roth, Nathalie Kayadjanian, and Caroline Vrana-Diaz for helpful feedback.

Conflicts of Interest: J.B. and T.V.S. are employees of the Foundation for Prader–Willi Research. J.M. and S.E.M. declare no conflicts of interest.

References

1. Cassidy, S.B.; Schwartz, S.; Miller, J.L.; Driscoll, D.J. Prader-Willi syndrome. *Genet. Med.* **2012**, *14*, 10–26. [CrossRef] [PubMed]
2. Lionti, T.; Reid, S.M.; White, S.M.; Rowell, M.M. A population-based profile of 160 Australians with Prader-Willi syndrome: Trends in diagnosis, birth prevalence and birth characteristics. *Am. J. Med. Genet. A* **2015**, *167*, 371–378. [CrossRef] [PubMed]
3. Driscoll, D.J.; Miller, J.L.; Schwartz, S.; Cassidy, S.B. Prader-Willi Syndrome. In *GeneReviews(R)*; Adam, M.P., Ardinger, H.H., Pagon, R.A., Wallace, S.E., Bean, L.J.H., Stephens, K., Amemiya, A., Eds.; University of Washington: Seattle, WA, USA, 1988; Last Revision: 14 December 2017.
4. Holm, V.A.; Cassidy, S.B.; Butler, M.G.; Hanchett, J.M.; Greenswag, L.R.; Whitman, B.Y.; Greenberg, F. Prader-Willi Syndrome: Consensus Diagnostic Criteria. *Pediatrics* **1993**, *91*, 398–402.
5. Chamberlain, S.J. RNAs of the human chromosome 15q11-q13 imprinted region. *Wiley Interdiscip. Rev. RNA* **2013**, *4*, 155–166. [CrossRef] [PubMed]
6. Angulo, M.A.; Butler, M.G.; Cataletto, M.E. Prader-Willi syndrome: A review of clinical, genetic, and endocrine findings. *J. Endocrinol. Investig.* **2015**, *38*, 1249–1263. [CrossRef] [PubMed]
7. Miller, J.L.; Lynn, C.H.; Driscoll, D.C.; Goldstone, A.P.; Gold, J.-A.; Kimonis, V.; Dykens, E.; Butler, M.G.; Shuster, J.J.; Driscoll, D.J. Nutritional Phases in Prader-Willi Syndrome. *Am. J. Med. Genet. Part A* **2011**, *155*, 1040–1049. [CrossRef] [PubMed]
8. Rice, L.J.; Gray, K.M.; Howlin, P.; Taffe, J.; Tonge, B.J.; Einfeld, S.L. The developmental trajectory of disruptive behavior in Down syndrome, fragile X syndrome, Prader-Willi syndrome and Williams syndrome. *Am. J. Med. Genet. Part C Semin. Med. Genet.* **2015**, *169*, 182–187. [CrossRef] [PubMed]
9. Yang, L.; Zhan, G.-D.; Ding, J.-J.; Wang, H.-J.; Ma, D.; Huang, G.-Y.; Zhou, W.-H. Psychiatric Illness and Intellectual Disability in the Prader–Willi Syndrome with Different Molecular Defects—A Meta Analysis. *PLoS ONE* **2013**, *8*, e72640. [CrossRef]

10. Bennett, J.A.; Germani, T.; Haqq, A.M.; Zwaigenbaum, L. Autism spectrum disorder in Prader-Willi syndrome: A systematic review. *Am. J. Med. Genet. Part A* **2015**, *167*, 2936–2944. [CrossRef]

11. Sinnema, M.; Boer, H.; Collin, P.; Maaskant, M.A.; Van Roozendaal, K.E.; Schrander-Stumpel, C.T.; Curfs, L.M. Psychiatric illness in a cohort of adults with Prader-Willi syndrome. *Res. Dev. Disabil.* **2011**, *32*, 1729–1735. [CrossRef]

12. Deal, C.L.; Tony, M.; Höybye, C.; Allen, D.B.; Tauber, M.; Christiansen, J.S.; Ambler, G.R.; Battista, R.; Beauloye, V.; Berall, G.; et al. Growth Hormone Research Society Workshop Summary: Consensus Guidelines for Recombinant Human Growth Hormone Therapy in Prader-Willi Syndrome. *J. Clin. Endocrinol. Metab.* **2013**, *98*, E1072–E1087. [CrossRef] [PubMed]

13. Goldstone, A.P.; Holland, A.J.; Hauffa, B.P.; Hokken-Koelega, A.C.; Tauber, M. Speakers Contributors at the Second Expert Meeting of the Comprehensive Care of Patients with PWS. Recommendations for the diagnosis and management of Prader-Willi syndrome. *J. Clin. Endocrinol. Metab.* **2008**, *93*, 4183–4197. [CrossRef] [PubMed]

14. McCandless, S.E. Clinical report-health supervision for children with Prader-Willi syndrome. *Pediatrics* **2011**, *127*, 195–204. [PubMed]

15. Tauber, M.; Mantoulan, C.; Copet, P.; Jauregui, J.; Demeer, G.; Diene, G.; Roge, B.; Laurier, V.; Ehlinger, V.; Arnaud, C.; et al. Oxytocin may be useful to increase trust in others and decrease disruptive behaviours in patients with Prader-Willi syndrome: A randomised placebo-controlled trial in 24 patients. *Orphanet J. Rare Dis.* **2011**, *6*, 47. [CrossRef] [PubMed]

16. Einfeld, S.L.; Smith, E.; McGregor, I.S.; Steinbeck, K.; Taffe, J.; Rice, L.J.; Horstead, S.K.; Rogers, N.; Hodge, M.A.; Guastella, A.J. A double-blind randomized controlled trial of oxytocin nasal spray in Prader Willi syndrome. *Am. J. Med. Genet. Part A* **2014**, *164*, 2232–2239. [CrossRef] [PubMed]

17. Kuppens, J.R.; Donze, S.H.; Hokken-Koelega, A.C. Promising effects of oxytocin on social and food-related behaviour in young children with Prader-Willi syndrome: A randomized, double-blind, controlled crossover trial. *Clin. Endocrinol.* **2016**, *85*, 979–987. [CrossRef] [PubMed]

18. Schwartz, L.; Holland, A.; Dykens, E.; Strong, T.; Roof, E.; Bohonowych, J. Prader-Willi syndrome mental health research strategy workshop proceedings: The state of the science and future directions. *Orphanet J. Rare Dis.* **2016**, *11*, 3. [CrossRef] [PubMed]

19. McCandless, S.E.; Yanovski, J.A.; Miller, J.; Fu, C.; Bird, L.M.; Salehi, P.; Chan, C.L.; Stafford, D.; Abuzzahab, M.J.; Viskochil, D.; et al. Effects of MetAP2 inhibition on hyperphagia and body weight in Prader-Willi syndrome: A randomized, double-blind, placebo-controlled trial. *Diabetes Obes. Metab.* **2017**, *19*, 1751–1761. [CrossRef]

20. Miller, J.L.; Strong, T.V.; Heinemann, J. Medication Trials for Hyperphagia and Food-Related Behaviors in Prader-Willi Syndrome. *Diseases* **2015**, *3*, 78–85. [CrossRef]

21. Rice, L.J.; Einfeld, S.L.; Hu, N.; Carter, C.S. A review of clinical trials of oxytocin in Prader-Willi syndrome. *Curr. Opin. Psychiatry* **2018**, *31*, 123–127. [CrossRef]

22. Dykens, E.M.; Miller, J.; Angulo, M.; Roof, E.; Reidy, M.; Hatoum, H.T.; Willey, R.; Bolton, G.; Körner, P. Intranasal carbetocin reduces hyperphagia in individuals with Prader-Willi syndrome. *JCI Insight* **2018**, *3*, 98333. [CrossRef] [PubMed]

23. Allas, S.; Caixàs, A.; Poitou, C.; Coupaye, M.; Thuilleaux, D.; Lorenzini, F.; Diene, G.; Crinò, A.; Illouz, F.; Grugni, G.; et al. AZP-531, an unacylated ghrelin analog, improves food-related behavior in patients with Prader-Willi syndrome: A randomized placebo-controlled trial. *PLoS ONE* **2018**, *13*, e0190849. [CrossRef] [PubMed]

24. Butler, M.G.; Kimonis, V.; Dykens, E.; Gold, J.A.; Miller, J.; Tamura, R.; Driscoll, D.J. Prader-Willi syndrome and early-onset morbid obesity NIH rare disease consortium: A review of natural history study. *Am. J. Med. Genet. A* **2018**, *176*, 368–375. [CrossRef] [PubMed]

25. Gliklich, R.E.; Dreyer, N.A.; Leavy, M.B. *Registries for Evaluating Patient Outcomes: A User's Guide*; Agency for Healthcare Research and Quality (US): Rockville, MD, USA, 2014.

26. McCarthy, J.; Lupo, P.J.; Kovar, E.; Rech, M.; Bostwick, B.; Scott, D.; Kraft, K.; Roscioli, T.; Charrow, J.; Vergano, S.A.S.; et al. Schaaf-Yang syndrome overview: Report of 78 individuals. *Am. J. Med. Genet. Part A* **2018**, *176*, 2564–2574. [CrossRef] [PubMed]

27. Butler, M.G.; Manzardo, A.M.; Heinemann, J.; Loker, C.; Loker, J. Causes of Death in Prader-Willi Syndrome: Prader-Willi Syndrome Association (USA) 40-Year Mortality Survey. *Genet. Med.* **2016**, *19*, 635–642. [CrossRef] [PubMed]
28. Azor, A.M.; Cole, J.H.; Holland, A.J.; Dumba, M.; Patel, M.C.; Sadlon, A.; Goldstone, A.P.; Manning, K.E. Increased brain age in adults with Prader-Willi syndrome. *NeuroImage Clin.* **2019**, *21*, 101664. [CrossRef] [PubMed]

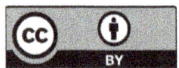 © 2019 by the authors. Licensee MDPI, Basel, Switzerland. This article is an open access article distributed under the terms and conditions of the Creative Commons Attribution (CC BY) license (http://creativecommons.org/licenses/by/4.0/).

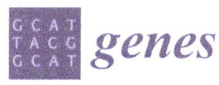

Article

Early Diagnosis in Prader–Willi Syndrome Reduces Obesity and Associated Co-Morbidities

Virginia E. Kimonis [1,2,*], Roy Tamura [3], June-Anne Gold [1,4], Nidhi Patel [1], Abhilasha Surampalli [1], Javeria Manazir [1], Jennifer L. Miller [5], Elizabeth Roof [6], Elisabeth Dykens [6], Merlin G. Butler [7] and Daniel J. Driscoll [5]

[1]   Division of Genetics and Genomic Medicine, Department of Pediatrics, University of California, Irvine, CA 92868, USA; juneannegold@gmail.com (J.-A.G.); nidhipatel.1992@gmail.com (N.P.); surampallia@gmail.com (A.S.); jmanazir@uci.edu (J.M.)
[2]   Children's Hospital of Orange County, Orange, CA 92868, USA
[3]   Health Informatics Institute, University of South Florida, Tampa, FL 33612, USA; Roy.Tamura@epi.usf.edu
[4]   Department of Pediatrics, Loma Linda University Medical School, Loma Linda, CA 92350, USA
[5]   Department of Pediatrics, University of Florida, Gainesville, FL 32610, USA; millejl@peds.ufl.edu (J.L.M.); driscdj@peds.ufl.edu (D.J.D.)
[6]   Vanderbilt Kennedy Center for Research on Human Development, Vanderbilt University, Nashville, TN 37203, USA; elizabeth.roof@Vanderbilt.edu (E.R.); elisabeth.m.dykens@Vanderbilt.edu (E.D.)
[7]   Departments of Psychiatry & Behavioral Sciences and Pediatrics, University of Kansas Medical Center, Kansas City, KS 66160, USA; mbutler4@kumc.edu
*   Correspondence: vkimonis@uci.edu; Tel.: +714-456-5791; Fax: +714-456-5330

Received: 28 September 2019; Accepted: 4 November 2019; Published: 6 November 2019

Abstract: Prader–Willi syndrome (PWS) is an imprinting genetic disorder characterized by lack of expression of genes on the paternal chromosome 15q11–q13 region. Growth hormone (GH) replacement positively influences stature and body composition in PWS. Our hypothesis was that early diagnosis delays onset of obesity in PWS. We studied 352 subjects with PWS, recruited from the NIH Rare Disease Clinical Research Network, to determine if age at diagnosis, ethnicity, gender, and PWS molecular class influenced the age they first become heavy, as determined by their primary care providers, and the age they first developed an increased appetite and began seeking food. The median ages that children with PWS became heavy were 10 years, 6 years and 4 years for age at diagnosis < 1 year, between 1 and 3 years, and greater than 3 years of age, respectively. The age of diagnosis and ethnicity were significant factors influencing when PWS children first became heavy ($p < 0.01$), however gender and the PWS molecular class had no influence. Early diagnosis delayed the onset of becoming heavy in individuals with PWS, permitting early GH and other treatment, thus reducing the risk of obesity-associated co-morbidities. Non-white individuals had an earlier onset of becoming heavy.

Keywords: Prader–Willi syndrome; age diagnosis; obesity; deletion; uniparental disomy

1. Introduction

1.1. Clinical Aspects of Prader–Willi Syndrome

Prader–Willi syndrome (PWS) affects about 1/15,000 individuals and is characterized by the lack of expression of genes on the paternal chromosome 15, located in the 15q11.2–q13 region [1–3]. The majority of imprinted genes in this region are involved in both RNA and protein processing of neuroregulators and hormones at the brain level. Disruptions in these genes negatively affect neuronal development, endocrine function and hormone levels, leading to the PWS phenotype [4–7]. Clinical features in the neonatal period include poor tone and suck, hypogonadism, feeding difficulty and failure to thrive. Later findings include a characteristic facial appearance, early-childhood onset of excessive hunger (hyperphagia), which can lead to morbid obesity if uncontrolled, mild intellectual disability, growth and other hormone deficiencies, leading to a short stature and small hands and feet, along with a distinctive behavioral phenotype, with temper tantrums, outbursts and self-injury (skin picking) [5,6,8]. Obesity related complications include cardiovascular problems, diabetes mellitus, hypertension, sleep apnea, gastric distension, necrosis, and choking as causes of death [4,9–12]. The diagnosis of PWS is often delayed, leading to excessive medical costs, parental anxiety and increased time before treatment with, e.g., growth hormone (GH) [13]. GH therapy in PWS allows for increased stature, muscle mass, strength and physical activity, thereby improving metabolic rate and energy expenditure, resulting in decreased fat mass and obesity status, particularly when administered at a young age [4,14–19]. When given at a young enough age, it improves the muscles used in sucking and feeding, enabling the avoidance of gastric tube placement. Although cognitive benefits of GH treatment have been identified in animal models and other patients with GH deficiencies, such ancillary effects of GH treatment in PWS have not been well studied. However, Dykens et al [20] showed the cognitive and adaptive advantages of early and continued GH treatment, and children with PWS who began treatment before 12 months of age had higher Nonverbal and Composite IQ scores than children who began treatment between 1 and 5 years of age. Most recently, Butler et al. [21] reported significantly higher IQ scores in the Vocabulary section of the Stanford–Binet test in the GH treated group when compared with non-GH treatment. These studies further emphasize the importance of earlier diagnosis and initiating treatment quickly.

1.2. Genetic Aspects of Prader–Willi Syndrome

Prader–Willi syndrome is a complex disorder of genomic imprinting caused by three main mechanisms, which ultimately results in a complete absence of paternally expressed genes in the 15q11.2–q13 region. The three PWS molecular genetic classes include a paternal deletion of the 15q11.2–q13 region (61% of cases), maternal uniparental disomy (UPD) 15 (36%), and an imprinting defect (ID) at 3% [22,23]. In the PWS chromosome region, the paternal gene copies are typically expressed, while the maternal alleles are silenced, due to a parent-of-origin specific imprinting process involving DNA methylation and other epigenetic factors during gametogenesis. The diagnosis of PWS is traditionally based on clinical suspicion and confirmed by a DNA methylation testing of chromosome 15, which detects 99% of individuals with PWS [4,6,24].

Driscoll et al. (2017) describes a comprehensive testing strategy to establish the specific genetic mechanism of an individual with DNA methylation analysis consistent with PWS [24]. Hartin et al. [25] provides an updated approach, using a genetic testing flow chart for PWS. The DNA methylation specific PCR (mPCR) test is the most rapid and cost-effective method to date in diagnosing PWS, however, it does not determine the specific PWS molecular classes. Chromosomal microarray analysis with SNP probes is currently the best method for identification of the individual PWS molecular classes, since it detects individuals with paternal 15q11–q13 deletions, segmental and total maternal isodisomy, and microdeletions of the imprinting center, however additional genetic testing is required in about 15% of patients in whom microarray results do not identify the genetic defect; the latter often requires parental DNA samples and chromosome 15 genotyping [22]. Methylation Specific -Multiplex Ligation-dependent Probe Amplification (MS-MLPA) of chromosome 15 and non-chromosome 15 polymorphic DNA markers may also be used to detect PWS once the diagnosis is under consideration [25–27]. In a study done by Bar et al. [28], the most common causes of delayed diagnosis in PWS were due to clinical features being missed in the neonatal period, as well as the use of fluorescence in situ hybridization (FISH) analysis for testing, which was the preferred method before the availability of methylation-specific PCR. FISH will only identify the 15q11–q13 deletion, which accounts for 60% of individuals with PWS, not maternal disomy 15 or imprinting defects. Next generation sequencing using chromosome 15 probes and, possibly, methylation-specific quantitative melting point analysis (MS-QMA) of imprinted genes in the chromosome 15 region, may become viable techniques in the future, to allow for more accurate and cost-efficient measures for early diagnosis, possibly including newborn screening [29,30].

2. Materials and Methods

The NIH-sponsored Rare Diseases Clinical Research Network (RDCRN) of the PWS/ Early Onset Morbidity (EMO) dataset was developed during the period 2008–2014, and data from the network were used in our study. Initially, the dataset was developed for natural history studies, characterization of diagnostic and therapeutic plans, and genotype–phenotype correlations in PWS. The RDCRN dataset has been utilized for several publications to date, which focused on the molecular and natural history, as well as the clinical characterization of PWS [5,25,31–34].

Our analysis was conducted on data collected from individuals with Prader–Willi syndrome recruited for the RDCRN Natural History 5202 protocol and stored at the Data Management Coordinating Center at the University of South Florida (Tampa), as described by Butler et al. [35]. The dataset included 355 individuals with genetically confirmed Prader–Willi syndrome, 37% of whom were diagnosed after the age of one year and 25% after the age of three years (with ages ranging from 1 month to 48 years). The age of diagnosis was elicited from the Natural History Form and approved by the local IRB Committees from the four participating clinic sites located in California, Kansas, Tennessee and Florida. If the data entry point was missing, then the age of diagnosis was defined as the age at which the last genetic test was performed on the enrolled subject.

Analysis

Three variables from the Natural History Form were analyzed: Age when child was first reported to become heavy; Age at which increased appetite first developed and Age the child first started to seek food. The age the child first became "heavy" (e.g., at or above the 85th percentile for weight for age and gender) was determined with input from the primary care providers and historical records for the majority of subjects enrolled. The majority of subjects between ages 2–20 years, who first became heavy during the trial, had a BMI above the 85th percentile for age and gender.

The variables were analyzed by the Cox proportional hazards model and by developing Kaplan–Meier curves, as undertaken in other reports on PWS (e.g., [36]). The earliest reported age for each of these variables was used as the endpoint age for each variable. Subjects who did not indicate an age for the variable were considered censored at their last recorded age. Because of the large variability in age at diagnosis (ranging from approximately 1 month to 48 years), the age of diagnosis was categorized into three categories, based on age distribution (<1 year, ≥1 years and <3 years, and ≥3 years) with the majority (62%) diagnosed at <1 year and 26% diagnosed at ≥3 years. In addition to age of diagnosis (categorized), ethnic background (white vs. non-white), gender, and PWS molecular class were included as covariates in the Cox hazard model and analyzed for statistical significance.

3. Results

Summaries of the number of subjects with PWS in each of the three age categories (<1 year, >1 years and <3 years, and ≥3 years) and other covariates are shown in Table 1. Kaplan–Meier curves for the age when the child first became heavy as determined by their primary care providers, age the child developed an increased appetite, and age the child began to actively seek food are shown in Figures 1–3, respectively. The Cox proportional hazards analyses for these three variables are shown in Table 2. For example, individuals with PWS having an imprinting defect had a hazard ratio (HR) of 1.45 of becoming heavy, compared to UPD15 or 15q11–q13 deletion molecular genetic classes, but the number of subjects tested with imprinting defects was low. The 15q11–q13 deletion group had the highest HR of 1.31 for an increased appetite, as well as for actively seeking food, with an HR of 1.14.

Both the age of diagnosis ($p < 0.001$) and race ($p = 0.004$) were significant factors influencing the age when the child was first reported to be heavy. The earlier the diagnosis of PWS, the later the age at which individuals became heavy. The estimated median age for when the child first became heavy was 10 years for an age of diagnosis of < 1 year, 6 years for an age of diagnosis between 1 and 3 years, and 4 years for an age of diagnosis greater than 3 years. Additional partitions of age of diagnosis ≥ 3 years category were also examined, but no evidence was found that further partitioning into separate categories produced significant statistical differences. Non-white individuals became heavier at an earlier age, compared with whites, with an estimated median age of 4 years for non-whites and a median age of 8 years for whites. However, age of diagnosis and race did not influence the age at which individuals first developed an increased appetite or began actively seeking food. In addition, our data analysis indicates that the age the individual became heavy, age of increased appetite and age of seeking food were not significantly different across the three PWS molecular classes (deletion, UPD or imprinting defects), except for a difference between the 15q11–q13 deletion and UPD15 subjects regarding increased appetite (Figures 1–3).

Table 1. Summary and frequency of Prader–Willi subjects in various categories.

Category	Frequency (%)
Age of Diagnosis (yrs.)	
Mean = 3.1	
Median = 0.3	
SD = 6.7	
Min =0.0	
Max = 48.0	
Age of Diagnosis Category	
<1 yr.	217 (62%)
≥1 yr. and <3 yrs.	42 (12%)
≥3 yrs.	93 (26%)
Gender	
Female	194 (55%)
Male	158 (45%)
Ethicity	
White	328 (93%)
Non-White	24 (7%)
Prader–Willi Molecular Class	
Deletion	216 (61%)
Imprinting Defect	11 (3%)
Uniparental Disomy	125 (36%)

Table 2. Cox proportional hazard analyses for age at which individuals first becoming heavy, age of increased appetite, and age individuals began actively seeking food.

	First Becoming Heavy	**Increased Appetite**	**Actively Seeking Food**
Effect	Hazard Ratio (95% CI) *p* value	Hazard Ratio (95% CI) *p* value	Hazard Ratio (95% CI) *p* value
Gender (ref = female)	0.99 (0.73, 1.33) 0.990	1.13 (0.88, 1.46) 0.332	1.09 (0.83, 1.44) 0.525
PWS Molecular Class			
Deletion vs. UPD	0.90 (0.66, 1.23) 0.499	1.31 (1.00, 1.72) 0.054	1.14 (0.85, 1.52) 0.393
ID vs. UPD	1.45 (0.69, 3.07) 0.326	0.72 (0.33, 1.58) 0.415	1.05 (0.50, 2.20) 0.893
Ethnicity (ref = white)	0.46 (0.28, 0.78) 0.004	0.76 (0.48, 1.21) 0.179	0.73 (0.44, 1.21) 0.224
Age of Diagnosis			
<1 vs. 1–3	0.67 (0.43, 1.04) 0.077	0.70 (0.47, 1.03) 0.067	0.72 (0.48, 1.09) 0.125
<1 vs. >3 yrs.	0.48 (0.35, 0.66) < 0.001	0.90 (0.67, 1.20) 0.456	1.05 (0.77, 1.43) 0.754

Bold represent labels for the material in the rows.

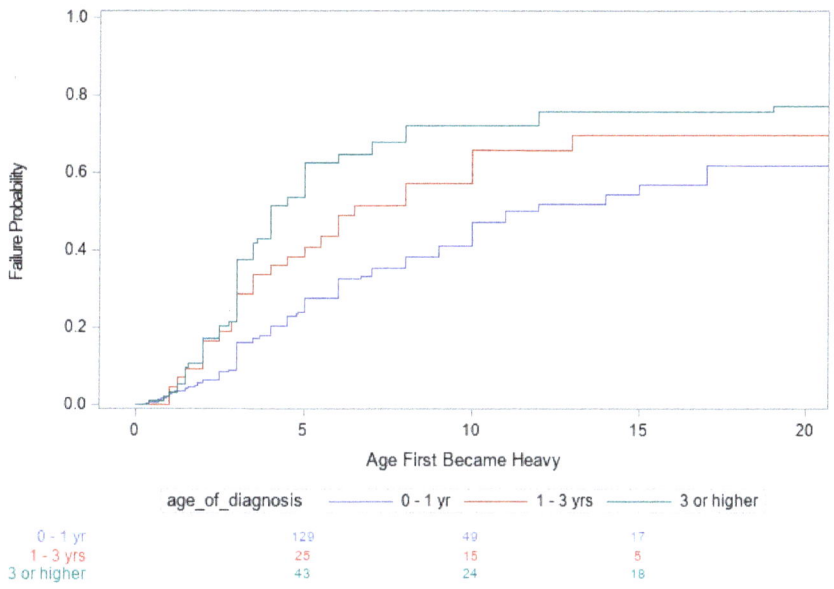

Figure 1. Kaplan–Meier Plot of the age individuals first become heavy.

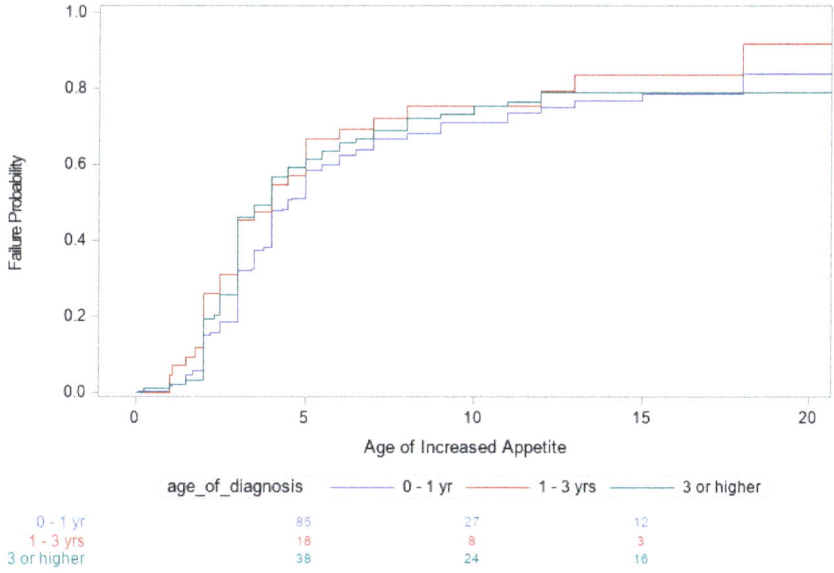

Figure 2. Kaplan–Meier Plot of ages individuals first developed an increased appetite.

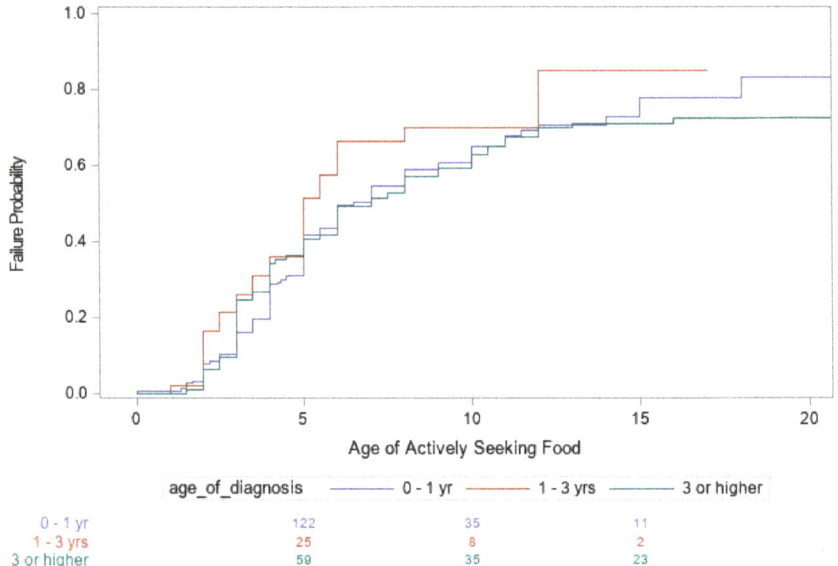

Figure 3. Kaplan–Meier Plot of the age individuals began to actively seek food.

4. Discussion

Early diagnosis of Prader–Willi syndrome, particularly in the newborn period, is critical for changing the lives of those with this disorder and further supported by our study results, showing that those with earlier diagnosis developed obesity at a later age. We firmly believe that early diagnosis in the first few weeks of the newborn period is critical for individuals with PWS to receive appropriate intervention and anticipatory guidance. This should happen at an early an age as possible. For example, GH treatment at an early age affords the opportunity to take proactive strategies for regulating caloric intake and delaying the onset and reducing the risk of early obesity, with associated co-morbidities such as diabetes, hypertension, and respiratory compromise. The earlier diagnosis would also impact the cost of medical care, by decreasing diagnostic evaluations and the length of hospital stays, as noted by Shoffstall et al. [13].

The typical time of diagnosis for individuals with PWS was noted approximately three decades ago to be between 7 and 9 years of age, depending on the genetic subtype (deletion vs. non-deletion status [8]). In our cohort of 352 analyzed subjects with PWS, the age of diagnosis in our younger subjects had decreased to a mean age of 3.1 years, but often not enough to avoid extensive and costly evaluations, with health concerns leading to ineffective medical care and treatment. We believe that it is critical to detect those with PWS in the newborn period, in order for treatment to begin as early as possible. Significant progress has been made in awareness and early diagnosis of PWS, but further efforts could be made to diagnose at earlier stages.

Better acceptance of expanded newborn screening programs nationwide regarding metabolic and genetic disorders may impact this problem. Early diagnosis and treatment can significantly improve prognosis in other disorders not readily detected at birth by routine physical examination, but sensitive, specific, inexpensive tests do exist, using expanded newborn screening programs with filter paper cards, a gold standard for newborn testing and diagnosis of genetic disorders [2]. As an example, on 21 May 2010, the Secretary of Health and Human Services added Severe Combined Immunodeficiency (SCID), an immune disorder with a frequency of 1/53,000 to the Recommended Uniform Newborn Screening Panel (RUSP) [1,3]. Pompe disease, another rare metabolic disorder was also added to the newborn screening list in several states. Since the clinical presentation and available treatment of PWS meets or fulfills the criteria for newborn screening, it is expected that newborn screening for PWS will become available in the future, depending on cost-effective genetic testing methods, where early diagnosis can impact medical care, treatment and quality of life [37]. Early diagnosis can also transform medical management of PWS, by eliminating extensive and expensive evaluations, along with the uncertainty generated by not having a diagnosis early in infancy. If the diagnosis is not made early, the patient is deprived of the benefits of optimal treatment and anticipatory strategies to avoid morbid obesity.

The benefits of lifelong GH therapy in infants, children and adults with PWS have been demonstrated in multiple well-designed and controlled studies [14,38–43]. For example, GH treatment for 2 years in children showed major increases in height and weight, and a decrease in body fat [44]. GH replacement therapy also improves linear growth velocity and, ultimately, height, and results in healthier body composition (increased lean body mass, decreased fat mass), muscle function and level of activity [4,40,45]. GH treatment in children with PWS ultimately improves growth, adult height and body composition, and nearly normalizes stature by 18 years of age, with a significant improvement in obesity status, as noted in PWS-specific standardized growth charts [10,18,46]. Evidence further supports treating PWS adults with GH, with it leading to increased muscle strength and physical activity, improved lipid levels and better quality of life measures after one year of treatment (e.g., [40]). The improvements with GH treatment are also demonstrated in bone mineral density [47,48]. When treatment occurs from infancy, facial appearance and body habitus also normalizes in conjunction with good dietary management, and there is an improvement in quality of life and psychosocial status in PWS individuals [45,49]. The benefits of initiating treatment before the age of 2 years are well recognized, and further improvement are possible, when the diagnosis and treatment is earlier particularly in the newborn period [50]. Early diagnosis, good dietary control, exercise and GH treatment with better therapeutic approaches [46,51] can reduce the risk and age of onset of obesity, and many of the associated co-morbidities, such as diabetes, hypertension, and respiratory compromise, common in PWS without early recognition and treatment. Despite significant advances in diagnosing PWS, the mean age of diagnosis is still delayed. As seen in our current study, there was a wide range of age at diagnosis, spanning birth–48.0 years. (mean ± SD = 3.1 yr. ± 6.7 yr.; median = 0.3 yr.).

We believe it is important for individuals to be diagnosed in the newborn period, to receive better treatment and appropriate, syndrome-specific medical care, beginning as early as the first few weeks of life. The current genetic testing methods (e.g., mPCR, high resolution chromosomal microarrays) which are useful for diagnosing PWS in the newborn period, would also have the added benefit of detecting the majority of newborns with Angelman syndrome (AS), as well. AS is caused by a maternal chromosome 15q11–q13 deletion, whereas PWS is associated with a paternal 15q11–q13 deletion. AS is associated with severe intellectual disability, electroencephalographic (EEG) abnormalities and epilepsy, limited or absent language development, an abnormal gait, inappropriate laughter and autistic behaviors, with a frequency of 1/12,000 [52,53]. The combined frequency for the two genomic imprinting disorders of PWS and AS would be about 1/6000. This frequency is more common than nearly all other disorders for which newborn screening is currently available. The benefits for early detection for Angelman syndrome would also be substantial, as early diagnosis avoids the unnecessary diagnostic odyssey (and expense), as seen in PWS, and anxiety that families experience prior to an accurate diagnosis, permitting early therapy with anticonvulsants and interventions with support. Early diagnosis, identifying abnormal DNA methylation, which has a 99% accuracy rate for the diagnosis of PWS and a 78% chance of accuracy identifying AS, would also allow for the detection of imprinting defects for both PWS or AS, which can be associated with a 50% recurrence risk, thereby permitting early and accurate genetic counseling [22,24,52]. Large-scale newborn screening programs for PWS/ Angelman syndrome would also give us a much more accurate frequency of the disorder, which may be more prevalent than we previously thought.

In summary, early diagnosis could lead to significant improvements, with decreased costs and better medical care of affected newborns (in both PWS and AS), leading to an enhanced quality of life.

More research is needed to further investigate the feasibility of lowering costs of testing, including DNA methylation analysis and its application in the newborn setting.

Author Contributions: Conceptualization, V.E.K.; Formal analysis, V.E.K., R.T. and D.J.D.; Funding acquisition, D.J.D.; Investigation, V.E.K., J.-A.G., J.L.M., E.D. and M.G.B.; Methodology, V.E.K., E.D., M.G.B. and D.J.D.; Project administration, V.E.K., J.-A.G. and E.R.; Resources, V.E.K. and M.G.B.; Supervision, V.E.K. and E.D.; Writing—Original draft, V.E.K. and J.M.; Writing—Review & editing, V.E.K., R.T., J.-A.G., N.P., A.S., J.M., J.L.M., E.R., E.D., M.G.B. and D.J.D.

Funding: This research was funded by NIH/NCATS Clinical and Translational Science Award University of Florida: UL1 TR000064. Prader-Willi Syndrome Association (USA); National Institutes of Health (NIH) Rare Disease Clinical Research Network (RDCRN): National Institutes of Health: U54 HD06122.

Acknowledgments: We thank the individuals with Prader–Willi syndrome, their families and their health care providers for their participation in the study. We acknowledge support from the Prader–Willi Syndrome Association (USA) and the Angelman, Rett and Prader–Willi Syndromes Consortium (U54 HD06122), which was part of the National Institutes of Health (NIH) Rare Disease Clinical Research Network (RDCRN) supported through collaboration between the NIH Office of Advancing Translational Science (NCATS), the National Institute of Child Health and Human Development (NICHD) and Data Management Coordinating Center of University of South Florida. We are very thankful for the invaluable help of the ICTS staff at the University of California-Irvine, as well as other institutions, for contributing their skills to the study. We thank Linda Freedkin for her assistance with the manuscript.

Conflicts of Interest: The authors declare no conflict of interest.

References

1. Baker, M.W.; Grossman, W.J.; Laessig, R.H.; Hoffman, G.L.; Brokopp, C.D.; Kurtycz, D.F.; Cogley, M.F.; Litsheim, T.J.; Katcher, M.L.; Routes, J.M. Development of a routine newborn screening protocol for severe combined immunodeficiency. *J. Allergy Clin. Immunol.* **2009**, *124*, 522–527. [CrossRef] [PubMed]

2. Routes, J.M.; Grossman, W.J.; Verbsky, J.; Laessig, R.H.; Hoffman, G.L.; Brokopp, C.D.; Baker, M.W. Statewide newborn screening for severe T-cell lymphopenia. *JAMA* **2009**, *302*, 2465–2470. [CrossRef] [PubMed]

3. Vogel, B.H.; Bonagura, V.; Weinberg, G.A.; Ballow, M.; Isabelle, J.; DiAntonio, L.; Parker, A.; Young, A.; Cunningham-Rundles, C.; Fong, C.T.; et al. Newborn screening for SCID in New York State: Experience from the first two years. *J. Clin. Immunol.* **2014**, *34*, 289–303. [CrossRef] [PubMed]

4. Butler, M.G. Management of obesity in Prader-Willi syndrome. *Nat. Clin. Pract. Endocrinol. Metab.* **2006**, *2*, 592–593. [CrossRef]

5. Butler, M.G.; Sturich, J.; Lee, J.; Myers, S.E.; Whitman, B.Y.; Gold, J.A.; Kimonis, V.; Scheimann, A.; Terrazas, N.; Driscoll, D.J. Growth standards of infants with Prader-Willi syndrome. *Pediatrics* **2011**, *127*, 687–695. [CrossRef] [PubMed]

6. Cassidy, S.B.; Schwartz, S.; Miller, J.L.; Driscoll, D.J. Prader-Willi syndrome. *Genet. Med.* **2012**, *14*, 10–26. [CrossRef]

7. Angulo, M.A.; Butler, M.G.; Cataletto, M.E. Prader-Willi syndrome: A review of clinical, genetic, and endocrine findings. *J. Endocrinol. Investig.* **2015**, *38*, 1249–1263. [CrossRef]

8. Butler, M.G. Prader-Willi syndrome: Current understanding of cause and diagnosis. *Am. J. Med. Genet.* **1990**, *35*, 319–332. [CrossRef]

9. Butler, M.G.; Manzardo, A.M.; Heinemann, J.; Loker, C.; Loker, J. Causes of death in Prader-Willi syndrome: Prader-Willi Syndrome Association (USA) 40-year mortality survey. *Genet. Med.* **2017**, *19*, 635–642. [CrossRef]

10. Butler, M.G. Single Gene and Syndromic Causes of Obesity: Illustrative Examples. *Prog. Mol. Biol. Transl. Sci.* **2016**, *140*, 1–45. [CrossRef]

11. Stevenson, D.A.; Heinemann, J.; Angulo, M.; Butler, M.G.; Loker, J.; Rupe, N.; Kendell, P.; Cassidy, S.B.; Scheimann, A. Gastric rupture and necrosis in Prader-Willi syndrome. *J. Pediatr. Gastroenterol. Nutr.* **2007**, *45*, 272–274. [CrossRef] [PubMed]

12. Stevenson, D.A.; Heinemann, J.; Angulo, M.; Butler, M.G.; Loker, J.; Rupe, N.; Kendell, P.; Clericuzio, C.L.; Scheimann, A.O. Deaths due to choking in Prader-Willi syndrome. *Am. J. Med. Genet. Part A* **2007**, *143*, 484–487. [CrossRef] [PubMed]

13. Shoffstall, A.J.; Gaebler, J.A.; Kreher, N.C.; Niecko, T.; Douglas, D.; Strong, T.V.; Miller, J.L.; Stafford, D.E.; Butler, M.G. The High Direct Medical Costs of Prader-Willi Syndrome. *J. Pediatr.* **2016**, *175*, 137–143. [CrossRef] [PubMed]

14. Lindgren, A.C.; Lindberg, A. Growth hormone treatment completely normalizes adult height and improves body composition in Prader-Willi syndrome: Experience from KIGS (Pfizer International Growth Database). *Horm. Res.* **2008**, *70*, 182–187. [CrossRef] [PubMed]

15. Nishi, Y.; Tanaka, T. Growth Hormone Treatment and Adverse Events. *Pediatr. Endocrinol. Rev.* **2017**, *14* (Suppl. 1), 235–239. [CrossRef]

16. Grugni, G.; Marzullo, P. Diagnosis and treatment of GH deficiency in Prader-Willi syndrome. *Best Pract. Res. Clin. Endocrinol. Metab.* **2016**, *30*, 785–794. [CrossRef]

17. Irizarry, K.A.; Miller, M.; Freemark, M.; Haqq, A.M. Prader Willi Syndrome: Genetics, Metabolomics, Hormonal Function, and New Approaches to Therapy. *Adv. Pediatr.* **2016**, *63*, 47–77. [CrossRef]

18. Butler, M.G.; Lee, J.; Cox, D.M.; Manzardo, A.M.; Gold, J.A.; Miller, J.L.; Roof, E.; Dykens, E.; Kimonis, V.; Driscoll, D.J. Growth Charts for Prader-Willi Syndrome During Growth Hormone Treatment. *Clin. Pediatr.* **2016**, *55*, 957–974. [CrossRef]

19. Heksch, R.; Kamboj, M.; Anglin, K.; Obrynba, K. Review of Prader-Willi syndrome: The endocrine approach. *Transl. Pediatr.* **2017**, *6*, 274–285. [CrossRef]

20. Dykens, E.M.; Roof, E.; Hunt-Hawkins, H. Cognitive and adaptive advantages of growth hormone treatment in children with Prader-Willi syndrome. *J. Child. Psychol. Psychiatry* **2017**, *58*, 64–74. [CrossRef]

21. Butler, M.G.; Matthews, N.A.; Patel, N.; Surampalli, A.; Gold, J.A.; Khare, M.; Thompson, T.; Cassidy, S.B.; Kimonis, V.E. Impact of genetic subtypes of Prader-Willi syndrome with growth hormone therapy on intelligence and body mass index. *Am. J. Med. Genet. Part A* **2019**, *179*, 1826–1835. [CrossRef] [PubMed]

22. Butler, M.G.; Hartin, S.N.; Hossain, W.A.; Manzardo, A.M.; Kimonis, V.; Dykens, E.; Gold, J.A.; Kim, S.J.; Weisensel, N.; Tamura, R.; et al. Molecular genetic classification in Prader-Willi syndrome: A multisite cohort study. *J. Med. Genet.* **2019**, *56*, 149–153. [CrossRef] [PubMed]

23. Manzardo, A.M.; Heinemann, J.; McManus, B.; Loker, C.; Loker, J.; Butler, M.G. Venous Thromboembolism in Prader-Willi Syndrome: A Questionnaire Survey. *Genes* **2019**, *10*. [CrossRef] [PubMed]

24. Driscoll, D.J.; Miller, J.L.; Schwartz, S.; Cassidy, S.B. Prader- Willi Syndrome. Available online: https://www.ncbi.nlm.nih.gov/books/NBK1330/ (accessed on 28 September 2019).

25. Henkhaus, R.S.; Kim, S.J.; Kimonis, V.E.; Gold, J.A.; Dykens, E.M.; Driscoll, D.J.; Butler, M.G. Methylation-specific multiplex ligation-dependent probe amplification and identification of deletion genetic subtypes in Prader-Willi syndrome. *Genet. Test. Mol. Biomark.* **2012**, *16*, 178–186. [CrossRef]

26. Hartin, S.N.; Hossain, W.A.; Francis, D.; Godler, D.E.; Barkataki, S.; Butler, M.G. Analysis of the Prader-Willi syndrome imprinting center using droplet digital PCR and next-generation whole-exome sequencing. *Mol. Genet. Genomic Med.* **2019**, *7*, e00575. [CrossRef] [PubMed]

27. Bittel, D.C.; Kibiryeva, N.; Butler, M.G. Methylation-specific multiplex ligation-dependent probe amplification analysis of subjects with chromosome 15 abnormalities. *Genet. Test.* **2007**, *11*, 467–475. [CrossRef] [PubMed]

28. Bar, C.; Diene, G.; Molinas, C.; Bieth, E.; Casper, C.; Tauber, M. Early diagnosis and care is achieved but should be improved in infants with Prader-Willi syndrome. *Orphanet J. Rare Dis.* **2017**, *12*, 118. [CrossRef] [PubMed]

29. Inaba, Y.; Schwartz, C.E.; Bui, Q.M.; Li, X.; Skinner, C.; Field, M.; Wotton, T.; Hagerman, R.J.; Francis, D.; Amor, D.J.; et al. Early detection of fragile X syndrome: Applications of a novel approach for improved quantitative methylation analysis in venous blood and newborn blood spots. *Clin. Chem.* **2014**, *60*, 963–973. [CrossRef]

30. Godler, D.E.; Inaba, Y.; Schwartz, C.E.; Bui, Q.M.; Shi, E.Z.; Li, X.; Herlihy, A.S.; Skinner, C.; Hagerman, R.J.; Francis, D.; et al. Detection of skewed X-chromosome inactivation in Fragile X syndrome and X chromosome aneuploidy using quantitative melt analysis. *Expert Rev. Mol. Med.* **2015**, *17*, e13. [CrossRef]

31. Butler, M.G.; Lee, J.; Manzardo, A.M.; Gold, J.A.; Miller, J.L.; Kimonis, V.; Driscoll, D.J. Growth charts for non-growth hormone treated Prader-Willi syndrome. *Pediatrics* **2015**, *135*, e126–e135. [CrossRef]

32. Butler, M.G.; Sturich, J.; Myers, S.E.; Gold, J.A.; Kimonis, V.; Driscoll, D.J. Is gestation in Prader-Willi syndrome affected by the genetic subtype? *J. Assist. Reprod. Genet.* **2009**, *26*, 461–466. [CrossRef] [PubMed]

33. Gold, J.A.; Ruth, C.; Osann, K.; Flodman, P.; McManus, B.; Lee, H.S.; Donkervoort, S.; Khare, M.; Roof, E.; Dykens, E.; et al. Frequency of Prader-Willi syndrome in births conceived via assisted reproductive technology. *Genet. Med.* **2014**, *16*, 164–169. [CrossRef] [PubMed]

34. Miller, J.L.; Lynn, C.H.; Driscoll, D.C.; Goldstone, A.P.; Gold, J.A.; Kimonis, V.; Dykens, E.; Butler, M.G.; Shuster, J.J.; Driscoll, D.J. Nutritional phases in Prader-Willi syndrome. *Am. J. Med. Genet. Part A* **2011**, *155*, 1040–1049. [CrossRef] [PubMed]

35. Butler, M.G.; Kimonis, V.; Dykens, E.; Gold, J.A.; Miller, J.; Tamura, R.; Driscoll, D.J. Prader-Willi syndrome and early-onset morbid obesity NIH rare disease consortium: A review of natural history study. *Am. J. Med. Genet. Part A* **2018**, *176*, 368–375. [CrossRef] [PubMed]

36. Manzardo, A.M.; Loker, J.; Heinemann, J.; Loker, C.; Butler, M.G. Survival trends from the Prader-Willi Syndrome Association (USA) 40-year mortality survey. *Genet. Med.* **2018**, *20*, 24–30. [CrossRef] [PubMed]

37. Mahmoud, R.; Singh, P.; Weiss, L.; Lakatos, A.; Oakes, M.; Hossain, W.; Butler, M.G.; Kimonis, V. Newborn screening for Prader-Willi syndrome is feasible: Early diagnosis for better outcomes. *Am. J. Med. Genet. Part A* **2019**, *179*, 29–36. [CrossRef] [PubMed]

38. Angulo, M.A.; Castro-Magana, M.; Lamerson, M.; Arguello, R.; Accacha, S.; Khan, A. Final adult height in children with Prader-Willi syndrome with and without human growth hormone treatment. *Am. J. Med. Genet. Part A* **2007**, *143*, 1456–1461. [CrossRef]

39. Carrel, A.L.; Myers, S.E.; Whitman, B.Y.; Allen, D.B. Sustained benefits of growth hormone on body composition, fat utilization, physical strength and agility, and growth in Prader-Willi syndrome are dose-dependent. *J. Pediatr. Endocrinol. Metab.* **2001**, *14*, 1097–1105. [CrossRef]

40. Butler, M.G.; Smith, B.K.; Lee, J.; Gibson, C.; Schmoll, C.; Moore, W.V.; Donnelly, J.E. Effects of growth hormone treatment in adults with Prader-Willi syndrome. *Growth Horm. IGF Res.* **2013**, *23*, 81–87. [CrossRef]

41. Carrel, A.L.; Myers, S.E.; Whitman, B.Y.; Eickhoff, J.; Allen, D.B. Long-term growth hormone therapy changes the natural history of body composition and motor function in children with prader-willi syndrome. *J. Clin. Endocrinol. Metab.* **2010**, *95*, 1131–1136. [CrossRef]

42. Mogul, H.R.; Lee, P.D.; Whitman, B.Y.; Zipf, W.B.; Frey, M.; Myers, S.; Cahan, M.; Pinyerd, B.; Southren, A.L. Growth hormone treatment of adults with Prader-Willi syndrome and growth hormone deficiency improves lean body mass, fractional body fat, and serum triiodothyronine without glucose impairment: Results from the United States multicenter trial. *J. Clin. Endocrinol. Metab.* **2008**, *93*, 1238–1245. [CrossRef] [PubMed]

43. Hoybye, C. Five-years growth hormone (GH) treatment in adults with Prader-Willi syndrome. *Acta Paediatr.* **2007**, *96*, 410–413. [CrossRef] [PubMed]

44. Myers, S.E.; Whitman, B.Y.; Carrel, A.L.; Moerchen, V.; Bekx, M.T.; Allen, D.B. Two years of growth hormone therapy in young children with Prader-Willi syndrome: Physical and neurodevelopmental benefits. *Am. J. Med. Genet. Part A* **2007**, *143*, 443–448. [CrossRef] [PubMed]

45. Butler, M.G.; Roberts, J.; Hayes, J.; Tan, X.; Manzardo, A.M. Growth hormone receptor (GHR) gene polymorphism and Prader-Willi syndrome. *Am. J. Med. Genet. Part A* **2013**, *161*, 1647–1653. [CrossRef]

46. Butler, M.G.; Manzardo, A.M.; Forster, J.L. Prader-Willi Syndrome: Clinical Genetics and Diagnostic Aspects with Treatment Approaches. *Curr. Pediatr. Rev.* **2016**, *12*, 136–166. [CrossRef]

47. Khare, M.; Gold, J.A.; Wencel, M.; Billimek, J.; Surampalli, A.; Duarte, B.; Pontello, A.; Galassetti, P.; Cassidy, S.; Kimonis, V.E. Effect of genetic subtypes and growth hormone treatment on bone mineral density in Prader-Willi syndrome. *J. Pediatr. Endocrinol. Metab.* **2014**, *27*, 511–518. [CrossRef]

48. Galassetti, P.; Saetrum Opgaard, O.; Cassidy, S.B.; Pontello, A. Nutrient intake and body composition variables in Prader-Willi syndrome—Effect of growth hormone supplementation and genetic subtype. *J. Pediatr. Endocrinol. Metab.* **2007**, *20*, 491–500. [CrossRef]

49. Whitman, B.Y.; Myers, S.; Carrel, A.; Allen, D. The behavioral impact of growth hormone treatment for children and adolescents with Prader-Willi syndrome: A 2-year, controlled study. *Pediatrics* **2002**, *109*, e35. [CrossRef]

50. Goldstone, A.P.; Holland, A.J.; Hauffa, B.P.; Hokken-Koelega, A.C.; Tauber, M. Recommendations for the diagnosis and management of Prader-Willi syndrome. *J. Clin. Endocrinol. Metab.* **2008**, *93*, 4183–4197. [CrossRef]

51. Butler, M.G.; Miller, J.L.; Forster, J.L. Prader-Willi Syndrome—Clinical Genetics, Diagnosis and Treatment Approaches: An Update. *Curr. Pediatr. Rev.* **2019**. [CrossRef]

52. Lossie, A.C.; Whitney, M.M.; Amidon, D.; Dong, H.J.; Chen, P.; Theriaque, D.; Hutson, A.; Nicholls, R.D.; Zori, R.T.; Williams, C.A.; et al. Distinct phenotypes distinguish the molecular classes of Angelman syndrome. *J. Med. Genet.* **2001**, *38*, 834–845. [CrossRef] [PubMed]

53. Dagli, A.I.; Mueller, J.; Williams, C.A. *Angelman Syndrome*; Adam, M.P., Ardinger, H.H., Pagon, R.A., Eds.; [Updated 2017 Dec 21]. GeneReviews®[Internet]; University of Washington: Seattle, WA, USA, 1993–2019. Available online: https://www.ncbi.nlm.nih.gov/books/NBK1144/ (accessed on 28 September 2019).

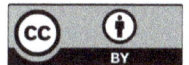 © 2019 by the authors. Licensee MDPI, Basel, Switzerland. This article is an open access article distributed under the terms and conditions of the Creative Commons Attribution (CC BY) license (http://creativecommons.org/licenses/by/4.0/).

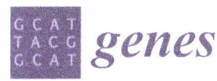

Concept Paper

Defining Mental and Behavioural Disorders in Genetically Determined Neurodevelopmental Syndromes with Particular Reference to Prader-Willi Syndrome

Anthony J. Holland, Lucie C.S. Aman and Joyce E. Whittington *

Department of Psychiatry, University of Cambridge, Cambridge CB2 8AH, UK; ajh1008@cam.ac.uk (A.J.H.); lcsa2@medschl.cam.ac.uk (L.C.S.A.)
* Correspondence: jew1000@cam.ac.uk; Tel.: +1-2234-65266

Received: 31 July 2019; Accepted: 3 December 2019; Published: 9 December 2019

Abstract: Genetically determined neurodevelopmental syndromes are frequently associated with a particular developmental trajectory, and with a cognitive profile and increased propensity to specific mental and behavioural disorders that are particular to, but not necessarily unique to the syndrome. How should these mental and behavioural disorders best be conceptualised given that similar symptoms are included in the definition of different mental disorders as listed in DSM-5 and ICD-10? In addition, a different conceptual framework, that of applied behavioural analysis, has been used to inform interventions for what are termed 'challenging behaviours' in contrast to types of interventions for those conditions meeting diagnostic criteria for a 'mental disorder'. These syndrome-specific developmental profiles and associated co-morbidities must be a direct or indirect consequence of the genetic abnormality associated with that syndrome, but the genetic loci associated with the syndrome may not be involved in the aetiology of similar symptoms in the general population. This being so, should we expect underlying brain mechanisms and treatments for specific psychopathology in one group to be effective in the other? Using Prader-Willi syndrome as an example, we propose that the conceptual thinking that informed the development of the Research Domain Criteria provides a model for taxonomy of psychiatric and behavioural disorders in genetically determined neurodevelopmental syndromes. This model brings together diagnostic, psychological and developmental approaches with the aim of matching specific behaviours to identifiable neural mechanisms.

Keywords: genetic syndrome; Prader-Willi syndrome; mental illness; psychosis; major depressive illness; obsessive-compulsive disorder; autism; eating disorder; skin picking

1. Introduction

Whilst abnormalities at a specific genetic locus can readily be linked to the presence of a specific physical illness (e.g., sickle cell anaemia and Huntington disease) establishing such similarly close relationships between single genes and particular behaviours and/or mental disorders has been much more elusive. The study of neurodevelopmental syndromes in which their genetics is known and the risk of specific behaviours and/or mental disorders are increased has the potential for providing new insights into the genetic influences on the aetiology of such problems. However, in order to investigate the mechanisms that underpin the rates of syndrome specific behavioural and psychiatric disorders it is important to be clear as to how these are best defined in a manner that more directly links them to known neural systems. Similarities in behaviour occur across neurodevelopmental syndromes: for example, intermittent aggressive or self-injurious behaviour. Just as there are likely to be different reasons for why a person has high blood sugar, so there are likely to be different reasons for why people engage in aggressive or self-injurious behaviour. However, there may be a common mechanism for similar behaviours within a specific syndrome. In each case the behaviours may have their own identifiable characteristics in terms of the age of onset, course, and the exact form of the behaviour. In clinical practice it is the diagnostic process and the specificity of the clinical history, physical examination, and investigations that enable the link to be made between reported symptoms or observed signs with the putative underlying pathology, and to treatment. Once the behavioural and psychiatric phenomenology are clearly defined, the question can be asked as to whether such phenomena are a consequence of abnormalities in the brain structure and function or whether the behaviour that is observed is better conceptualized as being primarily shaped by environmental contingencies. New treatments for such behaviours are unlikely to emerge from an understanding of the syndrome genetics alone but instead through an understanding of the unique impact of the syndrome genotype on brain development and neural function and the extent and nature of any interplay between the organic and the psychological.

We consider three conceptual frameworks for the description and/or classification of mental and behavioural disorders. These are: the diagnostic approach, applied behavioural analysis, and Research Domain Criteria. We consider how each approach can add to our understanding of such disorders, and why different approaches evolved. Firstly, dissatisfaction with the traditional DSM-5 [1] and ICD-10 [2] approach to classification and diagnosis (diagnostic approach) in respect of behavioural disorders, often termed 'challenging behaviours', has led to the application of applied behavioural analysis (ABA) to the understanding of such behaviours. However, this, in turn, fails to fully explain those behaviours that are prevalent in, and specific to, a given genetic syndrome. Now a new framework (Research Domain Criteria) has been proposed that we argue provides a better framework for understanding 'challenging behaviour' in the context of neurodevelopmental syndromes by seeking to match such behaviours to underlying neural mechanisms.

The aims of this paper are to explore these issues using Prader-Willi syndrome (PWS) as an example. We begin with a description of PWS, followed by a section on genetically determined neurodevelopmental syndromes, from which we have chosen PWS as a representative to illustrate our arguments. We then describe the three different models for the classification of mental and behavioural disorders, before showing that each can contribute to understanding and/or treating such disorders in PWS.

2. Prader-Willi Syndrome (PWS)

Prader-Willi Syndrome is a rare disorder with a birth incidence rate estimated at 1:25,000 [3–6] and UK prevalence around 1:50,000 [3]. The underlying cause of PWS is the loss of expression of maternally imprinted (paternally expressed) genes from the q11–q13 region of the paternally inherited chromosome 15. This can occur in one of two ways: part, or whole, of the region is deleted (deletion subtype); or two maternally marked chromosome 15 s, but no paternally marked chromosome, are inherited (maternal disomy subtype). There are two common deleted regions: Type 1 between breakpoints 1 and 3 and Type 2 between breakpoints 2 and 3. Maternally marked chromosomes in disomy subclasses are both inherited from the mother (mUPD) or one from the mother and one from the paternal grandmother (imprinting centre defect (IC defect)). The 15q11-q13 region contains both imprinted and non-imprinted genes (Figure 1), the imprinted genes *SNORD116* (human studies) and *MAGEL2* (mouse studies) being considered central to PWS.

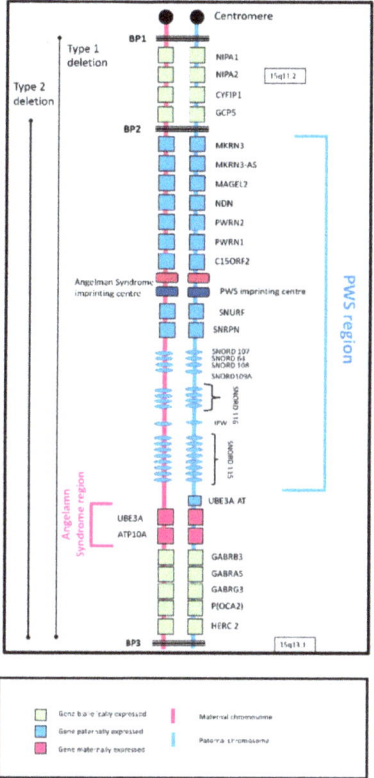

Figure 1. The genetics of Prader-Willi syndrome (PWS).

Although the underlying genetic abnormalities give a 'core' genotype, there are genetic differences between the subtypes, which give rise to observed phenotypic differences (see [7], Chapter 2 for more details of the genetics of PWS). As well as two copies of all non-imprinted genes, people with the maternal disomy subclasses will have two copies of paternally imprinted (maternally expressed) genes, while those with the deletion subtype and the general population have a single copy that is expressed. It has been argued that this may have implications for our understanding of the high risk for psychosis in those with PWS due to maternal disomy [8]. Non-imprinted genes have two intact copies in general but if one copy is deleted, as in deletion subtypes, a recessive gene is more likely to be expressed. Longer deletions (Type 1 vs. Type 2) also result in greater impairment [9].

3. The Behavioural Phenotype of PWS

The PWS genotype gives rise to a 'behavioural phenotype' with particular cognitive, social and behavioural characteristics and a risk for behavioural disorders and psychiatric problems [7] (Chapters 6 and 7). Initially there is pronounced hypotonia and failure to thrive, followed by developmental and cognitive delay, preoccupation with food and hyperphagia, and relative growth and sex hormone deficiency (short stature and impaired sexual development). Emerging behavioural problems include temper outbursts, repetitive and ritualistic behaviours, mood swings, and skin picking [10]. We note that the distributions of these behaviours in PWS are similar in shape to those in the general population but the distributions in PWS are shifted towards the more severe end of the general population distributions. Inactivity is characteristic and leisure time is typically spent in solitary pursuits such as jigsaw puzzles, word search puzzles, television viewing, and computer games [11]. In the teenage years and early twenties, or later, depression and/or psychosis develop in some people. Rates of depression in deletion subtypes tend to be similar to those in other forms of intellectual disability but less in maternal disomy subtypes. However, in people with PWS due to maternal disomy, rates of psychosis are much higher (60%–100% lifetime prevalence) but not in those with a 15q11-q13 deletion. This is considered further later in the paper.

The most prevalent disorder in PWS is the preoccupation with food and propensity to overeat, which in one form or another affects everyone with the syndrome. Hyperphagia develops in early childhood following a period of failure to thrive. It has features in common with anorexia (high ghrelin, low growth hormone, and absent menses), with bulimia (binge eating), with addiction (food seeking and stealing) and with obsessive-compulsive disorder (OCD; constantly thinking about it). However, it is present from infancy and on the basis of behavioural and neuroimaging studies it is generally acknowledged to be a defect of satiety [12–14]. It might be predicted that a reasonably direct path between genotype and phenotype will eventually be established. As of yet, however, no loss of function of genes known to be involved in feeding pathways has been observed and the link between genotype and this particular phenotype has not been explained.

Repetitive and ritualistic behaviours in PWS have been interpreted as OCD by some authors and as part of the syndrome of autism by others [15,16]. However, most people with PWS do not have OCD (there is an absence of distress or resistance to the behaviours as would be expected with true OCD). Although they may also have social impairments, the majority of people with PWS do not meet the full criteria for autism [17–21] but they do exhibit behaviours (hoarding, the need to ask or tell and insistence on routine) similar to those of typically developing young children [22]. One paper suggests that these behaviours in PWS are best conceptualised as a consequence of arrested development [23] given their similarities with what is observed as part of normal childhood development. It is unlikely therefore that there is a direct link between genes and this specific behavioural profile, rather it is the impact of the genotype on brain development more generally that leads to the increased prevalence of such behaviours.

Temper outbursts have been conceptualised similarly and have also been linked to insistence on routine as well as deficits in executive functioning and task-switching. These outbursts are characteristically triggered by change or a refusal of some specific request and follow a course that is likely to include the rapid onset of verbal outbursts and sometimes physical aggression, eventually resolving with expressions of regret and distress [24–26]. This pattern is similar to what is observed in young children. Observations of marked reductions in the frequency and severity of such behaviours by the use of vagus nerve stimulation might indicate that the mechanism resulting in the high risk for such behaviours is the presence of a low threshold of the autonomic nervous system to respond in a rapid flight/fight mode when faced with an actual or perceived threat [27,28]. Thus, the mechanism is one of impaired emotional regulation, potentially for developmental reasons. Observational studies indicate that external contingencies clearly have an important role to play but fundamentally, the underlying mechanism that increases the risk for such behaviours is a shift downwards in the threshold for responding in this 'fight' manner, as opposed to seeking to engage and de-escalate the situation through social engagement.

Skin picking has been variously interpreted as self-harm, obsessive compulsive behaviour, or as a direct consequence of the loss of the Necdin gene since, in the case of the last of these, abnormal grooming behaviour has been observed in Necdin knockout mice. The observation that such behaviours usually occur where there has been an insect bite or some irritation suggests that local factors may initiate the behaviour, which may lead to a local inflammatory response and further irritation. A high pain threshold also means that there is a reduced negative consequence to skin picking. Factor analysis studies show that skin picking is not found on the same factor as repetitive and ritualistic behaviours suggesting that such behaviour is not primarily driven by obsessionality [23,29]. Hall et al. [30] undertook a functional analysis and reported that skin picking occurred more commonly under conditions of low attention, suggesting an interactive model between a biological vulnerability and environmental contingencies and setting conditions.

The most striking finding on psychiatric illness in PWS is the rate of psychotic illness in the maternal disomy genetic subclasses (including both mUPD and imprinting centre defects). This has been estimated at 60%–100% lifetime prevalence [31–35]. This suggests a strong genetic component in the cause of psychotic symptoms in PWS. Moreover, since the rate of psychosis in the deletion subtypes is no more than that in people with intellectual disabilities, psychosis is not due to having the core PWS genotype and the causal gene or genes would have to be either more strongly expressed from the maternal chromosome 15 or imprinted. The search for such a gene has been unsuccessful to date [36].

Soni et al. [31] suggested a two-hit model to account for the differential rates of psychosis in PWS. They hypothesized that the genetics of PWS results, regardless of genetic type, in an increased propensity to affective disturbance with the 'second-hit', having a chromosome 15 mUPD, resulting in the markedly increased risk for psychosis. This would suggest that the increased propensity of those with mUPD to develop psychosis must be a combination of both the effects of the PWS genotype on neural development and circuits in the brain that serve mood regulation, as well as gene dosage effects from maternally expressed genes on chromosome 15, which result in aberrant functioning of neural circuits and in the emergence of abnormal mental experiences [8,27].

Deletion and mUPD Differences

Whilst this differential risk of psychotic illness must have a genetic basis this effect is likely to be mediated through differences in brain structure and function in those with the deletion compared with the maternal disomy form of PWS.

Cognitive function and brain structure have been shown to differ between PWS genetic subtypes, indicating potential differences in developmental pathways. The question remains as to whether such differences might in turn explain the differential risk for psychotic illness. PWS, irrespective of genetic type, is associated with mild to moderate intellectual disability, but differences in cognitive profiles between the subtypes have been identified. The studies typically report a full-scale IQ (FSIQ) relatively similar between genetic subtypes, but a slightly higher performance IQ (PIQ) in those with PWS due to a deletion, and a higher verbal IQ (VIQ) score but a greater impairment in processing speed in those with mUPD [37]. FSIQ seems more homogenous in those with deletion PWS with similar VIQ and PIQ, whereas those with mUPD have a higher average VIQ than PIQ [37–39]. Whittington et al. (2004) compared subtests scores across PWS genetic subtypes and a comparison mixed aetiology intellectual disability group [37]. The cognitive profile of the mUPD group differs from the deletion PWS and LD group, who have very similar profiles (Figure 2).

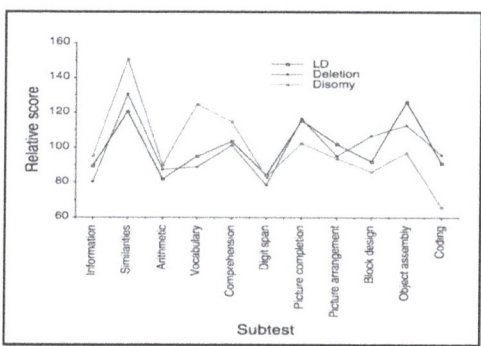

Figure 2. Weschler subtest profiles of mUPD, deletion PWS (delPWS), and learning disability groups from Whittington et al. 2004 [37].

From a neurophysiological angle, an encephalogram (EEG) study using a Go/No-Go task [40], found a reduced sensory processing speed in people with mUPD compared to those with deletion PWS. People with mUPD were reported to have significantly increased reaction times compared to those with deletion PWS and healthy controls, with deficits in both the N200 and P300 peaks related to early modality-specific inhibition and late general inhibition, respectively. Those with deletion PWS showed impairment only for N200 modulation. Another PWS study found a specific deficit in segregating human voices from a noisy background, and a failure to fully process sensory information before initiation of a behavioural response in PWS, again the deficit being greater in those with mUPD compared to those with deletion PWS [41]. A recent study in children with PWS has found significantly reduced white matter microstructure in most of the major white matter tracts in people with PWS due to mUPD compared to deletion PWS, similar to those reported in people with schizophrenia or those at ultra-high risk for psychosis [42,43]. The latter two populations have also been found to have an impaired processing speed [37,40,44]. Freedman et al. [45] observed compromised P50 sensory gating in patients with schizophrenia as well as some of their unaffected relatives, suggesting a role for such impairments in the aetiology of psychosis. Thus, impairments in both auditory processing and processing speed have been found in people with schizophrenia, those at risk for psychosis, and in people with PWS due to mUPD, suggesting at least partially common brain mechanisms and potential targets for treatment development.

4. Genetically Determined Neurodevelopmental Syndromes

Among the population of people with ID are groups with various genetically determined neurodevelopmental syndromes (Angelman, Cornelia de Lange, Cri-du-chat, Down, Fragile-X, Lesch Nyhan, Prader-Willi, Rett, Smith-Magenis, Tuberous sclerosis complex, Velocardiofacial, Williams, etc.). Individuals with these genetic syndromes have distinct phenotypes, including distinctive patterns of adaptive and maladaptive behaviours that distinguish one syndrome from others—referred to as the 'behavioural phenotype' of the syndrome [46]. In these cases the phenotypic behaviours and the characteristic phenomenology of the underlying mental state of the person may make up symptom clusters that then meet diagnostic criteria for a specific mental disorder, leading to a diagnosis, for example, of an anxiety disorder in an individual with Fragile-X or Williams syndrome [47]. In both of these syndromes 'anxiety' in different ways is common and the propensity to anxiety is considered to be characteristic of people with these syndromes. However, what is meant by saying that someone with one or other of these syndromes is 'anxious' and whether the underlying brain mechanisms between syndromes are similar or not (and therefore treatments may be similar) is far from clear but phenomenologically they appear to be different. Observed behaviours, such as self-injurious behaviour, may also be helpful diagnostically. For example, in the case of people with Lesch Nyhan syndrome (LNS) such behaviour is a key part of the phenotype of that syndrome. Its presence during childhood in males might well alert one to the diagnosis of this syndrome. In addition, the early onset, severity, and extent of this behaviour indicate that there is a direct link between the syndrome genotype and that aspect of the phenotype. In LNS the behaviour is universal, of early onset in life, and does not fit the criteria for other established mental disorders. This example highlights the importance to our understanding of the behavioural and mental health aspects of children and adults with neurodevelopmental syndromes to distinguish between: (1) whether a particular symptom (e.g., self-injurious behaviour) is a diagnostic feature of the syndrome itself; or (2) whether it is best understood as either a symptom of some additional co-morbid mental disorder; or (3) it is best understood through a different conceptual framework, such as that of the operant model of applied behavioural analysis. In this latter case the focus is on identifying external factors that predispose to, precipitate or are maintaining specific behaviours, or are internal or external setting conditions for such behaviours. As is considered in the case of PWS this is an important step in seeking to explore the relations between the syndrome genotype and its phenotype.

4.1. Diagnostic Criteria

Biomedical systems of classification, such as the DSM-5 and ICD-10, have done much to bring rigor into our definitions and understanding of mental disorder, a very necessary process if specific treatments are to be developed and tested. DSM-5 proposes that each of the mental disorders is defined by an agreed of symptoms or behaviours, not all of which are necessary and none of which is sufficient for a definite diagnosis (because they can appear in more than one such list). Characterised as a clinically significant behavioural or psychological syndrome or pattern that occurs in an individual that is associated with present distress or disability or with a significantly increased risk of death, pain, disability, or an important loss of freedom. This syndrome or pattern must not be merely an expectable and culturally sanctioned response to a particular event, such as a bereavement.

Mental disorder and mental illness may be difficult to define and diagnose and judgements have to be made as to what is clinically significant or an expectable culturally sanctioned event. There is no single definitive test for anxiety, depression, psychosis, bipolar disorder, or obsessive-compulsive disorder and there is an overlap of symptoms between diagnostic categories in the standard instruments DSM-5 and ICD 10. There is also a debate as to whether particular forms of mental disorder, such as autism spectrum conditions, are best considered as discrete (yes/no) or a continuum where a line divides those considered to have a positive diagnosis and are therefore 'atypical' from those considered to be 'typical'. This is similar to specific physical disorders, such as type 2 diabetes and hypertension—the recommendations as to where the cut off lies, above which some (kind of) treatment is recommended, changes over time. These difficulties are further compounded, in the case of people with intellectual disabilities; firstly because of the complexity associated with an atypical pattern of development; secondly, because the individuals concerned may have difficulty in communicating feelings and symptoms; and thirdly their level of functioning and behaviour may not conform to general expectations for their age. However, despite the limitations of this approach, the diagnosis of certain mental disorders, such as the major mental illnesses of bipolar disorder and schizophrenia, have, through the presence of a recognised grouping of specific characteristics come to imply some understanding as to likely causation, and this informs treatment and prognosis.

Prader-Willi syndrome, like other genetically determined neurodevelopmental syndromes, is considered to fall under the broad umbrella term of 'mental disorder'. PWS may be additionally classified as 'intellectual developmental disorder' if the necessary criteria are met. As we summarized above, PWS has an early clinical profile and developmental history that indicates involvement of different organ systems. These include the central nervous system, resulting in the presence of functional impairments and disabilities. In addition, for a significant proportion of children and adults with PWS, patterns of behaviour and particular mental states (the 'behavioural phenotype' of PWS) can be observed during their lifetime that also have a major impact on functioning. Some of these meet established diagnostic criteria for a co-morbid mental disorder and others do not. Psychosis (mainly in the disomy subtype) and depressive illness (mainly in the deletion subtype) do meet criteria, and this informs treatment by guiding as to the medications that might be tried. The question then arises as to how the additional behavioural phenomena are best conceptualised, characterised, and understood so that ultimately effective interventions are developed.

4.2. Applied Behavior Analysis

In contrast, another term, which is common in the intellectual disabilities literature, is that of 'challenging behaviour', attributed to Emerson [48] and defined as follows:

"Culturally abnormal behaviour(s) of such an intensity, frequency or duration that the physical safety of the person or others is likely to be placed in serious jeopardy, or behaviour which is likely to seriously limit use of, or result in the person being denied access to, ordinary community facilities."

Individual descriptions of challenging behaviour do not mimic the diagnostic process by attempting to group together specific signs or symptoms that characterises the behaviour in a manner that informs an understanding of causation or treatment. Whilst the presence of such behaviours may be an indication of some underlying and as yet undiagnosed mental disorder, the use of the term 'challenging behaviour' does not imply that the criteria for a specific mental disorder are met. The term is descriptive and is a marker for the level of impact of the behaviour and an indication that those providing support should seek to accommodate to the behaviours. In contrast to mental disorder, our more recent understanding of challenging behaviour, certainly as applied to people with intellectual disabilities, has been primarily led by the theoretical constructs of ABA. In this view, it is argued that such behaviours are under operant control and have come to have specific functions, such as avoiding demands or maintaining attention. In this context there has been a clear resistance to defining such behaviour as 'a mental disorder'. There remains an on-going tension between the biological and the psychological: what might be innate, what might be a disorder of cerebral function, what is learnt, and/or what is a consequence of factors in the physical and emotional environments that have shaped and reinforced these behaviours [49]. These and other conceptual issues are complex enough when applied to the typically developing population but can be even more problematic when it comes to children and adults with neurodevelopmental disorders. However, a failure to address some of these issues, as they apply to our understanding of mental health and behaviour disorders in children and adults with neurodevelopmental disorders, such as PWS, hinders research, impairs the development and trials of new and innovative treatments, and limits our ability to track a course from genotype to behavioural phenotype.

4.3. Research Domain Criteria (RDC)

More recently a different perspective and conceptual framework, that of Research Domain Criteria (RDC), has shifted the emphasis away from diagnoses using the DSM-5 system to linking psychopathology to discoveries in genetics and neuroscience. In this conceptual framework behavioural and psychiatric disorders are consider to arise as a consequence of disturbances in brain networks [50]. The system proposes five 'domains' to classify behaviour: negative valence, positive valence, cognitive processes, social processes, and arousal/regulatory systems. Using non-suicidal self-injurious behaviour as an example, it has been argued that diagnostic approaches fail as clinical characterisation does not map directly onto brain mechanisms whereas Research Domain Criteria seek to do that—whether they do is a matter for empirical study [51,52]. These different approaches, illustrated in Figure 3, each have their strength and utility.

The main strength of the RDC is that it seeks to classify by underlying brain mechanisms, rather than by lists of symptoms. In doing so it brings together psychological constructs, some of which are familiar to the ABA approach (reinforcement, reward, etc.); what is known about the neural basis of specific behaviours relevant to our understanding of PWS, such as hyperphagia (e.g., feeding pathways projecting from the hypothalamus to frontal areas of the brain); and specific neural circuits that underpin particular cognitions, such as executive functioning, the disruption of which may result in impairments in such tasks as attention shifting, planning, etc. This is particularly relevant to genetic syndromes, since a behaviour that is prevalent in and peculiar to a given syndrome must be directly or indirectly (for example, by its effect on regional brain development) connected to the genetics of that syndrome. Relevant to this approach, we note that in PWS functional proton emission tomography (fPET) and functional magnetic resonance imaging (fMRI) have been used to study the hyperphagia [14], attention switching as a trigger for temper outbursts [25], and skin picking behaviour [30].

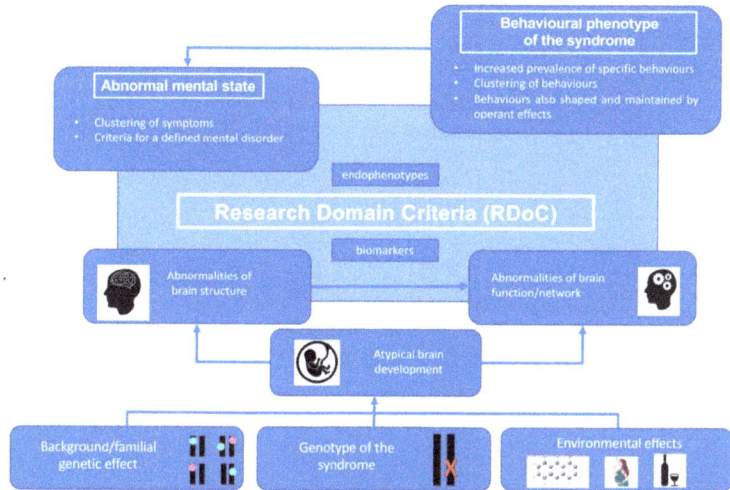

Figure 3. The genotype of the syndrome, as well as the background genetic and environmental effects, cause abnormalities in brain development, leading to abnormalities in brain structure and/or function. The top two boxes correspond to the diagnostic and applied behavioural analysis (ABA) approaches and the pale blue box to the Research Domain Criteria (RDC) approach.

5. Conclusions

The purpose behind establishing a diagnosis and of the diagnostic process, in general, is to arrive at an understanding of a particular syndrome, abnormal mental state, or behaviour. By accurately defining these different conditions through history taking, observation, and investigation, it is possible to compare with others who may have apparently similar conditions and to investigate causative mechanisms and, ultimately, to develop and test treatments. We propose that this fundamental proposition is still an appropriate clinical approach when it comes to neurodevelopmental syndromes, such as PWS, but that it must be more nuanced and involve different layers and models of understanding. The Research Domain Criteria takes this further and offers a different perspective seeking to link genes, brain, and behaviour [52]. This approach, in attempting to map behaviour to brain function, proposes using various neuroscience techniques to investigate the negative and positive valence of specific behaviours, the involvement of reward and other brain circuits, the role of social and sensory processing and underlying brain networks, and of the arousal systems of the brain. In order to develop our understanding of challenging behaviour, the need is to investigate whether, within and between groups of children and adults with different neurodevelopmental syndromes, specific aspects of the behaviour can be seen to cluster together and whether such behaviour can be mapped to dysfunction in particular neural systems, such as the reward circuits. What then are the key characteristics in the history, when observing challenging behaviour, that are important and which might then guide our understanding of mechanisms and ultimately of treatment?

We propose that:

Firstly, research needs to focus on the phenomenology of behaviours and mental states that are observed in those with neurodevelopmental syndromes. In the case of PWS this includes the hyperphagia, repetitive and ritualistic behaviours, temper outbursts, skin picking, and abnormal mental states. In order to move closer to understanding the causative mechanism and to establishing whether superficially similar behaviours across neurodevelopmental syndromes are likely to be similar or different, these behaviours and abnormal mental states need to be described in two major domains. One is the age of onset and course during development and over the lifetime. The other is an accurate description of the phenomenology. In the case of hyperphagia in PWS, for example, it includes the observations that the onset is in early childhood and persists probably throughout life, the severity of the behaviour and its consequences, the presence of food pre-occupations, food stealing, hoarding, etc. Similarly, with skin picking it would include age of onset, topography, course and phenomenology, and whether self-restraint is a feature. Detailed description would allow accurate comparisons of apparently similar phenomena within and across neurodevelopmental syndromes and in the typically developing population.

Secondly, the nature and clustering of the phenomenology and the observed behaviours and their course through time should be examined and the question asked as to whether or not they meet, or approximate to, established criteria for a known mental disorder. In the case of the repetitive and ritualistic behaviours in PWS this would clearly indicate that they are different from those observed in OCD, however, they are similar, but not identical, to those observed in people with autism spectrum disorders [19]. Thus, as a working hypothesis such behaviours may be best considered as of developmental origin rather than acquired during life. In contrast, the abnormal mental states that may appear in the teenage years or early adult life, particularly, in those with the mUPD form of PWS, may reasonably be called a psychotic illness even if it cannot be more narrowly defined as schizophrenia or bipolar disorder [53].

Thirdly, these behaviours or observed abnormalities of mental state should be considered from the perspective of causation. The question to be addressed is in essence which conceptual model of understanding best accounts for what is observed (phenomenology) and for the age of onset and the course over the lifespan. The models proposed are not mutually exclusive but we suggest that it is this process that is critical to understanding and which leads to informed intervention. Syndrome specific solutions may be required.

However, the approach put forward in the Research Domain Criteria is to ask the question: can particular behaviours, such as hyperphagia, be mapped against known neural networks and connections? By doing so, specific additional features in the history or on observation might be found to clump together and might be considered to have a common underlying mechanism and respond to a specific treatment. Such an approach will be informed by more detailed study using techniques such as neuroimaging. In PWS fPET and fMRI have been used to study the hyperphagia [14], attention switching as a trigger for temper outbursts [25], and skin picking behaviour [30]. This approach investigates the cerebral signature (endophenotype) that specifically underpins the behaviour in question and may well be able to determine whether similar behaviours across people with different syndromes have similar mechanisms. Whether similar behaviours but clustering together with different clinical features (e.g., self injurious behaviours with different topographies or with or without self restraint) have different mechanisms. In PWS, the hyperphagia may be best considered as a developmental abnormality characteristic of PWS that maps onto the functioning of the nuclei in the hypothalamus, and the connections and projections between the hypothalamus and the cortex that map onto areas of the brain that represent the conscious experiences of hunger and fullness. The repetitive and ritualistic behaviours and temper outbursts may be seen as a consequence of a more general abnormality of development resulting in poor emotional control and a low threshold for outbursts at minor real or perceived challenges that map onto the central connections of the autonomic nervous system and the limbic system. The abnormalities of the mental state, particularly observed in people with mUPD, which are a consequence of the development of a co-morbid mental illness might map to particular neural transmitter networks in the brain. For example, sensory processing is slower in those with mUPD, as it is in people at high risk for schizophrenia [8] and levels of cerebral GABA have been found, using magnetic resonance imaging (MRI), to be reduced in people with PWS [54]. One neuroimaging study has mapped skin picking to those areas of the brain (R insula and L precentral gyrus) mediating introceptive behaviours (itch and pain) [30].

In summary, we proposed that the diagnostic approach still has value in the identification of specific co-morbidities that may present with behavioural changes. In addition, we suggest that the Research Domain Criteria approach lends itself to the study of those behaviours, which severely impact on a person's life, where these behaviours are at present not easily categorised. Through an approach similar to that of the diagnostic process, these behaviours should be classified on the basis of their characteristics. This in turn may result in the identification of aetiologically distinct sub-groups of superficially similar behaviours. These may map to different neural networks and by implication will require different treatment approaches. The long-term aim is to be able to identify where specific abnormalities of gene expression impact on brain development and functioning in a manner that results in a recognisable and characteristic pattern—the behavioural phenotype of that syndrome.

Author Contributions: Main Argument, A.J.H.; PWS section, J.E.W.; Psychosis Section, L.C.S.A.

Funding: This research received no external funding.

Acknowledgments: We are grateful to Sam's Foundation and to the Foundation for Prader-Willi Research for funding our present research projects in PWS. We would also like to thank people with PWS who have helped with this research and their families and others who have given so generously of their time.

Conflicts of Interest: The authors declare no conflict of interest.

References

1. American Psychiatric Association. Task Force on DSM-V. In *Diagnostic and Statistical Manual of Mental Disorders: DSM-5*; American Psychiatric Association: New York, NY, USA, 2013.
2. WHO. ICD10. In *International Statistical Classification of Diseases and Related Health Problems*; WHO: Geneva, Switzerland, 2010.
3. Whittington, J.E.; Holland, A.J.; Webb, T.; Butler, J.; Clarke, D.; Boer, H. Population Prevalence and Estimated Birth Incidence and Mortality Rate for People with Prader-Willi Syndrome in One UK Health Region. *J. Med. Genet.* **2001**, *38*, 792–798. [CrossRef] [PubMed]
4. Vogels, A.; Van Den Ende, J.; Keymolen, K.; Mortier, G.; Devriendt, K.; Legius, E. Minimum prevalence, birth incidence and cause of death for Prader–Willi syndrome in Flanders. *Eur. J. Hum. Genet.* **2003**, *12*, 238–240. [CrossRef] [PubMed]
5. Smith, A.; Egan, J.; Ridley, G.; Haan, E.; Montgomery, P.; Williams, K.; Elliott, E. Birth Prevalence of Prader-Willi Syndrome in Australia. *Arch. Dis. Child.* **2003**, *88*, 263–264. [CrossRef] [PubMed]
6. Diene, G.; Mimoun, E.; Feigerlova, E.; Caula, S.; Molinas, C.; Grandjean, H.; Tauber, M. Endocrine Disorders in Children with Prader-Willi Syndrome—Data from 142 Children of the French Database. *Horm. Res. Paediatr.* **2010**, *74*, 121–128. [CrossRef]
7. Höybye, C. *Prader-Willi Syndrome*; Nova Science: New York, NY, USA, 2013.
8. Aman, L.C.S.; Manning, K.E.; Whittington, J.E.; Holland, A.J. Mechanistic Insights into the Genetics of Affective Psychosis from Prader-Willi Syndrome. *Lancet Psychiatry* **2018**, *5*, 370–378. [CrossRef]
9. Bittel, D.C.; Kibiryeva, N.; Butler, M.G. Expression of 4 Genes Between Chromosome 15 Breakpoints 1 and 2 and Behavioral Outcomes in Prader-Willi Syndrome. *Pediatrics* **2006**, *118*, e1276–e1283. [CrossRef]
10. Cassidy, S.B.; Schwartz, S.; Miller, J.L.; Driscoll, D.J. Prader-Willi syndrome. *Genet. Med.* **2012**, *14*, 10–26. [CrossRef]
11. Dykens, E.M. Leisure Activities in Prader-Wlli Syndrome: Implications for Health, Cognition and Adaptive Functioning. *J. Autism Dev. Disord.* **2014**, *44*, 294–302. [CrossRef]
12. Holland, A.J.; Treasure, J.; Coskeran, P.; Dallow, J.; Milton, N.; Hillhouse, E. Measurement of Excessive Appetite and Metabolic Changes in Prader-Willi Syndrome. *Int. J. Obes. Relat. Metab. Disord.* **1993**, *17*, 527–532.
13. Shapira, N.A.; Lessig, M.C.; He, A.G.; James, G.A.; Driscoll, D.J.; Liu, Y. Satiety Dysfunction in Prader-Willi Syndrome Demonstrated by FMRI. *J. Neurol. Neurosurg. Psychiatry* **2005**, *76*, 260–262. [CrossRef]
14. Hinton, E.C.; Holland, A.J.; Gellatly, M.S.N.; Soni, S.; Owen, A.M. An Investigation into Food Preferences and the Neural Basis of Food-Related Incentive Motivation in Prader-Willi Syndrome. *J. Intellect. Disabil. Res.* **2006**, *50*, 633–642. [CrossRef] [PubMed]
15. Dykens, E.M.; Leckman, J.F.; Cassidy, S.B. Obsessions and compulsions in Prader-Willi syndrome. *J. Child Psychol. Psychiatry* **1996**, *37*, 995–1002. [CrossRef] [PubMed]

16. Descheemaeker, M.J.; Govers, V.; Vermeulen, P.; Fryns, J.P. Pervasive developmental disorders in Prader-Willi syndrome: The Leuven experience in 59 subjects and controls. *Am. J. Med. Genet. A* **2006**, *140*, 1136–1142. [CrossRef] [PubMed]
17. Clarke, D.J.; Boer, H.; Whittington, J.; Holland, A.; Butler, J.; Webb, T. Prader-Willi Syndrome, Compulsive and Ritualistic Behaviours: The First Population-Based Survey. *Br. J. Psychiatry* **2002**, *180*, 358–362. [CrossRef] [PubMed]
18. Delorme, R.; Moreno-De-Luca, D.; Gennetier, A.; Maier, W.; Chaste, P.; Mössner, R.; Grabe, H.J.; Ruhrmann, S.; Falkai, P.; Mouren, M.C.; et al. Search for Copy Number Variants in Chromosomes 15q11-Q13 and 22q11.2 in Obsessive Compulsive Disorder. *BMC Med. Genet.* **2010**, *11*, 100. [CrossRef] [PubMed]
19. Greaves, N.; Prince, E.; Evans, D.W.; Charman, T. Repetitive and Ritualistic Behaviour in Children with Prader-Willi Syndrome and Children with Autism. *J. Intellect. Disabil. Res.* **2006**, *50*, 92–100. [CrossRef] [PubMed]
20. Flores, C.G.; Valcante, G.; Guter, S.; Zaytoun, A.; Wray, E.; Bell, L.; Jacob, S.; Lewis, M.H.; Driscoll, D.J.; Cook, E.H.; et al. Repetitive Behavior Profiles: Consistency across Autism Spectrum Disorder Cohorts and Divergence from Prader-Willi Syndrome. *J. Neurodev. Disord.* **2011**, *3*, 316. [CrossRef] [PubMed]
21. Dykens, E.M.; Roof, E.; Hunt-Hawkins, H.; Dankner, N.; Lee, E.B.; Shivers, C.M.; Daniell, C.; Kim, S.J. Diagnoses and Characteristics of Autism Spectrum Disorders in Children with Prader-Willi Syndrome. *J. Neurodev. Disord.* **2017**, *9*, 18. [CrossRef] [PubMed]
22. Evans, D.W.; Leckman, J.F.; Carter, A.; Reznick, J.S.; Henshaw, D.; King, R.A.; Pauls, D. Ritual, Habit, and Perfectionism: The Prevalence and Development of Compulsive-like Behavior in Normal Young Children. *Child Dev.* **1997**, *68*, 58–68. [CrossRef] [PubMed]
23. Holland, A.J.; Whittington, J.E.; Butler, J.; Webb, T.; Boer, H.; Clarke, D. Behavioral Phenotypes Associated with Specific Genetic Disorders: Evidence from a Population-Based Study of People with Prader-Willi Syndrome. *Psychol. Med.* **2003**, *33*, 141–153. [CrossRef]
24. Woodcock, K.; Oliver, C.; Humphreys, G. Associations between Repetitive Questioning, Resistance to Change, Temper Outbursts and Anxiety in Prader-Willi and Fragile-X Syndromes. *J. Intellect. Disabil. Res.* **2009**, *53*, 265–278. [CrossRef] [PubMed]
25. Woodcock, K.A.; Humphreys, G.W.; Oliver, C.; Hansen, P.C. Neural Correlates of Task Switching in Paternal 15q11-Q13 Deletion Prader-Willi Syndrome. *Brain Res.* **2010**, *1363*, 128–142. [CrossRef] [PubMed]
26. Woodcock, K.A.; Oliver, C.; Humphreys, G.W. The Relationship between Specific Cognitive Impairment and Behaviour in Prader-Willi Syndrome. *J. Intellect. Disabil. Res.* **2011**, *55*, 152–171. [CrossRef] [PubMed]
27. Manning, K.E.; McAllister, C.J.; Ring, H.A.; Finer, N.; Kelly, C.L.; Sylvester, K.P.; Fletcher, P.C.; Morrell, N.W.; Garnett, M.R.; Manford, M.R.; et al. Novel Insights into Maladaptive Behaviours in Prader-Willi Syndrome: Serendipitous Findings from an Open Trial of Vagus Nerve Stimulation. *J. Intellect. Disabil. Res.* **2015**, *60*, 149–155. [CrossRef]
28. Manning, K.E.; Beresford-Webb, J.A.; Aman, L.C.S.; Ring, H.A.; Watson, P.C.; Porges, S.W.; Oliver, C.; Jennings, S.R.; Holland, A.J. Transcutaneous Vagus Nerve Stimulation (t-VNS): A Novel Effective Treatment for Temper Outbursts in Adults with Prader-Willi Syndrome. *PLoS ONE* **2019**, *14*, e0223750. [CrossRef]
29. Feurer, D.; Dimitropoulos, A.; Stone, W.L.; Roof, E.; Butler, M.G.; Thompson, T. The Latent Variable Structure of the Compulsive Behaviour Checklist in People with Prader-Willi Syndrome. *J. Intellect. Disabil. Res.* **1998**, *42*, 472–480. [CrossRef]
30. Hall, S.S.; Hustyi, K.M.; Chui, C.; Hammond, J.L. Experimental Functional Analysis of Severe Skin-Picking Behavior in Prader-Willi Syndrome. *Res. Dev. Disabil.* **2014**, *35*, 2284–2292. [CrossRef]
31. Soni, S.; Whittington, J.; Holland, A.J.; Webb, T.; Maina, E.N.; Boer, H.; Clarke, D. The Phenomenology and Diagnosis of Psychiatric Illness in People with Prader–Willi Syndrome. *Psychol. Med.* **2008**, *38*, 1505–1514. [CrossRef]
32. Boer, H.; Holland, A.; Whittington, J.; Butler, J.; Webb, T.; Clarke, D. Psychotic Illness in People with Prader Willi Syndrome Due to Chromosome 15 Maternal Uniparental Disomy. *Lancet* **2002**, *359*, 135–136. [CrossRef]
33. Soni, S.; Whittington, J.; Holland, A.J.; Webb, T.; Maina, E.; Boer, H.; Clarke, D. The Course and Outcome of Psychiatric Illness in People with Prader-Willi Syndrome: Implications for Management and Treatment. *J. Intellect. Disabil. Res.* **2007**, *51*, 32–42. [CrossRef]
34. Vogels, A.; Matthijs, G.; Legius, E.; Devriendt, K.; Fryns, J.-P. Chromosome 15 Maternal Uniparental Disomy and Psychosis in Prader-Willi Syndrome. *J. Med. Genet.* **2003**, *40*, 72–73. [CrossRef] [PubMed]

35. Vogels, A.; De Hert, M.; Descheemaeker, M.J.; Govers, V.; Devriendt, K.; Legius, E.; Prinzie, P.; Fryns, J.P. Psychotic Disorders in Prader-Willi Syndrome. *Am. J. Med. Genet. A* **2004**, *127*, 238–243. [CrossRef] [PubMed]

36. Webb, T.; Maina, E.N.; Soni, S.; Whittington, J.; Boer, H.; Clarke, D.; Holland, A. In Search of the Psychosis Gene in People with Prader-Willi Syndrome. *Am. J. Med. Genet. Part A* **2008**, *146*, 843–853. [CrossRef] [PubMed]

37. Whittington, J.; Holland, A.; Webb, T.; Butler, J.; Clarke, D.; Boer, H. Cognitive Abilities and Genotype in a Population-Based Sample of People with Prader-Willi Syndrome. *J. Intellect. Disabil. Res.* **2004**, *48*, 172–187. [CrossRef] [PubMed]

38. Butler, M.G.; Bittel, D.C.; Kibiryeva, N.; Talebizadeh, Z.; Thompson, T. Behavioral Differences Among Subjects With Prader-Willi Syndrome and Type I or Type II Deletion and Maternal Disomy. *Pediatrics* **2004**, *113*, 565–573. [CrossRef] [PubMed]

39. Curfs, L.M.G.; Wiegers, A.M.; Sommers, J.R.M.; Borghgraef, M.; Fryns, J.P. Strengths and Weaknesses in the Cognitive Profile of Youngsters with Prader-Willi Syndrome. *Clin. Genet.* **1991**, *40*, 430–434. [CrossRef] [PubMed]

40. Stauder, J.E.A.; Boer, H.; Gerits, R.H.A.; Tummers, A.; Whittington, J.; Curfs, L.M.G. Differences in Behavioural Phenotype between Parental Deletion and Maternal Uniparental Disomy in Prader-Willi Syndrome: An ERP Study. *Clin. Neurophysiol.* **2005**, *116*, 1464–1470. [CrossRef]

41. Salles, J.; Strelnikov, K.; Carine, M.; Denise, T.; Laurier, V.; Molinas, C.; Tauber, M.; Barone, P. Deficits in Voice and Multisensory Processing in Patients with Prader-Willi Syndrome. *Neuropsychologia* **2016**, *85*, 137–147. [CrossRef] [PubMed]

42. Lukoshe, A.; van den Bosch, G.E.; van der Lugt, A.; Kushner, S.A.; Hokken-Koelega, A.C.; White, T. Aberrant White Matter Microstructure in Children and Adolescents With the Subtype of Prader–Willi Syndrome at High Risk for Psychosis. *Schizophr. Bull.* **2017**, *43*, 1090–1099. [CrossRef] [PubMed]

43. Roalf, D.R.; de la Garza, A.G.; Rosen, A.; Calkins, M.E.; Moore, T.M.; Quarmley, M.; Ruparel, K.; Xia, C.H.; Rupert, P.E.; Satterthwaite, T.D.; et al. Alterations in White Matter Microstructure in Individuals at Persistent Risk for Psychosis. *Mol. Psychiatry* **2019**, *24*. [CrossRef] [PubMed]

44. Karbasforoushan, H.; Duffy, B.; Blackford, J.U.; Woodward, N.D. Processing Speed Impairment in Schizophrenia Is Mediated by White Matter Integrity. *Psychol. Med.* **2015**, *45*, 109–120. [CrossRef] [PubMed]

45. Freedman, R.; Coon, H.; Myles-Worsley, M.; Orr-Urtreger, A.; Olincy, A.; Davis, A.; Polymeropoulos, M.; Holik, J.; Hopkins, J.; Hoff, M.; et al. Linkage of a Neurophysiological Deficit in Schizophrenia to a Chromosome 15 Locus. *Proc. Natl. Acad. Sci. USA* **1997**, *94*, 587–592. [CrossRef] [PubMed]

46. Flint, J. Implications of Genomic Imprinting for Psychiatric Genetics. *Psychol. Med.* **1992**, *22*, 5–10. [CrossRef] [PubMed]

47. Dykens, E.M. Anxiety, fears, and phobias in persons with Williams syndrome. *Dev. Neuropsychol.* **2003**, *23*, 291–316. [CrossRef]

48. Emerson, E. *Challenging Behaviour: Analysis and Intervention in People with Learning Disabilities*; Cambridge University Press: New York, NY, USA, 2001; ISBN 0-521-40485-1.

49. Stein, D.J.; Phillips, K.A.; Bolton, D.; Fulford, K.W.M.; Sadler, J.Z.; Kendler, K.S. What Is a Mental/Psychiatric Disorder? From DSM-IV to DSM-V. *Psychol. Med.* **2010**, *40*, 1759–1765. [CrossRef]

50. Sanislow, C.A.; Pine, D.S.; Quinn, K.J.; Kozak, M.J.; Garvey, M.A.; Heinssen, R.K.; Wang, P.S.E.; Cuthbert, B.N. Developing Constructs for Psychopathology Research: Research Domain Criteria. *J. Abnorm. Psychol.* **2010**. [CrossRef]

51. Westlund Schreiner, M.; Klimes-Dougan, B.; Begnel, E.D.; Cullen, K.R. Conceptualizing the Neurobiology of Non-Suicidal Self-Injury from the Perspective of the Research Domain Criteria Project. *Neurosci. Biobehav. Rev.* **2015**, *57*, 381–391. [CrossRef]

52. Cuthbert, B.N.; Insel, T.R. Toward the Future of Psychiatric Diagnosis: The Seven Pillars of RDoC. *BMC Med.* **2013**, *11*, 126. [CrossRef]

53. Bartolucci, G.; Younger, J. Tentative Classification of Neuropsychiatric Disturbances in Parader-Willi Syndrome. *J. Intellect. Disabil. Res.* **1994**, *38*, 621–629. [CrossRef]
54. Rice, L.J.; Lagopoulos, J.; Brammer, M.; Einfeld, S.L. Reduced gamma-aminobutyric acid is associated with emotional and behaviour problems in Prader-Willi syndrome. *Am. J. Med Genet Part B Neuropsychiatr. Genet.* **2016**, *171*, 1041–1048. [CrossRef]

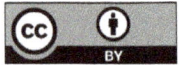 © 2019 by the authors. Licensee MDPI, Basel, Switzerland. This article is an open access article distributed under the terms and conditions of the Creative Commons Attribution (CC BY) license (http://creativecommons.org/licenses/by/4.0/).

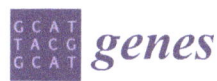

Article

Age Distribution, Comorbidities and Risk Factors for Thrombosis in Prader–Willi Syndrome

Merlin G. Butler [1,*,†], Aderonke Oyetunji [1,2,†] and Ann M. Manzardo [1]

[1] Departments of Psychiatry & Behavioral Sciences and Pediatrics, University of Kansas Medical Center, Kansas City, KS 66160, USA; aoyetunji@kumc.edu (A.O.); amanzardo@kumc.edu (A.M.M.)
[2] Department of Child Psychiatry, Truman Medical Centers, Kansas City, MO 64108, USA
*   Correspondence: mbutler4@kumc.edu; Tel.: +1-(913)-588-1800; Fax: +1-(913)-588-1305
†   Represents co-first authorship.

Received: 25 November 2019; Accepted: 1 January 2020; Published: 7 January 2020

Abstract: Prader–Willi syndrome (PWS) is an imprinting disorder caused by lack of expression of the paternally inherited 15q11.2–q13 chromosome region. The risk of death from obesity-related complications can worsen with age, but survival trends are improving. Comorbidities and their complications such as thrombosis or blood clots and venous thromboembolism (VTE) are uncommon but reported in PWS. Two phases of analyses were conducted in our study: unadjusted and adjusted frequency with odds ratios and a regression analysis of risk factors. Individuals with PWS or non-PWS controls with exogenous obesity were identified by specific International Classification of Diseases (ICD)-9 diagnostic codes reported on more than one occasion to confirm the diagnosis of PWS or exogenous obesity in available national health claims insurance datasets. The overall average age or average age per age interval (0–17 year, 18–64 year, and 65 year+) and gender distribution in each population were similar in 3136 patients with PWS and 3945 non-PWS controls for comparison purposes, with exogenous obesity identified from two insurance health claims dataset sources (i.e., commercial and Medicare advantage or Medicaid). For example, 65.1% of the 3136 patients with PWS were less than 18 years old (subadults), 33.2% were 18–64 years old (adults), and 1.7% were 65 years or older. After adjusting for comorbidities that were identified with diagnostic codes, we found that commercially insured PWS individuals across all age cohorts were 2.55 times more likely to experience pulmonary embolism (PE) or deep vein thrombosis (DVT) than for obese controls (p-value: 0.013; confidence interval (CI): 1.22–5.32). Medicaid-insured individuals across all age cohorts with PWS were 0.85 times more likely to experience PE or DVT than obese controls (p-value: 0.60; CI: 0.46–1.56), with no indicated age difference. Age and gender were statistically significant predictors of VTEs, and they were independent of insurance coverage. There was an increase in occurrence of thrombotic events across all age cohorts within the PWS patient population when compared with their obese counterparts, regardless of insurance type.

Keywords: Prader–Willi syndrome; insurance health claims; thrombosis; pulmonary embolism; deep venous thrombosis; individuals with exogenous obesity; confirmatory ICD-9 diagnostic codes

1. Introduction

Prader–Willi syndrome (PWS) is a neurodevelopmental genomic imprinting disorder that results from the absence of paternally expressed imprinted genes at the 15q11.2–q13 chromosome region due to a paternal deletion of this region (60% of cases), maternal uniparental disomy 15 (36%), or an imprinting defect (4%) [1]. PWS is a rare genetic disorder that is associated with an incidence between 1 in 10,000–30,000 live births with a specific phenotype, and it is considered to be the most common known genetic cause of obesity [2–4]. Reports have suggested an important association between obesity and early death in adults with PWS [4]. Comorbidities that are commonly associated with obesity in PWS include respiratory problems (pulmonary embolism, respiratory failure, and pulmonary hypertension) and deep venous thrombosis [5–9].

An increased risk of venous thromboembolisms (VTEs) was recently reported in PWS patients by using Prader–Willi syndrome Association (USA) syndrome-specific database of deaths between 1973 and 2015 [5,9]. Seven percent of all deaths in the reported PWS survey commonly found in adulthood were attributable to pulmonary embolism, which represented only a quarter of the most common causes of death that were related to respiratory failure [5,6]. However, the reported deaths that resulted from respiratory failure could be secondary to undiagnosed pulmonary embolism and may vary by gender and/or age of patient [5]. Death in infancy/young childhood was found to be related to respiratory failure—more so than obesity-related factors. Pulmonary thromboembolism and obesity-related complications were more commonly found in adolescents and adults, with females more likely to suffer from obesity-related morbidity [5,10]. Blood clots, venous thrombosis, and/or pulmonary are recognized as contributors to morbidity and mortality in PWS in the United States.

As PWS is estimated to affect over 500,000 people worldwide and risk factors including obesity are on the rise, there is no doubt that the associated, marked obesity in PWS predisposes patients to thrombosis [4]. In addition, a venous thrombosis survey reported by Manzardo et al. [6] was carried out in more than 1000 individuals with PWS in the United States with an age range of 0–63 years. This survey revealed the presence of thrombosis in 3% of cases, with the incidence greater in females than males. Thirty-three of the identified 38 clotting events occurred at ages greater than 17 years [6]. The occurrence of these events was associated with a greater age and an increased weight or obesity, as determined by the body mass index (BMI). The types of reported events included thrombosis or specified blood clots, deep venous thrombosis (DVT), and pulmonary embolism (PE). DVTs showed the highest percentage at 21%. Obesity was the most common finding that was associated with PE and that was identified in the previous PWS survey of blood clots reported by Manzardo et al. [6].

To further investigate the associated risk factors that play a role in blood clots and thrombotic events in living patients with PWS, we utilized two sources of national healthcare insurance claims datasets based on International Classification of Diseases (ICD)-9 diagnosis codes [11]. We aimed to identify thrombotic events and their occurrence in a large number of patients with PWS and non-PWS obese controls across all age groups, and we used key variables to analyze independent predictors/risk factors.

2. Materials and Methods

We used insurance health claims data from the MarketScan Research Databases for the years 2004–2014 as a source of data to carry out a preliminary record search of primary thrombosis and related blood clotting events in patients with Prader–Willi syndrome. The patients were identified from commercial or Medicare Advantage and Medicaid insurance groups. Individuals with exogenous obesity were also included as non-PWS controls as a comparison group. The Market Scan Research Databases contain de-identified health insurance enrollment information and fully-adjudicated claims data for all medical services and prescribed medications. As an example of the number of claim reports, approximately six million Medicaid enrollees from multiple states had more than 500 million claim records available for analysis [11]. The dataset provides a national cross-sectional and longitudinal view of demographics and enrollment among others in the United States.

Our study design applied a coding methodology and analysis plans by searching diagnostic ICD-9, Diagnosis Related Group (DRG), and Current Procedural Terminology (CPT) codes for key variables in the health insurance claims. The analyses focused on the occurrence of primary thrombosis events in 3136 patients with PWS and a non-PWS cohort with exogeneous obesity that consisted of 3945 individuals. These patients were identified by recorded ICD-9 codes (PWS, ICD-9 code 759.81; exogenous obesity, ICD-9 code 278.44) found on more than one occasion to confirm the diagnosis in both cohorts for inclusion.

Primary analyses in Phase I used contingency two-factor tables and the Chi-square test. Event rates were given as a percentage of patients that did/did not have a thrombosis or blood clotting code during their entire length of continuous enrollment over a ten-year period from 2004 to 2014. Odds ratios (ORs) with confidence intervals (CI) were calculated by using a logistic regression model with an offset term to adjust for differing lengths of continuous enrollment and follow-up between the two subject cohorts; these ORs are presented in terms of relative risk (PWS compared to non-PWS obese controls). The odds ratios were used to represent the occurrences of primary thrombosis events in the PWS versus non-PWS obese control populations that were identified in these health claims datasets.

Phase I quantified the occurrence of thrombosis events (did/did not have event) and calculated odds ratios though five prioritized analyses:

Analysis 1: PE and DVT codes

Analysis 2: PE and DVT and PWS confirmatory codes

Analysis 3: PE and DVT and other venous thrombosis codes

Analysis 4: PE and DVT and other venous thrombosis and PWS confirmatory codes

Analysis 5: Arterial thrombosis codes

Baseline comorbidity adjustment is considered an important component of research related to health services and clinical prognosis. When adjusting for comorbidities, investigators may consider comorbidities either individually or through the use of summary measures such as the Elixhauser comorbidity score, which is derived with regression estimates. A modified Elixhauser-adjusted method was used in this study, as previously described [12,13]. The Elixhauser- adjusted occurrences were primary thrombosis events and ORs that were calculated by using logistic regression models. Logistic regression models were adjusted for the 31 comorbidities contained in the Elixhauser comorbidities index. In Phase II, risk factors for thrombotic events were identified based on the Elixhauser comorbidities index by using a stepwise statistical selection approach to find a parsimonious model that incorporated 31 chronic diseases (which are discussed later) identified by ICD-9-CM codes (as well as age and gender as additional risk factors) deemed as comorbidities associated with thrombosis events in PWS [12,13] (see Figure 1). With significant risk factors/comorbidities identified as major contributors to primary thrombosis events, an unadjusted analysis of primary thrombosis events or blood clots was carried out in PWS patients relative to their obese non-PWS counterparts.

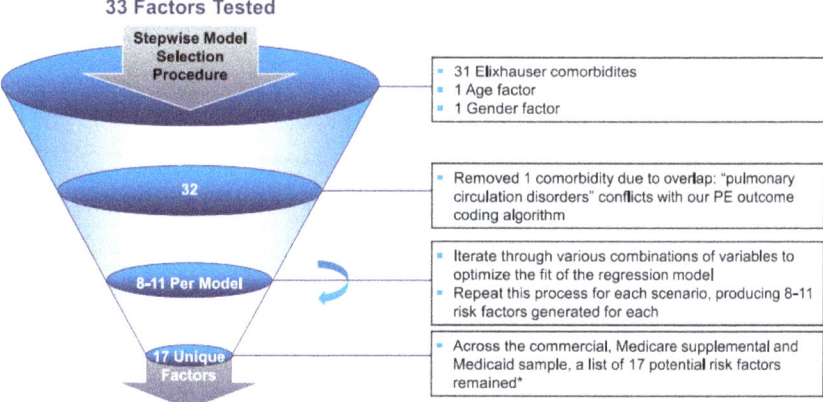

Figure 1. Iterative statistical stepwise approach to determine the risk factors that contributed significantly to thrombosis events.

3. Results

A total of 1821 patients with PWS were available for analysis from one of the groups of subjects with commercial or Medicare Advantage insurance coverage, of which 51% were males and 49% were females. In addition, 1315 patients with PWS had a second form of insurance coverage (e.g., Medicaid), of which 54% were males and 46% were females. Thus, a total number of 3136 PWS patients were studied with 52.5% males and 47.5% females (see Table 1). A total of 3945 non-PWS controls with exogenous obesity were identified using the two insurance coverage types, and they were selected to represent the average age and distribution with gender ratio seen in the PWS population for comparison purposes. When combined, a total number of 2042 (65.1%) patients with PWS had an age range of 0–17 years, 1040 (33.2%) patients were between the ages of 18 and 64 years, and 52 (1.7%) patients with PWS were 65 years and older. Furthermore, this health claims dataset was used to study the medical costs in PWS that were reported by Shoffstall et al. [10], who found higher medical costs in a five year subset (2009–2014) for PWS in comparison to non-PWS obese patients who were selected for comparison with a similar gender ratio and age distribution seen in three age cohorts [11]. Additionally, the age for the 1199 PWS subjects and 3945 non-PWS obese subjects were further grouped into eight categories beginning with 0–3 years, 2–4 years, 5–11 years, 12–17 years, 18–25 years, 26–40 years, 41–64 years and 65 years and older (see Figure 2).

Table 1. Ten year health insurance claims dataset (2004–2014) showing distribution of patients with Prader–Willi syndrome.

Prader–Willi Syndrome	Commercial and Medicare Advantage	Medicaid
N	N = 1821	N = 1315
Gender Distribution (%)		
Male	N = 921 (50.6)	N = 715 (54.4)
Female	N = 900 (49.4)	N = 600 (45.6)
Age Distribution (%)		
0–17 year	N = 1312 (72.0)	N = 731 (55.6)
18–64 year	N = 464 (25.5)	N = 576 (43.8)
65 year+	N = 45 (2.5)	N = 8 (0.6)

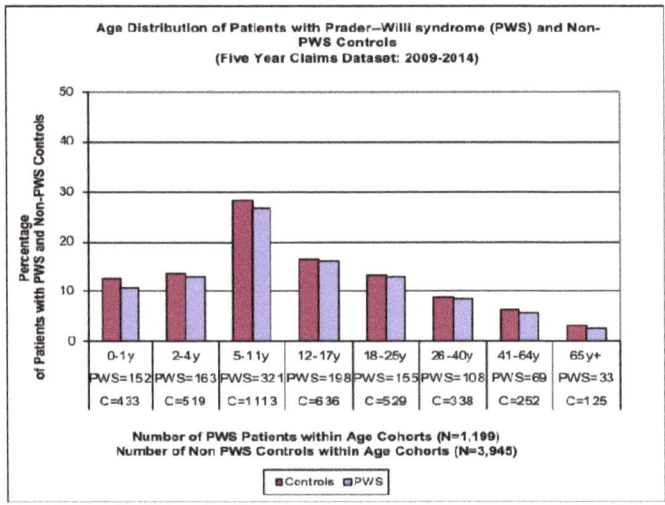

Figure 2. Age distribution bar graph of patients with Prader–Willi syndrome (PWS) and non-PWS obese controls.

Individuals with PWS experienced a higher overall frequency of thrombosis events than their similarly aged and gender-matched non-PWS obese counterparts across all analyses unadjusted for comorbidities. An addition of confirmatory codes to unadjusted thrombosis events caused a reduction in the total number of identified events, but the frequency of the events still trended higher across all age groups for all types of insurance coverage (see Figure 3).

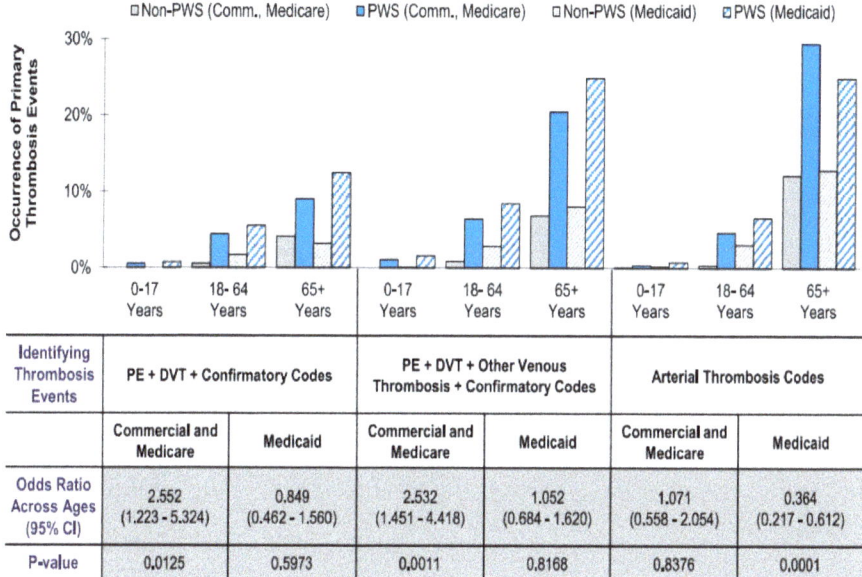

Identifying Thrombosis Events	PE + DVT + Confirmatory Codes		PE + DVT + Other Venous Thrombosis + Confirmatory Codes		Arterial Thrombosis Codes	
	Commercial and Medicare	Medicaid	Commercial and Medicare	Medicaid	Commercial and Medicare	Medicaid
Odds Ratio Across Ages (95% CI)	2.552 (1.223 - 5.324)	0.849 (0.462 - 1.560)	2.532 (1.451 - 4.418)	1.052 (0.684 - 1.620)	1.071 (0.558 - 2.054)	0.364 (0.217 - 0.612)
P-value	0.0125	0.5973	0.0011	0.8168	0.8376	0.0001

Figure 3. Adjusted primary thrombosis events of patients with Prader–Willi syndrome (PWS) in comparison to non-PWS obese patients across all age cohorts, insurances, and analyses.

Overall, there were more occurrences across all age cohorts for PE and DVT with confirmatory codes (Analysis 2); other occurrences included venous thrombosis (Analysis 4) and arterial thrombosis (Analysis 5) (see Figure 4A–C). Commercially insured individuals with PWS were also 4.98 times more likely to experience PE or DVT events than the obese controls (p-value < 0.0001). Meanwhile, 1.8% of the individuals experienced PE or DVT events compared to 0.3% for their similar non-PWS aged and gender-matched obese counterparts. For PE, DVT, and "other" venous thrombotic codes, 2.9% of the PWS individuals and 0.5% of the non-PWS individuals experienced thrombosis events with odds ratio of 5.13 (p-value < 0.0001). Arterial events (i.e., stroke and heart attacks) occurred in 2.2% of the PWS individuals and 0.5% of the non-PWS individuals; OR = 3.88 (p-value < 0.0001) (see Table 2A).

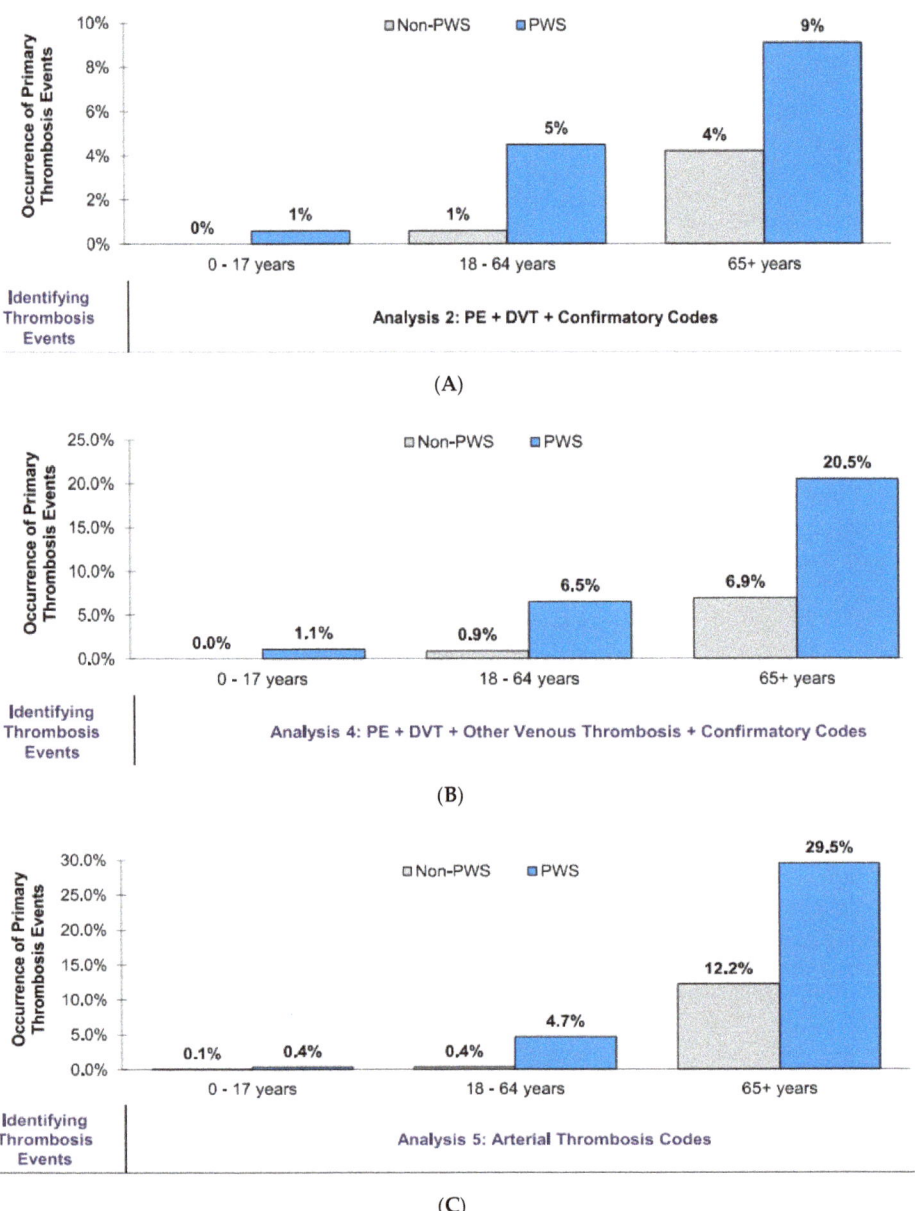

Figure 4. Primary thrombosis events in patients with Prader–Willi syndrome and non-PWS obese controls on commercial/Medicare coverage across all age cohorts with confirmatory codes in Analysis 2 (**A**), Analysis 4 (**B**) and Analysis 5 (**C**).

Table 2. Unadjusted primary thrombosis event occurrence in PWS subjects on commercial/Medicare and Medicaid coverage.

2A	% Experiencing Event		Odds Ratio (OR)	95% Lower Confidence Limit	95% Upper Confidence Limit	*p*-Value
Commercial/Medicare	PWS Subjects	Controls				
Analysis 1	2.10%	0.40%	4.3	2.5	7.2	<0.0001
Analysis 2	1.80%	0.30%	5	2.8	9	<0.0001
Analysis 3	3.80%	0.60%	5.3	3.5	8.1	<0.0001
Analysis 4	2.90%	0.50%	5.1	3.2	8.2	<0.0001
Analysis 5	2.20%	0.50%	3.9	2.3	6.5	<0.0001
2B	% Experiencing Event		Odds Ratio (OR)	95% Lower Confidence Limit	95% Upper Confidence Limit	*p*-Value
Medicaid	PWS Subjects	Controls				
Analysis 1	3.20%	0.80%	1.9	1.2	3	0.007
Analysis 2	3.00%	0.70%	1.9	1.2	3.2	0.007
Analysis 3	5.80%	1.50%	2	1.4	2.8	0.0002
Analysis 4	4.80%	1.30%	1.9	1.3	2.7	0.001
Analysis 5	3.50%	1.50%	1.1	0.8	1.7	0.47
Analysis 5	2.20%	0.50%	3.9	2.3	6.5	<0.0001

Analysis 1: PE and DVT codes. Analysis 2: PE and DVT codes and confirmatory codes. Analysis 3: PE and DVT codes and other venous thrombosis codes. Analysis 4: PE and DVT codes and other venous thrombosis codes and confirmatory codes. Analysis 5: arterial thrombosis codes. Selection Criteria: subjects with > = 1 year of continuous enrollment. Diagnosis criteria: At least two PWS diagnosis (ICD-9-CM 759.81) at any time during a subject's continuous enrollment period. *P*-values are based upon a Chi-square test.

In Phase 2, stepwise logistic regression identified 17 unique risk factors for PE or DVT out of the 31 chronic diseases modeled. The potential risk factors that were identified were, in alphabetical order, age cohort 18–64 (vs. 0–17), age cohort 65+ (vs. 0–17), AIDS/HIV, cardiac arrhythmias, chronic pulmonary disease, coagulopathy, congestive heart failure, deficiency anemia, diabetes uncomplicated, hypertension complicated, hypertension uncomplicated, male gender (vs. female), metastatic cancer, obesity, psychosis, rheumatoid arthritis/collagen, and solid tumor without metastasis (see Table 3).

Medicaid-insured individuals with PWS were 1.95 times more likely to experience PE or DVT events than the non-PWS obese controls (*p* = 0.0075), and 3.0% of these individuals experienced PE or DVT events compared to 0.7% of their similar non-PWS aged and gender-matched obese subjects. Including PE, DVT, and "other" venous thrombotic event codes, 4.8% of the PWS individuals and 1.3% of the non-PWS obese individuals experienced thrombosis events; OR = 1.88 (*p*-value = 0.0012).

Arterial events (i.e., stroke and heart attacks), occurred in 3.5% and 1.5% of the PWS and non-PWS cohorts, respectively. This difference was not statistically significant after controlling for differing lengths of enrollment (see Table 2B). However, this difference was statistically significant across all analyses for commercial/Medicare coverage, but it was not statistically significant for arterial thrombosis for Medicaid coverage (see Table 2A).

Table 3. Potential significant risk factors of thrombotic events.

		Commercial/Medicare Supplement		Medicaid		
		OR	*p*-Value		OR	*p*-Value
PE or DVT	Age Cohort 65+ (vs. 0–17)	11.0	<0.0001	Age Cohort 65+ (vs. 0–17)	6.2	0.02
	Age Cohort 18–64 (vs. 0–17)	6.2	<0.0001	Age Cohort 18–64 (vs. 0–17)	5.2	0.0001
	Cardiac Arrhythmia	3.0	0.002	Cardiac Arrhythmia	2.8	0.0005
	Coagulopathy	4.5	0.0005	Coagulopathy	8.4	<0.0001
	Male Gender (vs. Female)	2.3	0.01	Male Gender (vs. Female)	1.0	0.9
	Obesity	3.1	0.001	Hypertension Complicated	2.6	0.003
	AIDS/HIV	13.8	0.03	Solid Tumor without Metastasis	4.0	0.0002
	Diabetes Uncomplicated	2.6	0.006	Psychosis	1.9	0.03
PE, DVT or other thrombosis	Age Cohort 65+ (vs. 0–17)	4.9	0.0008	Age Cohort 65+ (vs. 0–17)	9.8	<0.0001
	Age Cohort 18–64 (vs. 0–17)	4.4	<0.0001	Age Cohort 18–64 (vs. 0–17)	4.6	<0.0001
	Cardiac Arrhythmia	2.2	0.007	Cardiac Arrhythmia	2.1	0.002
	Coagulopathy	4.8	<0.0001	Coagulopathy	7.3	<0.0001
	Male Gender (vs. Female)	1.6	0.08	Male Gender (vs. Female)	1.2	0.3
	Hypertension Complicated	3.6	<0.0001	Hypertension Complicated	2.1	0.004
	Solid Tumor without Metastasis	2.1	0.05	Obesity	1.7	0.05
	AIDS/HIV	10.9	0.01	Solid Tumor without Metastasis	2.2	0.05
	Deficiency Anemia	2.4	0.009	Congestive Heart Failure	1.7	0.05
	Chronic Pulmonary Disease	1.9	0.01	Metastatic Cancer	4.7	0.009
				Rheumatoid Arthritis/Collagen	2.5	0.006

Risk factors that were identified by using stepwise logistic regression modeling are shown above as significant in relation to thrombotic events in Prader–Willi syndrome, with the top risk factors being age cohorts (65+ years or age cohort 18–64 years versus 0–17 years in both cases), coagulopathy, cardiac arrhythmias, and male gender (vs. female).

4. Discussion

Patients with PWS continued to show a greater likelihood of experiencing thrombosis events than their similarly gender-matched obese counterparts across all age cohorts, regardless of insurance type after adjusting for comorbidities by evaluating PWS-specific contributions to thrombosis or blood clot events and by removing potentially confounding effects from comorbidities (see Figure 4). The inclusion of confirmatory codes to identify PE and DVT events provided a clearer picture of disparity across ages. In our study, all patients were identified and grouped into two insurance health claims datasets (commercial/Medicare and Medicaid). Patients with PWS who had commercial/Medicare coverage showed a higher occurrence of PE and DVT events than their similar aged and gender-matched counterparts across all age cohorts. Both PWS patients and obese controls in the 65+ year age cohort experienced the highest amount of PE and DVT events. With the inclusion of confirmatory PWS diagnostic codes, the PE and DVT events still had a higher occurrence in PWS patients than their obese counterparts (see Figure 3). Even though the number of events was lower in the PWS population, though not for the controls in the 18–64-year age cohort, the PWS patients in the 65+ year age cohort experienced a higher occurrence of events compared with their obese counterparts.

With other venous thrombotic events, PWS patients with commercial/Medicare coverage still had a higher occurrence of venous thrombotic events than their similarly-matched obese counterparts across all age cohorts despite the inclusion of confirmatory codes, which reduced the overall number of identified events, both in PWS patients and the controls. The occurrence of arterial thrombosis events in this same group of PWS patients was highest in the 65+ year age cohort when compared to the controls. The difference in the overall rate of occurrence between the PWS population and the controls was highest across all analyses with confirmatory codes in the 65+ year age cohort.

For patients with Medicaid coverage, the largest difference in the occurrence of PE and DVT events was seen in the 65+ year age cohort. As a function of advanced age, both PWS patients and obese controls had the highest occurrence of events. While the inclusion of confirmatory codes reduced the number of these same events that were identified in the 18–64-year age cohort, there was a higher occurrence in PWS patients than their similarly-matched obese counterparts across all age cohorts. For other venous thrombotic events, there was also a high occurrence rate in the 65+ year age cohort. In both analyses, differences may have been inflated by the smaller number of PWS patients compared to the obese controls, who were almost nine times more numerous (see Table 2). The inclusion of confirmatory codes reduced the number of events in the adult study population, but there was still a higher occurrence of these events in PWS patients than the controls. The occurrence of arterial thrombosis events was higher in the 65 year + age cohort than their non-PWS counterparts. These results were influenced by whether the model included comorbidities or not. These adjustments controlled for the given limitations of the claims data, permitting an assessment of the PWS-specific contribution to thrombosis event risk. For example, while the occurrence of arterial events (i.e., stroke and heart attacks) alone was higher for the commercially-insured individuals with PWS than the individuals in the obese control group (2.2% vs. 0.5%), when controlling for comorbidities, the difference was not statistically significant (OR = 1.071, *p*-value = 0.8375) (see Figure 3). After controlling for comorbidities, commercially insured subjects appeared 2.55 times more likely than the controls to have experienced a PE or DVT event (*p*-value = 0.013) but the difference in the frequency of events between the Medicaid-insured individuals and controls was not statistically significant. The results showed a trend of a higher frequency for thrombosis events in the PWS patients than the controls, but this was not always statistically different in all analyses. In the commercial and Medicare coverage, PWS patients had a difference in PE and DVT event frequency that was statistically significant when compared to obese non-PWS patients across all age groups, while in the Medicaid coverage group, the obese non-PWS controls experienced a higher occurrence of thrombosis events overall. Due to nuances of obesity coding in claims, we suspected a higher rate of false-negative detection of obesity, as well as a selection bias toward morbidly obese patients in the obese-positive cohorts. Statistically significant risk factors were also identified in PWS patients and appeared independently in all types of insurance coverage while using the Elixhauser comorbidities index.

Overall, survival in PWS is especially threatened by obesity, which is secondary to hyperphagia from a disturbance in the hypothalamic pathways of satiety control, irregularity in hormones that regulate food intake, and reduced energy expenditure in view of poor feeding and hypotonia [14,15]. Obesity is the most common cause of metabolic complications and can reduce the quality of life. Unfortunately, obesity and its complications are major contributors of increased mortality, especially in patients with PWS when compared with the general population [16,17].

With a shortened life expectancy that is attributed to the association of the level of intellectual disability and life-threatening complications in PWS that are related to hyperphagia and obesity, our study supports the trending decrease in the number of patients within the older age groups [18]. According to Manzardo et al. [10], the survival trends for patients diagnosed with PWS is on the rise when comparing recent era (post 2000 year) versus early era (pre 2000 year) mortality trends, thus suggesting a more optimistic future for PWS. However, the long-term survival trend shows clear gender- and disease-specific impacts, as supported by our findings that associated gender and disease are potential risk factors that can be targeted to improve and increase life spans (see Table 3).

A complication of obesity, especially in adults, is circulatory problems [19]. Butler et al. [5] reported that deaths due to obesity-related factors such as cardiovascular disease and pulmonary embolism that appear in childhood and increase throughout life, as opposed to other causes of death such as gastrointestinal infections which are generally more stable, at about a 10% mortality rate, throughout life. The increase in the occurrence rates of thrombotic events in the PWS population in our study showed an increasing rate over all age cohorts, with the highest occurrence in the 65+ years age cohort. However, thrombosis has been reported as a risk factor in PWS newborns with cerebral venous thrombosis [20]. Additionally, a study by Butler et al. [21] suggested that mean C-reactive protein values, indicators of inflammation, were higher in PWS subjects but similar to those seen in the non-PWS obese individuals with cardiovascular disease. This suggests that subjects with Prader–Willi syndrome and obese non-PWS subjects are at a similarly increased risk for complications of obesity including thrombosis. However, coagulopathy in PWS has been understudied. It is important to characterize the cause of venous vs. arterial blood clots in PWS in future studies. Disturbances in *F2* (thrombin), *F5* (coagulation factor 5) and other genes such as *PROC* (protein C), *SERPINC1* (serpin family C member 1) and *PROS1* (protein S) can produce both autosomal-dominant and autosomal-recessive patterns of inheritance of blood clots in families (https://www.omim.org), and more studies are required to possibly differentiate their role in arterial and venous thromboses impacted by age of onset in both PWS patients and obese controls.

More venous thromboses (e.g., VTEs) are reported than arterial thrombosis; however, these do occur, as illustrated by a clinical report from Kusuhara et al. [22] that highlighted a 19-year-old patient with PWS with a stroke and a brain MRI that revealed abnormal signal intensities in the left basal ganglia, including the right trigone of the lateral ventricle. An angiographic examination showed the occlusion of the bilateral proximal middle cerebral arteries with basal vessels, as well an occlusion of the left vertebral artery at its origin. This suggested that an arterial thrombosis event may have occurred, but it may have also resulted from atherosclerosis that secondary to the diagnosis of type 2 diabetes.

5. Conclusions

Thrombotic events in the PWS population, such as PE, DVT, other venous or arterial thromboses do occur but they are rare. Regardless of the type of insurance coverage and services received, the occurrence of thrombosis events or blood clots increased with age in PWS and is a leading cause of morbidity and mortality that is further increased by obesity. Survival trends can improve in patients with PWS if the associated risk factors for thrombosis events such as age, gender, coagulopathy, cardiac arrhythmias, and, especially, obesity and its related complications are targeted for proper management early and often throughout life, as thrombotic risk factors should be deeply considered together with comorbidities.

Author Contributions: Writing—original draft, A.O.; writing—review and editing, M.G.B. and A.M.M. All authors have read and agreed to the published version of the manuscript.

Funding: We acknowledge the funding provided by Zafgen Inc. (Boston, MA) for the database research and access to the data.

Acknowledgments: We would like to thank the families of patients with Prader–Willi syndrome who provided information found in the database. We acknowledge the support of Zafgen, Inc. (Boston, MA) to allow us to summarize and report on the database and the National Institute of Child Health and Human Development (NICHD) grant number HD02528.

Conflicts of Interest: M.G.B. was a site principal investigator for the Zafgen clinical trials on Prader-Willi syndrome.

References

1. Butler, M.G.; Hartin, S.N.; Hossain, W.A.; Manzardo, A.M.; Kimonis, V.; Dykens, E.; Gold, J.A.; Kim, S.J.; Weisensel, N.; Tamura, R.; et al. Molecular genetic classification in Prader-Willi syndrome: A multisite cohort study. *J. Med. Genet.* **2019**, *56*, 149–153. [CrossRef] [PubMed]

2. Butler, M.G. Prader-Willi syndrome: Current understanding of cause and diagnosis. *Am. J. Med. Genet.* **1990**, *35*, 319–332. [CrossRef] [PubMed]

3. Cassidy, S.B.; Schwartz, S.; Miller, J.L.; Driscoll, D.J. Prader-Willi syndrome. *Genet. Med. Off. J. Am. Coll. Med. Genet.* **2012**, *14*, 10–26. [CrossRef] [PubMed]

4. Butler, M.G. Single gene and syndromic causes of obesity: Illustrative examples. *Prog. Mol. Biol. Transl. Sci.* **2016**, *140*, 1–45. [CrossRef] [PubMed]

5. Butler, M.G.; Manzardo, A.M.; Heinemann, J.; Loker, C.; Loker, J. Causes of death in Prader-Willi syndrome: Prader-Willi syndrome association (USA) 40-year mortality survey. *Genet. Med. Off. J. Am. Coll. Med. Genet.* **2017**, *19*, 635–642. [CrossRef]

6. Manzardo, A.M.; Heinemann, J.; McManus, B.; Loker, C.; Loker, J.; Butler, M.G. Venous thromboembolism in Prader-Willi syndrome: A questionnaire survey. *Genes* **2019**, *10*, 550. [CrossRef]

7. Lionti, T.; Reid, S.M.; Rowell, M.M. Prader-Willi syndrome in Victoria: Mortality and causes of death. *J. Paediatr. Child Health* **2012**, *48*, 506–511. [CrossRef]

8. Einfeld, S.L.; Kavanagh, S.J.; Smith, A.; Evans, E.J.; Tonge, B.J.; Taffe, J. Mortality in Prader-Willi syndrome. *Am. J. Ment. Retard. AJMR* **2006**, *111*, 193–198. [CrossRef]

9. Hedgeman, E.; Ulrichsen, S.P.; Carter, S.; Kreher, N.C.; Malobisky, K.P.; Braun, M.M.; Fryzek, J.; Olsen, M.S. Long-term health outcomes in patients with Prader-Willi syndrome: A nationwide cohort study in denmark. *Int. J. Obes.* **2017**, *41*, 1531–1538. [CrossRef]

10. Manzardo, A.M.; Loker, J.; Heinemann, J.; Loker, C.; Butler, M.G. Survival trends from the Prader-Willi syndrome association (USA) 40-year mortality survey. *Genet. Med. Off. J. Am. Coll. Med. Genet.* **2018**, *20*, 24–30. [CrossRef]

11. Shoffstall, A.J.; Gaebler, J.A.; Kreher, N.C.; Niecko, T.; Douglas, D.; Strong, T.V.; Miller, J.L.; Stafford, D.E.; Butler, M.G. The high direct medical costs of Prader-Willi syndrome. *J. Pediatr.* **2016**, *175*, 137–143. [CrossRef] [PubMed]

12. Austin, S.R.; Wong, Y.-N.; Uzzo, R.G.; Beck, J.R.; Egleston, B.L. Why summary comorbidity measures such as the charlson comorbidity index and elixhauser score work. *Med. Care* **2015**, *53*, e65. [CrossRef] [PubMed]

13. Elixhauser, A.; Steiner, C.; Harris, D.R.; Coffey, R.M. Comorbidity measures for use with administrative data. *Med. Care* **1998**, *36*, 8–27. [CrossRef] [PubMed]

14. Butler, M.G.; Theodoro, M.F.; Bittel, D.C.; Donnelly, J.E. Energy expenditure and physical activity in Prader-Willi syndrome: Comparison with obese subjects. *Am. J. Med. Genet. Part A* **2007**, *143*, 449–459. [CrossRef]

15. Khan, M.J.; Gerasimidis, K.; Edwards, C.A.; Shaikh, M.G. Mechanisms of obesity in Prader-Willi syndrome. *Pediatr. Obes.* **2018**, *13*, 3–13. [CrossRef]

16. Proffitt, J.; Osann, K.; McManus, B.; Kimonis, V.E.; Heinemann, J.; Butler, M.G.; Stevenson, D.A.; Gold, J.-A. Contributing factors of mortality in Prader-Willi syndrome. *Am. J. Med. Genet. Part A* **2019**, *179*, 196–205. [CrossRef]

17. Eichinger, S.; Hron, G.; Bialonczyk, C.; Hirschl, M.; Minar, E.; Wagner, O.; Heinze, G.; Kyrle, P.A. Overweight, Obesity, and the risk of recurrent venous thromboembolism. *Arch. Intern. Med.* **2008**, *168*, 1678–1683. [CrossRef]

18. Butler, J.V.; Whittington, J.E.; Holland, A.J.; Boer, H.; Clarke, D.; Webb, T. Prevalence of, and risk factors for, physical Ill-Health in people with Prader-Willi syndrome: A population-based study. *Dev. Med. Child Neurol.* **2002**, *44*, 248–255. [CrossRef]

19. Vogels, A.; Van Den Ende, J.; Keymolen, K.; Mortier, G.; Devriendt, K.; Legius, E.; Fryns, J.P. Minimum prevalence, Birth incidence and cause of death for Prader-Willi syndrome in flanders. *Eur. J. Hum. Genet. EJHG* **2004**, *12*, 238–240. [CrossRef]

20. Beretta, L.; Hauschild, M.; Jeannet, P.-Y.; Addor, M.-C.; Maeder, P.; Truttmann, A.C. Atypical presentation of Prader-Willi syndrome with cerebral venous thrombosis: Association or fortuity? *Neuropediatrics* **2007**, *38*, 204–206. [CrossRef]

21. Butler, M.G.; Bittel, D.C.; Kibiryeva, N.; Garg, U. C-Reactive protein levels in subjects with Prader-Willi syndrome and obesity. *Genet. Med. Off. J. Am. Coll. Med. Genet.* **2006**, *8*, 243–248. [CrossRef] [PubMed]

22. Kusuhara, T.; Ayabe, M.; Hino, H.; Shoji, H.; Neshige, R. A case of Prader-Willi syndrome with bilateral middle cerebral artery occlusion and moyamoya phenomenon. *Rinsho Shinkeigaku* **1996**, *36*, 770–773. [PubMed]

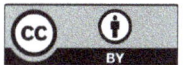 © 2020 by the authors. Licensee MDPI, Basel, Switzerland. This article is an open access article distributed under the terms and conditions of the Creative Commons Attribution (CC BY) license (http://creativecommons.org/licenses/by/4.0/).

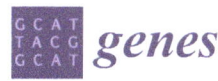

Case Report

Prader–Willi-Like Phenotype Caused by an Atypical 15q11.2 Microdeletion

Qiming Tan [1], Kathryn J. Potter [2], Lisa Cole Burnett [3], Camila E. Orsso [4], Mark Inman [5], Davis C. Ryman [3] and Andrea M. Haqq [1,4,*]

[1] Department of Pediatrics, University of Alberta, Edmonton, AB T6G 2E1, Canada; qtan3@ualberta.ca
[2] University of Alberta Hospital, Stollery Children's Hospital, Edmonton, AB T6G 2B7, Canada; Kathryn.Potter@albertahealthservices.ca
[3] Levo Therapeutics, Inc., Skokie, IL 60077, USA; lcburnett@levotx.com (L.C.B.); dryman@levotx.com (D.C.R.)
[4] Department of Agricultural, Food and Nutritional Science, University of Alberta, Edmonton, AB T6G 2E1, Canada; orsso@ualberta.ca
[5] Department of Pediatrics, University of Saskatchewan, Saskatoon, SK S7N 0W8, Canada; mark.inman@usask.ca
* Correspondence: haqq@ualberta.ca; Tel.: +1-(780)-492-0015

Received: 17 December 2019; Accepted: 22 January 2020; Published: 25 January 2020

Abstract: We report a 17-year-old boy who met most of the major Prader–Willi syndrome (PWS) diagnostic criteria, including infantile hypotonia and poor feeding followed by hyperphagia, early-onset morbid obesity, delayed development, and characteristic facial features. However, unlike many children with PWS, he had spontaneous onset of puberty and reached a tall adult stature without growth hormone replacement therapy. A phenotype-driven genetic analysis using exome sequencing identified a heterozygous microdeletion of 71 kb in size at chr15:25,296,613-25,367,633, genome build hg 19. This deletion does not affect the *SNURF-SNRPN* locus, but results in the loss of several of the PWS-associated non-coding RNA species, including the *SNORD116* cluster. We compared with six previous reports of patients with PWS who carried small atypical deletions encompassing the snoRNA *SNORD116* cluster. These patients share similar core symptoms of PWS while displaying some atypical features, suggesting that other genes in the region may make lesser phenotypic contributions. Altogether, these rare cases provide convincing evidence that loss of the paternal copy of the *SNORD116* snoRNA is sufficient to cause most of the major clinical features of PWS.

Keywords: Prader–Willi; 15q11.2; *SNORD116*; atypical microdeletion

1. Introduction

Prader–Willi syndrome (PWS) is an imprinted disorder affecting many organ systems, with a frequency of about 1 in 10,000 to 20,000 live births [1]. Major characteristics of PWS include infantile lethargy and hypotonia causing poor feeding and failure to thrive, followed by excess weight gain and onset of hyperphagia in early childhood, in addition to hypogonadism, short stature, delayed development, minor facial abnormalities, cognitive impairment, and behavioral and psychiatric disturbances [2]. PWS is caused by an absence of a functionally active paternal contribution in the chromosome 15q11.2-q13 region [2] via three distinct genetic mechanisms: large deletions (65–75%), maternal uniparental disomy (UPD; 20–30%), and imprinting defects (ID; 1–3%) [3]. More than 99% of cases can be easily detected by DNA methylation analysis of abnormal parent-specific imprinting within the Prader–Willi critical region on chromosome 15 [4]. The deletion class is subdivided into the typical Type 1 or Type 2 deletion, both of which are almost always de novo events [3]. The larger Type 1 deletion involves breakpoints (BP) BP1 and the distally located BP3 (~6 Mb), whereas Type 2 covers

BP2 to BP3 (~5.6 Mb). In rare cases, both larger and smaller deletions in PWS than typically described have been identified, which may show distinct phenotypic features [3].

Here, we report a 17-year-old boy who met six of the seven major revised clinical criteria for diagnosis of Prader–Willi syndrome, including neonatal hypotonia, feeding difficulties and failure to thrive as an infant, excess weight gain and hyperphagia by age 3, global developmental delay, and dysmorphic facial features. Unlike many children with PWS, from age 4 onward, his height followed the 90–95th percentiles, and he had spontaneous onset of puberty by age 15. Methylation analysis of the *SNURF-SNRPN* exon 1 region showed a normal pattern in the proband. However, further genetic analysis using exome sequencing identified a heterozygous microdeletion of 71 kb in size, spanning at least chr15:25296613-25367633 (genome build hg 19; Figure 1). This deletion results in the loss of several of the PWS-associated non-coding RNA species, including the *SNORD116* cluster. In the literature, only six PWS cases that were caused by small atypical deletions spanning snoRNAs at 15q11.2 have been reported before, with deletion sizes ranging from 80 to 236 kb (see Table 1), all of which overlap the *SNORD116* region [5–10]. Altogether, these rare cases provide further insights into genotype–phenotype correlations.

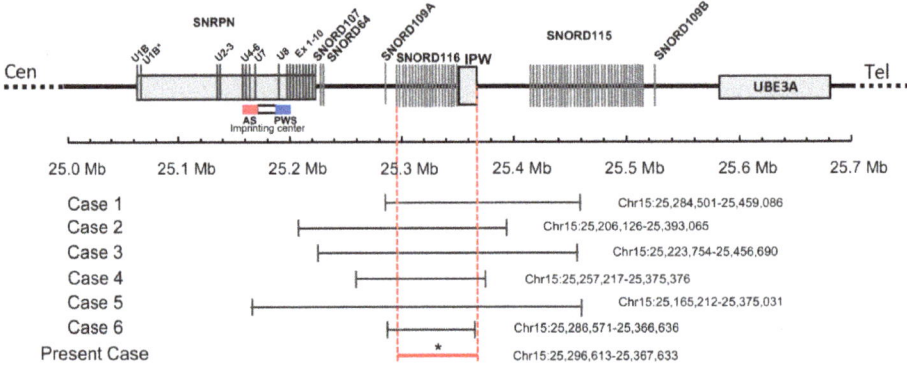

Figure 1. Schematic map of the 15q11.2 region between the *SNRPN* and *UBE3A* genes, which is represented at scale with physical distance in Mb. The reported deletions are shown at the bottom drawn to scale and depicting genomic coordinates for build hg19. * The exact breakpoints of the deletion in the present case are not available. The minimal critical region spans from 25296613bp to 25367633pb as shown by the red horizontal line.

Table 1. Comparison of present case with previously published cases with *SNORD116* microdeletion.

	Case 1 [5]	Case 2 [6]	Case 3 [7]	Case 4 [8]	Case 5 [9]	Case 6 [10]	Present case
Deletion size (kbp)	175	187	236	118	210	80	71
Ethnicity	Caucasian	South Asian Indian	African-American	Caucasian	Caucasian	Caucasian	Caucasian
Gender	Male	Male	Male	Female	Female	Male	Male
Birth weight (g)	3218	2800	3020	2780	3334	2710	3140
Birth length (cm)	54.5	N/A	53	48	54.6	49	51
Age at examination (years)	4.8	19.5	11	23	26	18	17
Clinical features							
Hypotonia	+	+	+	+	+	+	+
Infantile feeding problems/FTT	+	+	+	+	+	−	+
Tube feeding	+	−	+	+	−	−	+
Start of excess weight gain (months)	18	24	6	18	30	Between 48–72	36
Hyperphagia	+	+	+	+	+	+	+
Overweight/Obesity	+	+	+	+	+	+	+
Distinctive facial features	+	N/A	+	+	+	+	+
Hypogonadism	+	+	+	+	N/A	+	−
Developmental delay	+	+	+	+	+	+	+
Mental retardation	+	+	+	+	N/A	−	−
Behavioral problems	+	+	+	+	+	−	+
Skin picking	+	+	−	+	+	−	+
Sleep disturbances/ apnea	+	N/A	+	+	N/A	−	+
Short stature	−	+	+	+	+	−	−
Small hands/feet for height	+	+	−	N/A	+	−	−
Eye abnormalities	−	N/A	+	N/A	N/A	+	−

FTT: failure to thrive; N/A: not available; +: present PWS characteristic; −: absent PWS characteristic.

2. Materials and Methods

Given that the patient's rare phenotype had remained unexplained, clinical-grade exome sequencing with deletion and duplication analysis was done (Fulgent Genetics, Temple City, California, CA, USA) [11]. Rare variant and del/dup analysis of 4637 genes was guided by the phenotype, focusing on genes annotated to intellectual delay, hypotonia, obesity, and other features matching the patient's clinical presentation. Genomic DNA was isolated from whole blood using an automated DNA extraction machine (AnaPrep system, BioChain, Newark, DE, United States). DNA was sheared and barcoded using the Illumina TrusightOne Kit, and enriched for the coding exons of targeted genes using hybrid capture technology. Prepared DNA libraries were then sequenced using the Next Generation Sequencing technology.

Following alignment, variants were called in regions of at least 10× coverage. For this specimen, 99.3% and 98.3% of the coding regions and splicing junctions of the genes listed had achieved coverage of at least 10× and 20×, respectively. Regions that did not reach 10× coverage were not evaluated, unless they could be filled in by targeted Sanger sequencing assays. Variants were annotated using locus-specific databases, literature searches, and manual curation. The *SNORD116* cluster deletion was identified by Fulgent Genetics' proprietary copy number detection algorithm and pipeline; precise breakpoints could not be established using this pipeline. Only variants classified as pathogenic, likely-pathogenic, or of unknown significance, which were thought to be related to the patient's phenotype, were reported [12]. Any reported variants that had quality scores less than 500 (roughly 40× of the coverage for a heterozygous variant) were confirmed by Sanger sequencing. All genes listed were evaluated for large deletions and/or duplications in regions of the genes with significant pseudogenes.

Additionally, real-time quantitative polymerase chain reaction (qPCR) analyses were done to quantify *SNORD116* allele number in the patient and his parents. DNA was amplified for the targeted region of the *SNORD116* microdeletion and quantified using a QuantStudio 6 instrument. Detection of PCR products was enabled by the inclusion of a fluorescent reporter molecule in each reaction well that yielded increased fluorescence in real time as product DNA accumulated. Signal strength for the reactions targeting *SNORD116* were compared to control genes and control individuals, to assess the presence of the haploid versus diploid copy number.

3. Results

3.1. Clinical History

A Caucasian boy was born at 38 weeks' gestation through cesarean section, with appropriate weight (3140 g; 18th percentile, Z = −0.9) and length (51 cm; 50th percentile, Z = 0.0) for gestational age [13]. There were no complications during pregnancy. The patient received resuscitation after birth due to marked hypotonia and low respiratory effort. He stayed in the neonatal intensive care unit for three weeks and required nasogastric (NG) tube feeding because of prominent hypotonia, extreme lethargy, and severe failure to thrive as an infant. A gastrostomy tube (G-tube) was placed as a result of aspiration pneumonia at 6 months of age, and reversed at age 3. He had global development delay and walked at 20 months. He started to say "mama" and "dada" at 18 months and speak in sentences at 40 months of age. In Grade 7, difficulties in learning, especially in reading and mathematics, were present. Due to poor academic performance in school and his history of medical concerns, he was referred for a psycho-educational assessment. The Wechsler Intelligence Scale for Children®Fifth Edition test results indicated that he had processing speed deficits (Processing Speed Index = 6th percentile), interfering with the encoding, process and retrieval of information; however, his overall cognitive ability was in the average range (53rd percentile). Nevertheless, he was mainstreamed in normal education programs. He was noted to have central sleep apnea since birth and has been on bilevel positive airway pressure therapy (BiPAP) since the age of 6. He had orchidopexy surgeries when he was 22 and 30 months of age and had a tonsillectomy and adenoidectomy at age 3.

Hyperphagia and excess weight gain were first noted at age 3 years. The boy experienced an unrelenting feeling of hunger but did not often engage in food-seeking behaviors. From age 4 onward, his body weight and body mass index (BMI) remained above the 97th percentile for age. Strict control of food access and energy-restricted diets (1000–1200 calories per day) had stabilized his BMI at 28.45 kg/m^2 (97.8%, Z = 2.01; Figure S1). Meanwhile, his height followed the 90–95th percentiles, and he reached a tall adult stature (181.4 cm, 81.0%, Z = 0.88; mid-parental height is 181.5 cm) without the use of growth hormone (GH) replacement therapy, which is atypical for PWS. His hands (19 cm) and feet (27 cm) are of normal size. He exhibited characteristic facial features, including a narrow bitemporal diameter of the skull, almond shaped eyes, and a thin and down-turned upper lip. The boy had ongoing behavioral problems including rigidity and intolerance of changes in routine. He also presented with frequent skin picking to the point of bleeding. Levothyroxine was given from age 14 years 11 months to 17 years for his fatigue and possible central hypothyroidism (FreeT4 = 10.1 pmol/L). Fluoxetine was used to treat his depression, anxiety, obsessive compulsive disorder (OCD), and suicidal thoughts. He was prescribed atomoxetine for attention deficit hyperactivity disorder (ADHD), depression, social anxiety disorder, and autism spectrum disorder (Level 1). Lamotrigine was given as a mood stabilizing adjunct for his major depression. In addition, he was in regular consultation with a psychiatrist for behavioral and emotional management.

The patient was referred to our clinic at age 15, by which his puberty was complete. Unlike many children with PWS, he had spontaneous onset of puberty. He had Tanner 5 pubic hair and his testes were 20 mL bilaterally. Previous urology notes indicated that he was in puberty at age 11.5. His left testis was >3–4 mL (~Tanner 2). At age 12 years 9 months, he had Tanner 4 pubic hair; his left testis was 10 mL and the right one was not-palpable. Laboratory results showed normal thyroid function on levothyroxine (low-normal Free T4 = 10.1–12.7 pmol/L), as well as normal hemoglobin A1C, morning cortisol, and fasting lipid profile; testosterone level was consistent with puberty. There was no history or symptoms of diabetes or adrenal insufficiency. He had no issues with headaches or vision problems. His parents were healthy; they previously had a baby girl who was stillborn at 38 weeks. The patient's older brother and younger sister were healthy with no known genetic diagnosis.

His maternal and paternal grandfathers were obese, but there is no known family history of morbid obesity, genetic syndromes, hypotonia, or mental retardation.

3.2. Genetic Findings

Because of his neonatal hypotonia, the boy had diagnostic testing targeting the PWS critical region. However, DNA methylation analysis of the PWS-imprinting center showed a normal methylation pattern, and chromosome analysis showed a normal male karyotype. Testing for spinal muscular atrophy (SMA) and myotonic dystrophy type 1 were also negative. In addition, his muscle biopsy and brain magnetic resonance imaging (MRI) were normal. He was re-referred for genetic counseling at age 6 years because his phenotype was more suggestive of PWS than of any other recognizable disorder, and testing for the fragile X expansion was negative. The patient was assessed as having the phenotype of PWS without a genetic confirmation. Neuromuscular workup between ages 12 and 13, done because of ongoing hypotonia, was normal. Following that, clinical-grade exome sequencing was performed, and this identified the *SNORD116* microdeletion.

A heterozygous deletion distal to the *SNRPN* gene in the PWS critical region at 15q11.2 was identified in the submitted specimen. The exact breakpoints of this deletion were not discernible from the present analysis. The deletion spans the following region in the GRCh37/hg19 build of the human genome: chr15: 25296613-25367633. This deletion does not affect the *SNURF-SNRPN* locus; however, it leads to the loss of a number of non-coding RNA species which have been implicated in PWS, or a PWS-like phenotype, including the *SNORD116* cluster (PubMed: 19498035, 20588305, 18500341). Subsequent parental testing showed that the parents did not carry this microdeletion, suggesting that the microdeletion found in the patient was de novo and had occurred on the paternally transmitted allele.

4. Discussion

We describe here a rare atypical case, in which a 71 kb microdeletion at 15q11.2 involving the *SNORD116* complex results in a Prader–Willi-like phenotype. The patient exhibited many of the major clinical diagnostic criteria for PWS [14], including neonatal and infantile hypotonia, feeding difficulties that required tube feeding for the first 3 years of life, followed by the onset of excess weight gain and hyperphagia, global developmental delay, and characteristic facial features. Additional features included sleep apnea, behavioral problems, skin picking, and speech delay. Hypogonadism is a common clinical feature of PWS but not seen in this patient. Individuals with PWS commonly fail to spontaneously complete puberty. They have a typical pattern of growth, which is characterized by decreased height velocity in childhood, absence of a pubertal growth spurt, and compromised final adult height [15]. Interestingly, this patient had spontaneous progression through puberty and reached a tall adult stature without GH treatment.

The minimal critical region for PWS is proposed to be approximately 95 kb in size (at chr15:25280000-25375000, genome build hg 19) containing two C/D box snoRNAs: the *SNORD116* cluster and *SNORD109A*, as the only putative functional genes [9]. In review of the regions of deletion in the present and previously described cases that cause the key characteristics of the PWS phenotype, the *SNORD116* cluster, *SNORD109A* and the Imprinted in Prader–Willi (*IPW*) exons were found to be consistently deleted. Additionally, in four of the seven subjects, at least one of the adjacent genes, including the *SNURF-SNRPN* locus, *SNORD107*, *SNORD64*, *SNORD108*, and *SNORD115* cluster, was also deleted [5–7,9]. The microdeletion in our patient is very similar to the cases reported by Bieth et al. [8] and Fontana et al. [10]. The deletion in Bieth's subject was 118 kb in size, encompassing the *SNORD109A* gene, the whole *SNORD116* cluster, and the non-coding exons of the *IPW* transcript. The subject in Fontana's report had an 80 kb microdeletion that was restricted to the *SNORD109A* gene, the complete *SNORD116* cluster, and the first 2 exons and part of exon 3 of the *IPW* gene. The two subjects and our patient shared a core phenotype, which is characterized by neonatal hypotonia, excess weight gain, hyperphagia, global development delay, and distinctive facial features, pointing towards a causative role for the genes in the minimal critical region in the broader phenotype of typical PWS. Further, in animal models of PWS, knockout *Snord116* mice displayed cognitive deficits [16], growth retardation [17], hyperphagia, and marked obesity [18]. However, the role of *SNORD109A* in the clinical manifestations of PWS has not been examined as no mouse orthologs have been identified for this gene [19]. Nevertheless, the current findings demonstrate that the deficiency of *SNORD116* snoRNA is sufficient to result in hyperphagia, obesity, developmental delay, and other clinical manifestations associated with PWS, while additional genes in the region may contribute.

The microdeletion in our patient is the shortest among those in the six previously reported subjects; these patients, however, showed no obvious clinical differences. Some features appear to be less constant in these individuals compared to those with typical PWS deletions. Patients with PWS commonly fail to spontaneously complete puberty. Impaired linear growth is frequently observed in PWS with approximately 90% of affected individuals being short in stature without GH treatment. Like those with the typical genetic lesions seen in PWS, the subjects reported by de Smith et al. [6], Bieth et al. [8], and Hassan et al. [9] had delayed or incomplete puberty and short adult heights (below the 25th percentile). Interestingly, our patient had spontaneous puberty and reached an adult height above the 95th percentile. The subject with PWS reported by Fontana et al. [10] had delayed puberty but his adult stature was within the normal range (174 cm; between the 25th and 50th percentile). He also had normal sized hands and feet and intellectual development (intelligence quotient (IQ) of 80) with mild learning disability, which is very similar to our patient. There were no feeding problems during infancy. He had no sleep disturbances, skin picking or other behavioral problems. Of note, in our patient and the ones reported by Bieth et al. [8] and Fontana et al. [10], food-related behavioral problems (e.g., foraging and sneaking) were milder than typically seen in individuals with PWS. They had the lowest BMIs at 31, 28.45, and 25.1, respectively (through dietary restriction), with a range of 39–50 for the other subjects. These atypical findings indicate that certain genes in the PWS critical region may make more subtle contributions to traits, resulting in a milder phenotype.

In summary, we report on a patient with a Prader–Willi-like phenotype caused by an atypical microdeletion in the PWS critical region. Our findings provide further evidence that deletion of the *SNORD116* region is sufficient to cause the key characteristics of PWS, although some atypical features, including tall stature and spontaneous complete puberty, suggest that other genes in the region may make lesser phenotypic contributions. More research is needed to better understand the role of *SNORD116* in human energy homeostasis and growth.

Supplementary Materials: The following are available online at http://www.mdpi.com/2073-4425/11/2/128/s1, Figure S1: (a) BMI curve and (b) height and weight evolution plotted on World Health Organization Growth Charts for Canada.

Author Contributions: Writing—original draft preparation, Q.T.; supervision, A.M.H.; software, C.E.O.; All authors have read and agreed to the published version of the manuscript.

Funding: Q.T. is supported by the W. Garfield Weston Foundation. C.E.O. is a recipient of the 2018 Alberta SPOR Graduate Studentship in Patient-Oriented Research, which is jointly funded by Alberta Innovates and the Canadian Institutes of Health Research.

Acknowledgments: The authors acknowledge the assistance of William T. Gibson (University of British Columbia and BC Children's Hospital Research Institute), who provided helpful discussions and editorial suggestions during the final submission stage. The authors also thank Levo Therapeutics for their contribution to publication.

Conflicts of Interest: The authors declare no conflict of interest.

Diagnostic Testing: DNA-level diagnostics were performed by Fulgent Genetics (Temple City, California).

References

1. Butler, M.G. Prader-Willi syndrome: Current understanding of cause and diagnosis. *Am. J. Med. Genet.* **1990**, *35*, 319–332. [CrossRef] [PubMed]

2. Irizarry, K.A.; Miller, M.; Freemark, M.; Haqq, A.M. Prader-Willi syndrome: Genetics, metabolomics, hormonal function, and new approaches to therapy. *Adv. Pediatr.* **2016**, *63*, 47–77. [CrossRef] [PubMed]

3. Kim, S.J.; Miller, J.L.; Kuipers, P.J.; German, J.R.; Beaudet, A.L.; Sahoo, T.; Driscoll, D.J. Unique and atypical deletions in Prader-Willi syndrome reveal distinct phenotypes. *Eur. J. Hum. Genet.* **2012**, *20*, 283–290. [CrossRef] [PubMed]

4. Ramsden, S.C.; Clayton-Smith, J.; Birch, R.; Buiting, K. Practice guidelines for the molecular analysis of Prader-Willi and Angelman syndromes. *BMC Med. Genet.* **2010**, *11*, 70. [CrossRef] [PubMed]

5. Sahoo, T.; del Gaudio, D.; German, J.R.; Shinawi, M.; Peters, S.U.; Person, R.E.; Garnica, A.; Cheung, S.W.; Beaudet, A.L. Prader-Willi phenotype caused by paternal deficiency for the HBII-85 C/D box small nucleolar RNA cluster. *Nat. Genet.* **2008**, *40*, 719–721. [CrossRef] [PubMed]

6. de Smith, A.J.; Purmann, C.; Walters, R.G.; Ellis, R.J.; Holder, S.E.; Van Haelst, M.M.; Brady, A.F.; Fairbrother, U.L.; Dattani, M.; Keogh, J.M. A deletion of the HBII-85 class of small nucleolar RNAs (snoRNAs) is associated with hyperphagia, obesity and hypogonadism. *Hum. Mol. Genet.* **2009**, *18*, 3257–3265. [CrossRef] [PubMed]

7. Duker, A.L.; Ballif, B.C.; Bawle, E.V.; Person, R.E.; Mahadevan, S.; Alliman, S.; Thompson, R.; Traylor, R.; Bejjani, B.A.; Shaffer, L.G. Paternally inherited microdeletion at 15q11.2 confirms a significant role for the SNORD116 C/D box snoRNA cluster in Prader-Willi syndrome. *Eur. J. Hum. Genet.* **2010**, *18*, 1196–1201. [CrossRef] [PubMed]

8. Bieth, E.; Eddiry, S.; Gaston, V.; Lorenzini, F.; Buffet, A.; Conte Auriol, F.; Molinas, C.; Cailley, D.; Rooryck, C.; Arveiler, B. Highly restricted deletion of the SNORD116 region is implicated in Prader-Willi syndrome. *Eur. J. Hum. Genet.* **2015**, *23*, 252–255. [CrossRef] [PubMed]

9. Hassan, M.; Butler, M.G. Prader-Willi syndrome and atypical submicroscopic 15q11-q13 deletions with or without imprinting defects. *Eur. J. Med. Genet.* **2016**, *59*, 584–589. [CrossRef] [PubMed]

10. Fontana, P.; Grasso, M.; Acquaviva, F.; Gennaro, E.; Galli, M.L.; Falco, M.; Scarano, F.; Scarano, G.; Lonardo, F. SNORD116 deletions cause Prader-Willi syndrome with a mild phenotype and macrocephaly. *Clin. Genet.* **2017**, *92*, 440–443. [CrossRef] [PubMed]

11. Fulgent Genetics. Clinical Exome. Available online: https://fulgentdiagnostics.com/Clinical-Exome (accessed on 21 January 2020).

12. Richards, C.S.; Bale, S.; Bellissimo, D.B.; Das, S.; Grody, W.W.; Hegde, M.R.; Lyon, E.; Ward, B.E.; Molecular Subcommittee of the ACMG Laboratory Quality Assurance Committee. ACMG recommendations for standards for interpretation and reporting of sequence variations: Revisions 2007. *Genet. Med.* **2008**, *10*, 294–300. [CrossRef] [PubMed]

13. World Health Organization. *WHO Child Growth Standards: Length/ Height-For-Age, Weight-For-Age, Weight-For-Height and Body Mass Index- For-Age: Methods and Development*; World Health Organization: Geneva, Switzerland, 2006; Available online: https://www.who.int/childgrowth/standards/technical_report/en/ (accessed on 1 December 2019).

14. Butler, M.G.; Miller, J.L.; Forster, J.L. Prader-Willi syndrome—Clinical genetics, diagnosis and treatment approaches: An update. *Curr. Pediatr. Rev.* **2019**, *15*. [CrossRef] [PubMed]

15. Grugni, G.; Sartorio, A.; Crinò, A. Growth hormone therapy for Prader-Willi syndrome: Challenges and solutions. *Ther. Clin. Risk Manag.* **2016**, *12*, 873–881. [CrossRef]

16. Adhikari, A.; Copping, N.A.; Onaga, B.; Pride, M.C.; Coulson, R.L.; Yang, M.; Yasui, D.H.; LaSalle, J.M.; Silverman, J.L. Cognitive deficits in the Snord116 deletion mouse model for Prader-Willi syndrome. *Neurobiol. Learn. Mem.* **2018**, 106874. [CrossRef] [PubMed]

17. Ding, F.; Li, H.H.; Zhang, S.; Solomon, N.M.; Camper, S.A.; Cohen, P.; Francke, U. SnoRNA Snord116 (Pwcr1/MBII-85) deletion causes growth deficiency and hyperphagia in mice. *PLoS ONE* **2008**, *3*, e1709. [CrossRef] [PubMed]

18. Polex-Wolf, J.; Lam, B.Y.; Larder, R.; Tadross, J.; Rimmington, D.; Bosch, F.; Cenzano, V.J.; Ayuso, E.; Ma, M.K.; Rainbow, K. Hypothalamic loss of Snord116 recapitulates the hyperphagia of Prader-Willi syndrome. *J. Clin. Invest.* **2018**, *128*, 960–969. [CrossRef] [PubMed]

19. Spikol, E.D.; Laverriere, C.E.; Robnett, M.; Carter, G.; Wolfe, E.M.; Glasgow, E. Zebrafish models of Prader-Willi syndrome: Fast track to pharmacotherapeutics. *Diseases* **2016**, *4*, 13. [CrossRef] [PubMed]

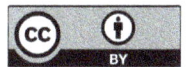 © 2020 by the authors. Licensee MDPI, Basel, Switzerland. This article is an open access article distributed under the terms and conditions of the Creative Commons Attribution (CC BY) license (http://creativecommons.org/licenses/by/4.0/).

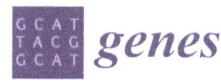

Article

Food and Non-Food-Related Behavior across Settings in Children with Prader–Willi Syndrome

Marie G. Gantz *, Sara M. Andrews and Anne C. Wheeler

RTI International, Research Triangle Park, NC 27709, USA; sandrews@rti.org (S.M.A.);
acwheeler@rti.org (A.C.W.)
* Correspondence: mgantz@rti.org; Tel.: +1-919-597-5110

Received: 7 December 2019; Accepted: 13 February 2020; Published: 17 February 2020

Abstract: This study sought to describe food- and non-food-related behaviors of children aged 3 to 18 years with Prader–Willi syndrome (PWS) in home and school settings, as assessed by 86 parents and 63 teachers using 7 subscales of the Global Assessment of Individual's Behavior (GAIB). General Behavior Problem, Non-Food-Related Behavior Problem, and Non-Food-Related Obsessive Speech and Compulsive Behavior (OS/CB) scores did not differ significantly between parent and teacher reports. Food-Related Behavior Problem scores were higher in parent versus teacher reports when the mother had less than a college education (difference of 13.6 points, 95% Confidence Interval (CI) 5.1 to 22). Parents assigned higher Food-Related OS/CB scores than teachers (difference of 5.7 points, 95% CI 2.4 to 9.0). Although teachers reported fewer Food-Related OS/CB, they scored overall OS/CB higher for interfering with daily activities compared with parents (difference of 0.9 points, 95% CI 0.4 to 1.4). Understanding how behaviors manifest in home and school settings, and how they vary with socio-demographic and patient characteristics can help inform strategies to reduce behavior problems and improve outcomes.

Keywords: Prader–Willi syndrome; food-related behavior; childhood

1. Introduction

Prader–Willi syndrome (PWS), a genetic disorder caused by a lack of expression on paternal chromosome 15 (15q11-q13) [1,2], manifests as a result of three causes: paternal deletion, maternal uniparental disomy (UPD), or imprinting defect. The most common subtype is the paternal deletion, which accounts for approximately 70 percent of all PWS cases [2,3]. Paternal deletions are classified as Type I (TI) or Type II (TII), based on the size of the deletion [2,4]. UPD accounts for approximately 25 percent of PWS cases, and imprinting defects are the cause of approximately 5 percent of cases [2,5].

Although the most notable clinical feature of PWS is hyperphagia, which can begin in early childhood and can lead to obesity and related health issues [2,5,6], behavioral challenges are also common. The behavioral phenotype of PWS generally includes food-seeking behaviors, tantrums, repetitive speech, obsessions, compulsions, and self-injurious behaviors, such as skin picking, as well as internalizing problems such as feelings of negative self-worth, withdrawal, and sadness [5,7–10].

Behavioral challenges vary across age and PWS subtype. In infancy, there are more physical than behavioral concerns, including hypotonia, feeding difficulties, failure to thrive, hypogonadism, lethargy, and decreased interest in feeding [11,12]. Early childhood often brings a significant increase in both externalizing (tantrums, aggression, stealing, etc.) and internalizing (anxiety and depression, skin picking, etc.) behaviors [10,13]. Intellectual disabilities (IDs) and social difficulties become more apparent as children progress through the school-age years. Most individuals with PWS have mild to moderate ID and, even among those with higher IQs, learning and social problems are common [14–16]. Many children with PWS have difficulties relating to peers and often prefer to be with older or younger

Genes **2020**, *11*, 204; doi:10.3390/genes11020204   www.mdpi.com/journal/genes

groups of children [7]. In addition, children with PWS may withdraw into more solitary activities, such as word searches and jigsaw puzzles, rather than engaging in social activities [7]. During early and late adulthood, severe psychiatric illness, such as depression and affective psychosis may develop, especially in those with UPD [17–20]. Maladaptive and compulsive behaviors that began in childhood, such as overeating, hoarding, and tantrums may be elevated into middle adulthood but have been reported to greatly diminish in older adulthood [10,21].

While physical, cognitive, and behavioral concerns are almost universally reported in PWS, there is some evidence to suggest the manifestation of these concerns differs by subtype. Compared to individuals with UPD, individuals with the deletion subtype have been found to demonstrate more compulsive behavior [9,22–24], which has been implicated in both social and academic challenges. Within the deletion subtypes, some have reported no significant difference in behavior between TI and TII deletion [21,25], and those who have found a difference between the two differ in their report on which deletion subtype exhibits more severe compulsive behavior [23,26].

Due the extreme hyperphagia characteristic of PWS, many of the behaviors typically seen in individuals with PWS are food related (i.e., seeking and hoarding food, impulsivity, repetitive requests for food). However, many of the behaviors described by parents include non-food-related concerns as well, such as hoarding non-food items, needing to ask or tell something, ordering and arranging objects, and repeating rituals [27,28].

As most studies examining PWS phenotypic expression have depended on parent report, there is a dearth of information regarding specific differences in food- and non-food-related behaviors at school compared to the home environment. Although, to date, no studies have specifically compared behaviors at home versus at school, several aspects of the PWS phenotype suggest there may be significant differences in behaviors in these two settings. For example, research suggests that behavioral outbursts in children with PWS often occur in conjunction with unexpected changes in settings or routines, which is likely to pose a problem at school [29–31]. There is some evidence that children with TII deletions especially may struggle with compulsive behaviors that relate to specific academic areas while those with TI deletions may have more compulsions related to social activities and grooming [24], suggesting behavioral challenges may differ between subtypes at school as well as at home. Furthermore, individuals with PWS may experience more social problems at school as a result of increased exposure to and relationships with peers [7,24,32]. Conversely, the structured setting and increase in distractions may result in a reduction of food-related behavior problems compared to the home setting where there may be more access to food and where most meals are likely to take place.

The goals of this study were to explore in greater detail the food- and non-food-related behavior patterns of children with PWS as assessed by parents for the home setting and by teachers for the school setting. Associations between behavior scores and participant characteristics including PWS genetic subtype were also explored.

2. Materials and Methods

2.1. Participants

Children with PWS between the ages of 3 and 18 years participated in this study as part of a larger project exploring development, learning, and behavioral profiles in children with PWS. Parents or primary caregivers of the children were invited to participate through one of four means: (1) the Prader–Willi Clinic located at a university medical center; (2) invitations on list-servs and websites serving families and educators of children with PWS; (3) through national organizations for individuals and families of individuals with PWS; (4) and through invitational letters distributed at the annual Prader–Willi Syndrome Association conference. Parents distributed the questionnaires to their child's primary teacher, who returned the completed forms directly to the researchers.

2.2. Procedures

The study was approved by the institutional review board of the University of North Carolina, Chapel Hill, UNC IRB # 05-2572. Parents of all subjects gave their informed consent for their child's inclusion in the study, and children provided assent, as appropriate. After receiving verbal consent, parents were sent packets, which included parent and teacher consent forms, release forms for the school and doctor, parent and teacher rating forms, and several rating scales including a demographic form and the Global Assessment of Individual's Behaviors [33]. The packet also included letters explaining the study, directions for completing forms and rating scales, and self-addressed and stamped envelopes for returning the documents. Parents were asked to provide teachers with the letter and forms to be completed and mailed individually for their child's assessment. For a subsample of children, Stanford–Binet Abbreviated Brief IQ scores [34] were obtained during a research-based visit to the university clinic. PWS diagnosis and subtype were reported by parents and confirmed via genetic report. For most participants, these reports included follow-up testing to determine subtype; however, for 17 participants, only the methylation test confirming PWS was available.

2.3. Measures

2.3.1. Global Assessment of Individual's Behavior (GAIB)

The Global Assessment of Individual's Behavior (GAIB) [33] is a rating instrument that is designed to assess and identify behavior problems typically associated with PWS. The GAIB-PWS was adapted from the Nisonger Child Behavior Rating Form (CBRF), a rating scale which was normed on children and adolescents with developmental disabilities [35]. The GAIB is comprised of 7 subscales: Social Competence (10 items with values ranging from 0 = "Not True" to 3 = "Always True"), General Behavior Problems (40 items with values ranging from 0 = "Not a Problem" to 3 = "Major Problem"), Food-Related Behavior Problems (24 items with values ranging from 0 = "Not a Problem" to 3 = "Major Problem"), Non-Food-Related Behavior Problems (24 items with values ranging from 0 = "Not a Problem" to 3 = "Major Problem"), Food-Related Obsessive Speech and Compulsive Behavior (OS/CB) (16 items with values ranging from 0 = "Not a Problem" to 3 = "Major Problem"), Non-food-Related OS/CB (16 items with values ranging from 0 = "Not a Problem" to 3 = "Major Problem"), and Level of Interference of OS/CB with Daily Function (Interference) (4 items with values of 0 = "No" or 1 = "Yes"). These scales were designed primarily as a clinical measure to help assess the relative challenges across different areas of behaviors, for example, to compare food- versus non-food-related behaviors in order to optimize behavior management techniques.

Due to the highly specific nature of this rating scale (designed specifically for children with PWS), norms are not available to provide a comparison to our sample. Rather, the data provided by this measure are used to examine differences with respect to clinically relevant demographic characteristics (age, sex, race, maternal education), PWS genetic subtype, and teacher and parent report.

2.3.2. Cognitive Functioning

For participants who were seen in clinic, estimated cognitive function was obtained through administration of the Abbreviated Brief IQ (ABIQ) scale of the Stanford Binet Intelligence Scales 5th edition [34]. The ABIQ is composed of two subtests—one focused on verbal reasoning and the other on nonverbal reasoning. Although not as comprehensive as the full-scale IQ, the ABIQ provides a reliable estimate of cognitive functioning, with correlations with the full-scale IQ ranging from 0.81 to 0.85 [34,36]. The ABIQ was administered by a licensed psychologist with expertise in assessment of children with developmental disabilities.

2.4. Statistical Analysis

Demographic characteristics were described as percentages or as means and standard deviations (SD) for children with GAIB assessments completed by parents, teachers, or both. Characteristics were compared between participants who had both parent and teacher assessments versus only one assessment using t tests or Chi-square tests.

Raw scores were calculated for the 7 subscales of the GAIB by summing the scores for all component items. If a teacher did not provide an answer to the General Behavior Problems item "trouble sleeping at night," the value was imputed as the average of the non-missing subscale items. For all subscales other than Interference, if only one question was missing (other than the "trouble sleeping" item), it was imputed to be the average value of the other items in the subscale. If more than one component question was missing an answer, the subscale was not calculated. Mean (with SD) and median (with interquartile range) scores were calculated for parent and teacher reports.

General linear mixed models were created to compare parent and teacher scores, adjusting for patient characteristics considered to be clinically important: age, sex, race (categories of white, black, other/unknown), maternal education (categories of less than college degree, college graduate, unknown), and genetic subtype (categories of deletion, UPD/imprinting, unknown). Race, maternal education, and genetic subtype were collapsed for modeling because of small numbers in some categories. Models accounted for the within-subject correlation between parent and teacher assessments using a compound symmetry covariance structure. To assess whether there were differences between parent and teacher reports within subgroups, interactions between evaluator (parent or teacher) and other covariates were assessed, and those that were statistically significant at the $\alpha <0.05$ level were retained in the final models. For scores that differed between subgroups, individual questions were examined to provide insight into which items contributed the most to those differences, but this was considered exploratory and statistical tests are not reported.

Food-related and non-food-related scores for behavior problems and OS/CB were compared separately for parent and teacher reports using general linear mixed models that accounted for within-subject correlation between food and non-food scores using a compound symmetry covariance structure. Associations between GAIB scores and the ABIQ scale were assessed using Pearson correlation.

Throughout the analysis, p values <0.05 were considered statistically significant. No adjustments were made for multiple testing; thus, the results should be interpreted cautiously.

3. Results

Between February 2007 and February 2010, 149 GAIB forms were completed: 86 parent assessments, and 63 teacher assessments. GAIB assessments were returned by both parents and teachers for 49 children. One hundred children were represented—of whom, 48 were male, 82 were white, and 47 had mothers with college degrees (Table 1). The average age was 9.9 years (standard deviation 4.3). The PWS genetic subtype was known for 83 children, with 55 deletions, 27 UPD cases, and 1 imprinting error. The subsets of children with GAIB parent reports, teacher reports, or both were representative of the 100 children with any assessment, with no meaningful differences between those with one versus two raters (Table S1).

Table 1. Characteristics of Study Participants.

Characteristic	Category	All Children (N = 100)	Parent (N = 86)	Teacher (N = 63)	Parent and Teacher (N = 49)
Age at Assessment	Mean (SD)	9.9 (4.3)	9.9 (4.4)	9.1 (3.9)	8.9 (4.0)
Male		48 (48.0%)	44 (51.2%)	30 (47.6%)	26 (53.1%)
Race	White	82 (82.0%)	74 (86.0%)	50 (79.4%)	42 (85.7%)
	Black	2 (2.0%)	2 (2.3%)	2 (3.2%)	2 (4.1%)
	Hispanic	5 (5.0%)	3 (3.5%)	4 (6.3%)	2 (4.1%)
	Bi-Racial	4 (4.0%)	3 (3.5%)	2 (3.2%)	1 (2.0%)
	Other or Unknown	7 (7.0%)	4 (4.7%)	5 (7.9%)	2 (4.1%)
Maternal Education Level	HS Graduate or Less	9 (9.0%)	8 (9.3%)	7 (11.1%)	6 (12.2%)
	Some College	25 (25.0%)	23 (26.7%)	16 (25.4%)	14 (28.6%)
	College Graduate	30 (30.0%)	27 (31.4%)	20 (31.7%)	17 (34.7%)
	Graduate Degree	17 (17.0%)	15 (17.4%)	8 (12.7%)	6 (12.2%)
	Unknown	19 (19.0%)	13 (15.1%)	12 (19.0%)	6 (12.2%)

Table 1. *Cont.*

Characteristic	Category	All Children (N = 100)	Parent (N = 86)	Teacher (N = 63)	Parent and Teacher (N = 49)
PWS Genetic Subtype	Deletion Type I	9 (9.0%)	8 (9.3%)	7 (11.1%)	6 (12.2%)
	Deletion Type II	15 (15.0%)	15 (17.4%)	8 (12.7%)	8 (16.3%)
	Deletion Type Unknown	31 (31.0%)	25 (29.1%)	19 (30.2%)	13 (26.5%)
	UPD	27 (27.0%)	25 (29.1%)	14 (22.2%)	12 (24.5%)
	Imprinting	1 (1.0%)	1 (1.2%)	1 (1.6%)	1 (2.0%)
	Unknown	17 (17.0%)	12 (14.0%)	14 (22.2%)	9 (18.4%)

SD: Standard Deviation; HS: High School; UPD: Maternal Uniparental Disomy.

For parent-reported GAIB questionnaires, the amount of missing data for individual questions was relatively low, and subscales could be calculated for between 78/86 (91%) and 84/86 (98%) of returned forms (depending on the subscale) (Table 2). Teacher-completed questionnaires had higher amounts of missing data for some subscales, and the total number of calculated scores ranged from 54/63 (86%) to 61/63 (97%).

Table 2. Raw Global Assessment of Individual's Behavior (GAIB) Subscale Scores.

Statistic Type	Parent	Teacher
Social Competence		
N	84	59
Mean (SD)	17.5 (5.4)	16.9 (4.3)
Median (IQR)	18 (14, 21)	16.7 (15, 18.9)
General Behavior Problems		
N	82	61
Mean (SD)	25 (17.4)	25.5 (16.5)
Median (IQR)	22.5 (12, 35)	23 (15, 31.8)
Food-Related Behavior Problems		
N	82	61
Mean (SD)	23.6 (19.4)	15.6 (16.3)
Median (IQR)	17 (8.3, 35)	10 (1, 26)
Non-Food-Related Behavior Problems		
N	80	57
Mean (SD)	23.5 (16)	24.1 (16.1)
Median (IQR)	20.5 (12, 32.5)	21.5 (11.5, 32)
Food-Related Obsessive Speech and Compulsive Behavior		
N	78	55
Mean (SD)	11.7 (11.3)	5.8 (6.3)
Median (IQR)	7 (3, 19)	3.5 (0, 10)
Non-Food-Related Obsessive Speech and Compulsive Behavior		
N	81	54
Mean (SD)	14.2 (10.5)	11 (8.1)
Median (IQR)	12 (6, 21)	8 (4.5, 17)
Level of Interference of Obsessive Speech and Compulsive Behavior with Daily Function		
N	81	58
Mean (SD)	2 (1.6)	3 (1.5)
Median (IQR)	2 (1, 4)	4 (2, 4)

N: Number; IQR: Interquartile Range.

3.1. Associations Between GAIB Scores and Patient Characteristics

In modeling results, older age at the time of assessment was associated with a lower score for Social Competence (mean −0.4 points, 95% CI −0.6 to −0.2, for each 1 year increase in age), and higher scores for General Behavior Problems (1.2 points, 95% CI 0.5 to 1.9, for each 1 year increase in age),

Food-Related Behavior Problems (1.8 points, 95% CI 1.1 to 2.4), Non-Food-Related Behavior Problems (1.6 points, 95% CI 0.9 to 2.3), and Food-Related OS/CB (0.4 points, 95% CI 0.03 to 0.8) (Table 3).

Table 3. Model Results for GAIB Subscales.

Model Effect	Category	Estimate (95% CI)	*P* value
Social Competence			
Age at Assessment	Increase of 1 Year	−0.4 (−0.6, −0.2)	<0.001
Sex (Average Effect)	Female vs. Male	−0.5 (−2.3, 1.4)	0.6
Race	Non-White vs. White	0.1 (−2.8, 3)	0.94
Maternal Education	< College Grad vs. College Grad	0.5 (−1.5, 2.6)	0.61
PWS Genetic Type	UPD/Imprinting vs. Deletion	−0.2 (−2.4, 1.9)	0.83
Evaluator (Average Effect)	Parent vs. Teacher	0.9 (−0.4, 2.3)	0.18
Evaluator*Sex Interaction	Parent vs. Teacher (Females)	−0.5 (−2.4, 1.5)	0.65
Evaluator*Sex Interaction	Parent vs. Teacher (Males)	2.3 (0.4, 4.3)	0.018
Evaluator*Sex Interaction	Female vs. Male (Parent Assessment)	−1.9 (−4, 0.2)	0.08
Evaluator*Sex Interaction	Female vs. Male (Teacher Assessment)	0.9 (−1.6, 3.4)	0.47
General Behavior Problems			
Age at Assessment	Increase of 1 Year	1.2 (0.5, 1.9)	<0.001
Sex	Female vs. Male	4.3 (−1.3, 9.8)	0.13
Race	Non-White vs. White	5.9 (−3.2, 15)	0.2
Maternal Education	< College Grad vs. College Grad	2.7 (−3.5, 8.8)	0.39
PWS Genetic Type	UPD/Imprinting vs. Deletion	1.2 (−5.4, 7.7)	0.73
Evaluator	Parent vs. Teacher	−0.5 (−5.8, 4.8)	0.86
Food-Related Behavior Problems			
Age at Assessment	Increase of 1 Year	1.8 (1.1, 2.4)	<0.001
Sex	Female vs. Male	3.3 (−2.3, 8.9)	0.25
Race	Non-White vs. White	7.8 (−1.4, 17)	0.1
Maternal Education (Average Effect)	< College Grad vs. College Grad	4.6 (−1.7, 11)	0.15
PWS Genetic Type	UPD/Imprinting vs. Deletion	2.7 (−3.9, 9.3)	0.42
Evaluator (Average Effect)	Parent vs. Teacher	8.9 (3.2, 14.6)	0.002
Evaluator*Education Interaction	Parent vs. Teacher (Mother < College Grad)	13.6 (5.1, 22)	0.002
Evaluator*Education Interaction	Parent vs. Teacher (Mother is College Grad)	−0.3 (−7.9, 7.2)	0.93
Non-Food-Related Behavior Problems			
Age at Assessment	Increase of 1 Year	1.6 (0.9, 2.3)	<0.001
Sex	Female vs. Male	2 (−3.5, 7.5)	0.46
Race	Non-White vs. White	−0.3 (−9.2, 8.7)	0.95
Maternal Education	< College Grad vs. College Grad	−0.1 (−6.3, 6)	0.96
PWS Genetic Type	UPD/Imprinting vs. Deletion	3.5 (−3, 9.9)	0.29
Evaluator	Parent vs. Teacher	−2 (−6.6, 2.7)	0.4
Food-Related Obsessive Speech and Compulsive Behavior			
Age at Assessment	Increase of 1 Year	0.4 (0, 0.8)	0.028
Sex	Female vs. Male	3.3 (0, 6.6)	0.049
Race	Non−White vs. White	4.7 (−0.6, 10)	0.08
Maternal Education	< College Grad vs. College Grad	1 (−2.7, 4.6)	0.59
PWS Genetic Type	UPD/Imprinting vs. Deletion	−1.8 (−5.7, 2.1)	0.36
Evaluator	Parent vs. Teacher	5.7 (2.4, 9)	<0.001
Non-Food-Related Obsessive Speech and Compulsive Behavior			
Age at Assessment	Increase of 1 Year	0.3 (−0.1, 0.7)	0.2
Sex	Female vs. Male	1.4 (−2.2, 5)	0.43
Race	Non-White vs. White	3.4 (−2.4, 9.3)	0.25
Maternal Education	< College Grad vs. College Grad	−0.2 (−4.2, 3.8)	0.92
PWS Genetic Type	UPD/Imprinting vs. Deletion	−1.6 (−5.9, 2.7)	0.45
Evaluator	Parent vs. Teacher	3.2 (0, 6.4)	0.05
Level of Interference of Obsessive Speech and Compulsive Behavior with Daily Function			
Age at Assessment	Increase of 1 Year	0 (0, 0.1)	0.17
Sex	Female vs. Male	0.2 (−0.4, 0.8)	0.48
Race	Non-White vs. White	0.8 (−0.2, 1.7)	0.11
Maternal Education	< College Grad vs. College Grad	0 (−0.7, 0.6)	0.92
PWS Genetic Type	UPD/Imprinting vs. Deletion	−0.3 (−0.9, 0.4)	0.42
Evaluator	Parent vs. Teacher	−0.9 (−1.4, −0.4)	<0.001

CI: Confidence Interval; PWS: Prader–Willi syndrome.

3.2. Differences Between Parent- and Teacher-Reported GAIB Scores

General Behavior Problem, Non-Food-Related Behavior Problem, and Non-Food-Related OS/CB scores did not differ significantly between parent and teacher reports (Table 3).

For Social Competence, there was an interaction between evaluator and sex (p value = 0.046), such that for boys, parents reported higher Social Competence than teachers (difference of 2.3 points, 95% CI 0.4 to 4.3). The individual items with the largest differences were "complied with rules or demands", "initiated positive social interactions", and "shared with or helped others."

For Food-Related Behavior Problem scores, there was a statistical interaction between evaluator and maternal education (p value = 0.032). Further investigation revealed that parent scores were higher than teacher scores when maternal education was less than college graduate (difference of 13.6 points, 95% CI 5.1 to 22) (Table 3). The items with the largest differences were those related to crying, frustration, anger, and irritability, along with talking too much or too loudly, and difficulty transitioning activities.

For Food-Related OS/CB scores, parents assigned higher scores than teachers (difference of 5.7 points, 95% CI 2.4 to 9.0), and girls had higher scores than boys (difference of 3.3 points, 95% CI 0.02 to 6.6) (Table 3). Differences between parent and teacher reports were largest for GAIB items related to repetitive speech and questioning, as well as "insisted on closing or opening doors or cupboards." Differences between girls and boys were largest for excessively cleaning body parts and for hiding or hoarding objects.

Interference scores given by parents were lower than teacher reports, averaged over all children (difference of −0.9 points, 95% CI −1.4 to −0.4) (Table 3). Teachers reported more interference with social activities or regular routines, and more interference for greater than one hour per day.

3.3. Food-Related Compared to Non-Food-Related GAIB Scores

Parent-reported Food-Related Behavior Problem scores were higher than Non-Food-Related scores when the mother had less than a college degree (difference of 5.8, 95% CI 0.7 to 10.8) and lower than Non-Food-Related scores when the mother was a college graduate (difference of −5.1 points, 95% CI −9.5 to −0.8) (Table 4).

For parent-reported OS/CB scores, the difference between Food-Related and Non-Food-Related scores increased with age (difference of 0.3 points for each increase of 1 year, 95% CI 0.04 to 0.6), and there was a difference in Food-Related versus Non-Food-Related scores for boys (difference of −3.8, 95% CI −5.4 to −2.2) but not girls (Table 4).

In teacher assessments, Food-Related scores were lower than Non-Food-Related scores for Behavior Problems (difference of −9.3 points, 95% CI −13.8 to −4.8) and for OS/CB (difference of −5.3 points, 95% CI −7.2 to −3.4) (Table 5). Averaging over Food-Related and Non-Food-Related Behavior Problem scores, teachers gave higher scores to students with UPD or imprinting PWS subtypes compared to those with deletions (difference of 7.8 points, 95% CI 0.3 to 15.4).

Table 4. Model Results Comparing Food- and Non-Food-Related Scores for Parent-Reported GAIB Subscales.

Model Effect	Category	Estimate (95% CI)	*p* Value
Behavior			
Age at Assessment	Increase of 1 Year	1.7 (1, 2.5)	<0.001
Sex	Female vs. Male	2.7 (−3.7, 9.1)	0.4
Race	Non-White vs. White	2.5 (−9.1, 14.1)	0.67
Maternal Education (Average Effect)	<College Grad vs. College Grad	6.2 (−0.8, 13.3)	0.08
PWS Genetic Type	UPD/Imprinting vs. Deletion	−0.3 (−7.6, 7)	0.93
Score Type (Average Effect)	Food vs. Non-Food	1.5 (−2, 4.9)	0.39
Score Type*Education Interaction [1]	Food vs. Non-Food (Mother < College Grad)	5.8 (0.7, 10.8)	0.026
Score Type*Education Interaction [1]	Food vs. Non-Food (Mother is College Grad)	−5.1 (−9.5, −0.8)	0.022
Obsessive Speech and Compulsive Behavior			
Age at Assessment (Average Effect)	Increase of 1 Year	0.2 (−0.3, 0.7)	0.45
Sex (Average Effect)	Female vs. Male	4 (−0.5, 8.6)	0.08
Race	Non-White vs. White	6.9 (−1.4, 15.3)	0.1
Maternal Education	<College Grad vs. College Grad	1.9 (−3.1, 7)	0.44
PWS Genetic Type	UPD/Imprinting vs. Deletion	−2.4 (−7.8, 3)	0.38
Score Type (Average Effect)	Food vs. Non-Food	−2.4 (−3.5, −1.3)	<0.001
Score Type*Sex Interaction [2]	Food vs. Non-Food (Females)	−1 (−2.6, 0.5)	0.2
Score Type*Sex Interaction [2]	Food vs. Non-Food (Males)	−3.8 (−5.4, −2.2)	<0.001
Score Type*Age at Assessment [2]	Food vs. Non-Food (for Each 1-Year Increase in Age)	0.3 (0, 0.6)	0.022

[1] P value for interaction between score type (food or non-food) and maternal education was 0.005. [2] P values for interaction with score type (food or non-food) were 0.023 for age and 0.016 for sex.

Table 5. Model Results Comparing Food- and Non-Food-Related Scores for Teacher-Reported GAIB Subscales.

Model Effect	Category	Estimate (95% CI)	*p* Value
Behavior			
Age at Assessment	Increase of 1 Year	1.3 (0.4, 2.2)	0.007
Sex	Female vs. Male	1.3 (−5, 7.5)	0.69
Race	Non-White vs. White	7 (−3, 16.9)	0.16
Maternal Education	<College Grad vs. College Grad	−2.5 (−9.4, 4.4)	0.47
PWS Genetic Type	UPD/Imprinting vs. Deletion	7.8 (0.3, 15.4)	0.043
Score Type	Food vs. Non-Food	−9.3 (−13.8, −4.8)	<0.001
Obsessive Speech and Compulsive Behavior			
Age at Assessment	Increase of 1 Year	0.3 (−0.1, 0.8)	0.17
Sex	Female vs. Male	−0.2 (−3.7, 3.3)	0.93
Race	Non-White vs. White	1.6 (−3.8, 7.1)	0.55
Maternal Education	<College Grad vs. College Grad	−1.5 (−5.5, 2.4)	0.44
PWS Genetic Type	UPD/Imprinting vs. Deletion	−0.2 (−4.6, 4.2)	0.93
Score Type	Food vs. Non-Food	−5.3 (−7.2, −3.4)	<0.001

3.4. Associations Between GAIB Scores and Stanford–Binet Abbreviated Brief IQ

In general, the ABIQ scale was negatively correlated with behavior problems. Pearson correlations were statistically significant between ABIQ and teacher-reported Food-Related Behavior Problems (correlation −0.42, *p* value = 0.017) and parent-reported General Behavior Problems (correlation −0.39, *p* value = 0.024) and Non-Food-Related Behavior Problems (correlation −0.36, *p* value = 0.044) (Table 6).

Table 6. Correlation between GAIB Subscales and Stanford–Binet Abbreviated Brief IQ.

Statistic Type	Parent	Teacher
Social Competence		
N	37	30
Pearson Correlation	0.06	0.33
p value	0.71	0.07
General Behavior Problems		
N	34	31
Pearson Correlation	−0.39	−0.16
p value	**0.024**	0.4
Food-Related Behavior Problems		
N	33	31
Pearson Correlation	−0.2	−0.42
p value	0.27	**0.017**
Non-Food-Related Behavior Problems		
N	32	28
Pearson Correlation	−0.36	−0.02
p value	**0.044**	0.91
Food-Related Obsessive Speech and Compulsive Behavior		
N	34	27
Pearson Correlation	−0.34	−0.17
p value	0.05	0.39
Non-Food-Related Obsessive Speech and Compulsive Behavior		
N	34	26
Pearson Correlation	−0.3	0.05
p value	0.09	0.8
Level of Interference of Obsessive Speech and Compulsive Behavior with Daily Function		
N	35	30
Pearson Correlation	−0.32	−0.21
p value	0.06	0.26

4. Discussion

This study sought to expand understanding of behavioral concerns in children with PWS by including specific examination of food- versus non-food-related behaviors in different settings (home versus school). Results suggested that child age is the greatest predictor of behavior problems as assessed by parents and teachers, with older children exhibiting more behavioral challenges than younger children. This finding is consistent with previous literature describing an increase in behavior challenges in children with PWS through childhood, adolescence, and young adulthood, with a decrease occurring only once the individual reaches later adulthood [10,21]. The increasing difference with age between parent-reported scores for food- and non-food-related behavior problems is also consistent with the progression of PWS through stages of increased food interest, culminating in the onset of hyperphagia at a median age of 8 years [6].

Two subscales revealed sex-related differences. For boys, higher social competence was reported by parents than teachers. In the home environment, children may be more comfortable exhibiting characteristics such as socialization and helpfulness. Girls scored higher than boys for food-related obsessive speech and compulsive behaviors including hiding or hoarding. At least one other study has found that food-related behaviors differ based on both sex and genetic subtype of PWS, with less severe behavior reported in males within the UPD subtype [37]. More research studies focused on potential sex-based differences in behavioral phenotypes of PWS are needed.

While non-food-related subscales were similar in parent and teacher reports, food-related behaviors were more likely to be noted as problematic by parents compared to teachers. These findings suggest that the food-seeking behaviors of children with PWS may be less problematic in the school setting than at home. Mothers with less education reported more food-related behavior problems such as crying, frustration, anger, difficulty transitioning, and repetitive speech than teachers, and they scored food-related behaviors as more problematic than non-food-related behaviors. In contrast, mothers with more education reported fewer food-related than non-food-related behavior problems, suggesting a complex environmental picture. It could be that mothers with lower education levels are at a disadvantage with respect to resources for managing the home environment for their child with PWS. More exploration into how families with varying education and socio-economic backgrounds manage their child's PWS may be warranted in order to identify the best mechanisms for providing appropriate supports.

Although teachers reported fewer food-related obsessive speech and compulsive behaviors compared to parents, teachers reported that when the behaviors occurred, they caused more interference with daily routines than was reported by parents. This is not surprising given expectations for maintaining order and adhering to schedules in the classroom, which may lead to more opportunities for obsessive speech and compulsive behaviors to be disruptive. However, it also speaks to the potential for unique challenges for children with PWS within the school setting. If obsessive speech and compulsive behaviors result in reduced ability to manage the school day, the ability to learn and appropriately interact with peers is compromised.

Higher estimated IQ was associated with less parent-reported general and non-food-related behavior problems, and less teacher-reported food-related behavior problems. It may be that it is easier to structure the school setting and provide distractions from food for children who are less cognitively impaired.

In this study, the only difference observed between the genetic subtypes was that teachers gave higher Behavior Problems scores to children with UPD compared to those with a deletion subtype when food- and non-food-related scores were combined in analysis. Other studies have generally found greater compulsive behavior in deletion [9,22,24] and more autistic behaviors in UPD [25,38,39]. Given the body of literature showing consistent differences in behaviors between UPD and deletion subtypes and some studies reporting differences between the two deletion subtypes [9,22–26], we expected to see more genetic subtype differences. However, our largest category for genetic subtypes was deletion type unknown as seen in Table 1. Thus, our findings could be associated with the small sample size in our study, with the largest genetic subtype group being comprised of deletion type unknown, or with the nature of the measure used to assess behavior. Regarding the latter, the GAIB is not designed to identify co-morbid psychiatric conditions or increased symptomology relative to other children. Rather it is designed to assess specific behaviors known to be of high prevalence in children with PWS, with specific attention to identifying which behaviors are food- and non-food-related. It could be that while general behavior problems differ in frequency and severity between genetic subtypes, when it comes to specific PWS behaviors, this is not the case. However, given our small sample size, additional research is warranted to confirm this hypothesis. Another possibility is that significant differences are more likely to be observed within subtypes in adolescence and early adulthood. Dykens et al. (2004) reported that young adults in their 20s scored highest on measures of maladaptive and compulsive behavior compared to other age groups [10]. Most studies that have reported behavioral differences between genetic subgroups have assessed young adults, with mean age in early to mid-20s [9,23,24,26], whereas the mean age of our study population was 9.9 years.

There are several aspects of this study that limit our ability to make broad conclusions regarding the results. First, the GAIB is not a validated measure with published norms or psychometrics, which limits our ability to generalize these findings to compare with other behavioral studies. Furthermore, while the GAIB provides important information on behaviors specific to PWS, results cannot be compared to other populations. Therefore, we are unable to draw any conclusions regarding the similarities or differences in behavioral profiles of children with PWS versus those without PWS. Also, while our sample is large relative to other studies of this rare neurogenetic condition, our power to detect differences, especially between genetic subtypes, was limited by the sample size, and we did not have sufficient numbers to compare TI and TII deletions. We were also unable to collect several important variables, including degree of obesity and other co-morbid conditions, which may have provided additional insight into how and why these behaviors manifest. Additional, larger studies with more complete genetic subtype information and data on obesity, hyperphagia, and co-morbid conditions are needed to further understand food- and non-food-related behaviors in home and school settings.

This study is the first that we know of that specifically examines food-related and non-food-related behaviors across home and school settings in children with PWS. Understanding how these behaviors manifest across different settings can help inform strategies to reduce behavior problems and improve outcomes.

Supplementary Materials: The following are available online at http://www.mdpi.com/2073-4425/11/2/204/s1. Table S1: Characteristics of Study Participants with 1 versus 2 Assessments

Author Contributions: Conceptualization, A.C.W.; formal analysis, M.G.G. and A.C.W.; funding acquisition, A.C.W.; methodology, M.G.G. and A.C.W.; project administration, A.C.W.; supervision, A.C.W.; writing—original draft, M.G.G., S.M.A. and A.C.W.; writing—review and editing, M.G.G., S.M.A. and A.C.W. All authors have read and agreed to the published version of the manuscript.

Funding: This research was funded by the Foundation for Prader Willi Research and support for manuscript preparation was provided by RTI International.

Acknowledgments: We would like to acknowledge the following people who were involved in the implementation of this study at the University of North Carolina, Chapel Hill: Stephen Hooper, Donna Yerby, Carly Hoffend Gasior, and Kristy Ten Haagen. We greatly appreciate the children with PWS and their parents and teachers for their time and the invaluable information they provided.

Conflicts of Interest: The authors declare no conflict of interest. The funders supported the recruitment of participants, but were not involved in the design, of the study, data collection or analysis or preparation of the manuscript.

References

1. Bittel, D.C.; Butler, M.G. Prader–Willi syndrome: Clinical genetics, cytogenetics and molecular biology. *Expert Rev. Mol. Med.* **2005**, *7*, 1–20. [CrossRef] [PubMed]
2. Butler, M.G.; Manzardo, A.M.; Forster, J.L. Prader-Willi Syndrome: Clinical Genetics and Diagnostic Aspects with Treatment Approaches. *Curr. Pediatr. Rev.* **2016**, *12*, 136–166. [CrossRef] [PubMed]
3. Ledbetter, D.H.; Riccardi, V.M.; Airhart, S.D.; Strobel, R.J.; Keenan, B.S.; Crawford, J.D. Deletions of chromosome 15 as a cause of the Prader-Willi syndrome. *N. Engl. J. Med.* **1981**, *304*, 325–329. [CrossRef] [PubMed]
4. Butler, M.G.; Fischer, W.; Kibiryeva, N.; Bittel, D.C. Array comparative genomic hybridization (aCGH) analysis in Prader-Willi syndrome. *Am. J. Med. Genet. A* **2008**, *146*, 854–860. [CrossRef] [PubMed]
5. Cassidy, S.B.; Schwartz, S.; Miller, J.L.; Driscoll, D.J. Prader-Willi syndrome. *Genet. Med.* **2012**, *14*, 10–26. [CrossRef] [PubMed]
6. Miller, J.L.; Lynn, C.H.; Driscoll, D.C.; Goldstone, A.P.; Gold, J.A.; Kimonis, V.; Dykens, E.; Butler, M.G.; Shuster, J.J.; Driscoll, D.J. Nutritional phases in Prader-Willi syndrome. *Am. J. Med. Genet. A* **2011**, *155*, 1040–1049. [CrossRef]
7. Whittington, J.; Holland, A. Neurobehavioral phenotype in Prader-Willi syndrome. *Am. J. Med. Genet. C Semin. Med. Genet.* **2010**, *154*, 438–447. [CrossRef]
8. Ho, A.Y.; Dimitropoulos, A. Clinical management of behavioral characteristics of Prader-Willi syndrome. *Neuropsychiatr. Dis. Treat.* **2010**, *6*, 107–118. [CrossRef]
9. Hartley, S.L.; Maclean, W.E., Jr.; Butler, M.G.; Zarcone, J.; Thompson, T. Maladaptive behaviors and risk factors among the genetic subtypes of Prader-Willi syndrome. *Am. J. Med. Genet. A* **2005**, *136*, 140–145. [CrossRef]
10. Dykens, E.M. Maladaptive and compulsive behavior in Prader-Willi syndrome: New insights from older adults. *Am. J. Ment. Retard* **2004**, *109*, 142–153. [CrossRef]
11. Maggio, M.; Corsello, M.; Piccione, M.; Piro, E.; Giuffrè, M.; Liotta, A. Neonatal presentation of Prader Willi syndrome. Personal records. *Minerva Pediatr.* **2008**, *59*, 817–823.

12. Butler, M.G. Prader-Willi Syndrome: Obesity due to Genomic Imprinting. *Curr. Genom.* **2011**, *12*, 204–215. [CrossRef] [PubMed]

13. Skokauskas, N.; Sweeny, E.; Meehan, J.; Gallagher, L. Mental health problems in children with prader-willi syndrome. *J. Can. Acad. Child Adolesc. Psychiatry* **2012**, *21*, 194–203. [CrossRef]

14. Whittington, J.; Holland, A. Cognition in people with Prader-Willi syndrome: Insights into genetic influences on cognitive and social development. *Neurosci. Biobehav. Rev.* **2017**, *72*, 153–167. [CrossRef] [PubMed]

15. Gross-Tsur, V.; Landau, Y.E.; Benarroch, F.; Wertman-Elad, R.; Shalev, R.S. Cognition, Attention, and Behavior in Prader-Willi Syndrome. *J. Child Neurol.* **2001**, *16*, 288–290. [CrossRef]

16. Roof, E.; Stone, W.; MacLean, W.; Feurer, I.D.; Thompson, T.; Butler, M.G. Intellectual characteristics of Prader-Willi syndrome: Comparison of genetic subtypes. *J. Intellect. Disabil. Res.* **2000**, *44 Pt 1*, 25–30. [CrossRef]

17. Boer, H.; Holland, A.; Whittington, J.; Butler, J.; Webb, T.; Clarke, D. Psychotic illness in people with Prader Willi syndrome due to chromosome 15 maternal uniparental disomy. *Lancet* **2002**, *359*, 135–136. [CrossRef]

18. Whittington, J.; Holland, A. A review of psychiatric conceptions of mental and behavioural disorders in Prader-Willi syndrome. *Neurosci. Biobehav. Rev.* **2018**, *95*, 396–405. [CrossRef]

19. Soni, S.; Whittington, J.; Holland, A.J.; Webb, T.; Maina, E.N.; Boer, H.; Clarke, D. The phenomenology and diagnosis of psychiatric illness in people with Prader-Willi syndrome. *Psychol. Med.* **2008**, *38*, 1505–1514. [CrossRef]

20. Vogels, A.; De Hert, M.; Descheemaeker, M.J.; Govers, V.; Devriendt, K.; Legius, E.; Prinzie, P.; Fryns, J.P. Psychotic disorders in Prader-Willi syndrome. *Am. J. Med. Genet. A* **2004**, *127*, 238–243. [CrossRef]

21. Dykens, E.; Roof, E. Behavior in Prader-Willi syndrome: Relationship to genetic subtypes and age. *J. Child Psychol. Psychiatry* **2008**, *49*, 1001–1008. [CrossRef] [PubMed]

22. Dykens, E.M.; Cassidy, S.B.; King, B.H. Maladaptive behavior differences in Prader-Willi syndrome due to paternal deletion versus maternal uniparental disomy. *Am. J. Ment. Retard.* **1999**, *104*, 67–77. [CrossRef]

23. Novell-Alsina, R.; Esteba-Castillo, S.; Caixas, A.; Gabau, E.; Gimenez-Palop, O.; Pujol, J.; Deus, J.; Torrents-Rodas, D. Compulsions in Prader-Willi syndrome: Occurrence and severity as a function of genetic subtype. *Actas Esp. Psiquiatr.* **2019**, *47*, 79–87.

24. Zarcone, J.; Napolitano, D.; Peterson, C.; Breidbord, J.; Ferraioli, S.; Caruso-Anderson, M.; Holsen, L.; Butler, M.G.; Thompson, T. The relationship between compulsive behaviour and academic achievement across the three genetic subtypes of Prader-Willi syndrome. *J. Intellect. Disabil. Res.* **2007**, *51*, 478–487. [CrossRef] [PubMed]

25. Milner, K.M.; Craig, E.E.; Thompson, R.J.; Veltman, M.W.; Thomas, N.S.; Roberts, S.; Bellamy, M.; Curran, S.R.; Sporikou, C.M.; Bolton, P.F. Prader-Willi syndrome: Intellectual abilities and behavioural features by genetic subtype. *J. Child Psychol. Psychiatry* **2005**, *46*, 1089–1096. [CrossRef] [PubMed]

26. Butler, M.G.; Bittel, D.C.; Kibiryeva, N.; Talebizadeh, Z.; Thompson, T. Behavioral differences among subjects with Prader-Willi syndrome and type I or type II deletion and maternal disomy. *Pediatrics* **2004**, *113*, 565–573. [CrossRef] [PubMed]

27. Dimitropoulos, A.; Blackford, J.; Walden, T.; Thompson, T. Compulsive behavior in Prader-Willi syndrome: Examining severity in early childhood. *Res. Dev. Disabil.* **2006**, *27*, 190–202. [CrossRef]

28. Dykens, E.M.; Leckman, J.F.; Cassidy, S.B. Obsessions and compulsions in Prader-Willi syndrome. *J. Child Psychol. Psychiatry* **1996**, *37*, 995–1002. [CrossRef]

29. Tunnicliffe, P.; Woodcock, K.; Bull, L.; Oliver, C.; Penhallow, J. Temper outbursts in Prader-Willi syndrome: Causes, behavioural and emotional sequence and responses by carers. *J. Intellect. Disabil. Res.* **2014**, *58*, 134–150. [CrossRef]

30. Woodcock, K.A.; Oliver, C.; Humphreys, G.W. The relationship between specific cognitive impairment and behaviour in Prader-Willi syndrome. *J. Intellect. Disabil. Res.* **2011**, *55*, 152–171. [CrossRef]

31. Woodcock, K.; Oliver, C.; Humphreys, G. Associations between repetitive questioning, resistance to change, temper outbursts and anxiety in Prader-Willi and Fragile-X syndromes. *J. Intellect. Disabil. Res.* **2009**, *53*, 265–278. [CrossRef] [PubMed]

32. Dykens, E.M.; Roof, E.; Hunt-Hawkins, H.; Daniell, C.; Jurgensmeyer, S. Profiles and trajectories of impaired social cognition in people with Prader-Willi syndrome. *PLoS ONE* **2019**, *14*, e0223162. [CrossRef] [PubMed]

33. Tasse, M.J.; Havercamp, S.M.; Mandal, R.L. *Global Assessment of Individual Behavior-Prader Willi Syndrome*; University of North Carolina: Chapel Hill, NC, USA, 2002.

34. Roid, G.H. *Stanford Binet Intelligence Scales*, 5th ed.; Riverside Pub.: Itasca, IL, USA, 2003.

35. Aman, M.G.; Tasse, M.J.; Rojahn, J.; Hammer, D. The Nisonger CBRF: A child behavior rating form for children with developmental disabilities. *Res. Dev. Disabil.* **1996**, *17*, 41–57. [CrossRef]

36. Roid, G.H. *Essentials of Stanford-Binet Intelligence Scales (SB5) Assessment*; John Wiley & Sons: Hoboken, NJ, USA, 2004.

37. Gito, M.; Ihara, H.; Ogata, H.; Sayama, M.; Murakami, N.; Nagai, T.; Ayabe, T.; Oto, Y.; Shimoda, K. Gender Differences in the Behavioral Symptom Severity of Prader-Willi Syndrome. *Behav. Neurol.* **2015**, 294127. [CrossRef] [PubMed]

38. Veltman, M.W.; Thompson, R.J.; Roberts, S.E.; Thomas, N.S.; Whittington, J.; Bolton, P.F. Prader-Willi syndrome—A study comparing deletion and uniparental disomy cases with reference to autism spectrum disorders. *Eur. Child Adolesc. Psychiatry* **2004**, *13*, 42–50. [CrossRef] [PubMed]

39. Dimitropoulos, A.; Ho, A.; Feldman, B. Social responsiveness and competence in Prader-Willi syndrome: Direct comparison to autism spectrum disorder. *J. Autism Dev. Disord.* **2013**, *43*, 103–113. [CrossRef] [PubMed]

© 2020 by the authors. Licensee MDPI, Basel, Switzerland. This article is an open access article distributed under the terms and conditions of the Creative Commons Attribution (CC BY) license (http://creativecommons.org/licenses/by/4.0/).

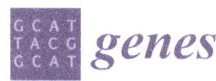

Review

Clinical Observations and Treatment Approaches for Scoliosis in Prader–Willi Syndrome

Harold J.P. van Bosse [1,*] and Merlin G. Butler [2]

[1] Shriners Hospital for Children, 3551 North Broad Street, Philadelphia, PA 19140, USA
[2] Departments of Psychiatry & Behavioral Sciences and Pediatrics, University of Kansas Medical Center, Kansas City, KS 66160, USA; mbutler4@kumc.edu
* Correspondence: Hvanbosse@shrinenet.org

Received: 22 January 2020; Accepted: 25 February 2020; Published: 28 February 2020

Abstract: Prader–Willi syndrome (PWS) is recognized as the first example of genomic imprinting, generally due to a de novo paternal 15q11-q13 deletion. PWS is considered the most common genetic cause of marked obesity in humans. Scoliosis, kyphosis, and kyphoscoliosis are commonly seen in children and adolescents with PWS with a prevalence of spinal deformities cited between 15% to 86%. Childhood risk is 70% or higher, until skeletal maturity, with a bimodal age distribution with one peak before 4 years of age and the other nearing adolescence. As few reports are available on treating scoliosis in PWS, we described clinical observations, risk factors, therapeutic approaches and opinions regarding orthopedic care based on 20 years of clinical experience. Treatments include diligent radiographic screening, starting once a child can sit independently, ongoing physical therapy, and options for spine casting, bracing and surgery, depending on the size of the curve, and the child's age. Similarly, there are different surgical choices including a spinal fusion at or near skeletal maturity, versus a construct that allows continued growth while controlling the curve for younger patients. A clear understanding of the risks involved in surgically treating children with PWS is important and will be discussed.

Keywords: Prader–Willi syndrome; scoliosis; kyphosis; spinal deformities; junctional kyphosis; risk factors; treatment options; surgery; bracing

1. Introduction

Prader–Willi syndrome (PWS), a rare syndrome caused by errors in genomic imprinting, is considered the most common genetic cause of marked obesity in humans [1]. It occurs in about one in 15,000 to 30,000 births with an estimated 400,000 affected individuals worldwide [2]. PWS characteristics at birth and infancy include hypotonia with a poor suck reflex leading to feeding difficulties, and failure to thrive [3,4]; hypogonadism and hypogenitalism are present, associated with varying deficiencies in growth, thyroid and sex hormones; developmental and cognitive delays range between mild and severe. Small hands and feet, short stature, and mild facial dysmorphic features are recognized, especially in children lacking growth hormone treatment. Behavioral problems arise at different stages of childhood, including skin picking, temper tantrums and outbursts, obsessive compulsions and food seeking (hyperphagia). If not externally controlled, the hyperphagia, along with decreased physical activity and a low metabolic rate, can lead to obesity; the obesity itself is often life-threatening.

PWS results from loss of gene expression of the paternally derived chromosome 15q11-q13, most commonly (60%) due to a deletion of the region. The second most common cause (35%) is maternal disomy of chromosome 15 (UPD), where both copies of the chromosome are maternally inherited without a paternal copy. The remaining cases have an error in the center that controls the activity of the region's imprinted genes or from translocations or inversions involving chromosome 15 [5].

Children and adults with the deletion form of PWS are more prone to self-injury, compulsions and lower cognition than those with maternal disomy 15 [6,7]. In comparison, those with maternal disomy 15 are at a greater risk of autistic features and psychosis during late adolescence or early adulthood [1].

Scoliosis, kyphosis, and kyphoscoliosis are commonly seen in children and adolescents with PWS. Spinal deformities are measured using the Cobb angle method, where lines are drawn along the endplates of the uppermost and lowermost vertebra contained in a curve, and the curve value is measured as the angle between these two endplate lines. A typical child of any age has virtually no measurable deviation from a straight spine. Curves under 10° are considered not to be scoliotic. Curves between 10° and 20° are closely observed, but treatment is usually withheld until a curve shows obvious progression or is larger than 20°–25°. The prevalence of spinal deformities is cited between 15% and 86% [8–13]. For example, a 2007 survey in the USA of caregivers of persons with PWS by the Prader–Willi Syndrome Association ((PWSA (USA)) found that 40% of 1603 respondents were positive for scoliosis and/or kyphosis. This is similar to studies reviewed earlier by Butler in 1990 [3] in summarizing 538 patients found in the literature prior to growth hormone treatment with 44% having scoliosis. In the PWSA (USA) survey, the female to male ratio for those with minor curves was 1.23:1, and 2.3:1 for curves requiring treatment (bracing or surgery). Females had about a 10% higher chance of developing scoliosis, but both sexes had an equal risk of curve progression. As for the PWS genetic classes, those with maternal disomy 15 appeared to have a slightly higher risk of developing scoliosis, but no PWS genetic type had a higher risk of progression. The survey also identified two peak age incidences for spine deformities, at 0–24 months, and the second at 73–96 months, indicating a bimodal age distribution. The 40% prevalence rate is probably an underestimate, as many participants were included before they reached skeletal maturity, and scoliosis was identified by caretakers' knowledge of a spine deformity rather than on spine radiographs. In studies that used radiographs and stratified by age, an overall higher prevalence was found. Odent et al. found an overall rate of 43%, but 68% for those that reached skeletal maturity [14]. Nagai et al noted 22% of patients 5 years or younger had scoliosis, 25% for those 6–11 years, and 68% for those over 12 years of age [12]. Similarly, de Lind van Wijngaarden et al. reported a prevalence of 23% for infants, 29% for juveniles, and 12 of 15 adolescents (80%) [8]. These studies support a bimodal age pattern for scoliosis in PWS, with 23% of patients developing curves before their 4th birthday, likely due to hypotonia. Relatively few patients were found in the juvenile period (2–6%), and some may have had curves missed during the infant period. Near adolescence, a second substantial curve onset occurs with approximately 45% of children. Overall, the cumulative risk of developing a spine deformity appears to be about 70%.

Patients with PWS can exhibit both the C-shape and the S-shaped curves. The C-shape is primarily a sign of the underlying hypotonia where the child will list asymmetrically to the side. As the child gains strength, they are able to compensate above and below the initial curve, thereby functional centering the head over the pelvis. This converts the curve to an S-shape. The C-shaped curve may be referred to as uncompensated while the S-shaped curves are compensated.

Reasons for treating spine deformities in PWS are not so much related to body image; although children and adults with PWS are body-conscientious, most do not display the same self-awareness as seen in their peers. The decreased respiratory status of children and adults is the more important issue, with elements of sleep apnea (both obstructive and central), weak respiratory musculature, and nocturnal hypoventilation [15–18]. Scoliosis and/or kyphosis are often indicated as significant co-morbidities for respiratory compromise, by virtue of associated chest deformities, although conclusive proof is still lacking [10,19–23]. People with PWS have a decreased life expectancy, with survivorship analysis varying from 87% at 35 years to 71% at 40 years of age, and a mortality rate of 99% by 60 years [24–26]. Cor pulmonale and respiratory failure are the most common causes of death [24,27]; hence, diagnosing and treating scoliosis early is of the utmost importance.

The lifetime risk of an individual with PWS developing scoliosis is remarkably high, approximately 70%. Screening should start after the child begins sitting independently and continue on a regular basis until skeletal maturity. Given the lack of vertebral rotation related to the curve, radiographic monitoring is recommended on a yearly basis for children under 4 years of age. The curves seem to result from the characteristic hypotonia, particularly in the younger children. Interestingly, more than half of the curves occur in the adolescent period which is also the most common age group seen in idiopathic scoliosis. In idiopathic adolescent scoliosis, a number of associated chromosome abnormalities have been reported (e.g., 1p36.32, 2q36.1, 8q12, 10q24.31, 17q25.3, and 19p13.3) that may involve genes affecting growth and musculoskeletal development [28]. For example, next-generation sequencing, genotyping, linkage analysis, GWAS and gene expression studies in tissues have identified 23 genes that are related to scoliosis [29–34]. These genes code for extracellular matrix proteins, collagen, bone formation, mineralization and metabolism, growth and sex hormones, and homeobox genes required for differentiation of skeletal elements and structural integrity of the vertebrae. Eight of these 23 genes are located in those associated chromosome regions identified to be disturbed in humans with scoliosis (Online Mandelian Inheritance in Man (OMIM), www.omim.org). It is unclear how causative any of these genes are to the spinal deformity in PWS, and none of the identified genes are on chromosome 15, let alone in the PWS region. However, the genetics of scoliosis in PWS has been poorly studied. Interestingly, both *NIPA1* and *NIPA2* genes are located in the 15q11.2 BP1–BP2 region and the encoded proteins are involved as magnesium or cation transporters with bone morphogenetic protein (BMP) production, signaling pathways or BMP receptors, along with transforming growth factors and their receptors thereby influencing cartilage and bone formation (GeneCards.org; OMIM). [35]. One could speculate that disturbances could impact differentiation of myoblasts and osteoblasts, calcium regulation and bone mineralization, maintenance of neuromuscular junctions and formation of cartilage and bone mass in PWS. The multifactorial nature of scoliosis may also indicate that allelic differences on other chromosomes are necessary for development of scoliosis in children with PWS.

2. Clinical Observations and Treatment

2.1. Clinical Experiences and Treatment for Scoliosis in Prader–Willi Syndrome

As there are few reports on treating scoliosis in PWS, a major focus of this report is to describe the best treatment strategies for spine deformities in children with PWS based on 20 years of clinical experience. Clinical observations, risk factors, therapeutic approaches and opinions regarding orthopedic care will be divided into subsections in this report.

2.1.1. Physical Therapy

All children with PWS, except the most atypical, need ongoing therapy services starting as a neonate. Since children with PWS are initially stronger in their extremities rather than their core, emphasis first is on trunk strengthening and sensory integration. Developmental milestones in PWS are delayed with ambulation not occurring until 27 months on average [36]. Although there is a strong temptation to have these children upright, unsupported upright sitting should be delayed until the child has the strength to pull themselves to a sitting position spontaneously. This should prevent initiation of a spine deformity due to a hypotonic slouch when sitting prior to physiological readiness (Figure 1). A reclined seated position (~about 60°) will allow for feeding and appropriate interactions, while preventing postural droop. Similarly, once a child is sitting, emphasis then should be placed on quadruped stance and crawling, while also developing standing skills. Solid ankle-foot-orthoses will stabilize ankle weakness and hyperlaxity. At risk children may also benefit from hippotherapy for spine strengthening and balance at a suitable age.

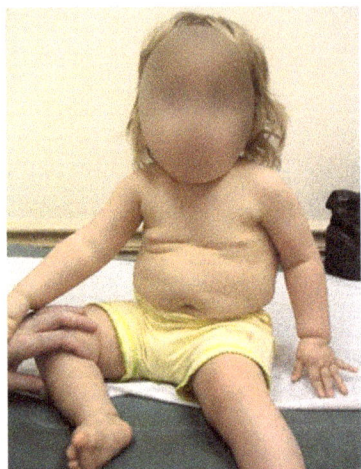

Figure 1. 18-month-old female with Prader–Willi syndrome (PWS) maternal disomy of chromosome 15 (UPD) type, displaying the typical hypotonic sitting position.

2.1.2. Screening

Scoliosis in infants and children with PWS is more difficult to diagnose clinically compared to children with idiopathic scoliosis [37]. The spine in patients with PWS exhibits much less rotation relative to curve size, resulting in diminished posterior rib asymmetry. Because the incidence of scoliosis is high in the infantile period in PWS, routine radiographic screening is important for early recognition of children at risk. In the uncommon case of a child showing obvious signs of a spinal asymmetry at an early age, the finding should be appropriately evaluated radiographically. But in the routine case, screening radiographs are first performed once a child can sit unassisted and are done yearly as seated or standing spine films until about 4 years of age. The risk of developing a curve thereafter is relatively small until the child nears adolescence. Any deviation from straight should probably be followed by a physician experienced in treating pediatric spine deformities, so they can verify measurements, and set a schedule for clinical and radiographic follow-up.

2.1.3. Serial Spinal Casting

Serial casting for spine deformities in infants and young children has had a resurgence of interest after Mehta published her article in 2005 [38] and others [39]. Spine casting is done on a special Risser table, where the child, under general anesthesia, has traction applied through a head halter traction and crisscrossing pelvis straps. The table top can then be lowered, so that the patient is suspended by transverse bars at the level of the shoulders and pelvis, which allows for full circumferential exposure of the trunk and chest. Casting material is applied, and the appropriate maneuver of chest derotation and sagittal translation for curve correction is performed (Figure 2). The cast is changed every 2 months for those younger than 2 years, every 3 months for those between 2 and 3 years of age, and every 4 months for those over 3 years.

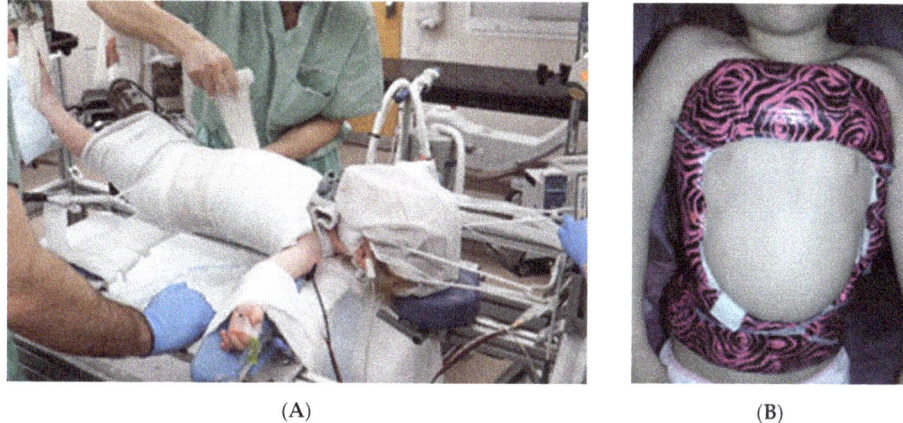

(A)   (B)

Figure 2. (**A**) Patient on the Risser casting table. Note the straps from the head halter traction, as well as the pelvis traction straps visible lateral to the patients left hip. (**B**) Patient in a spine cast.

Although there is the occasional case where an infantile curve spontaneously resolves, most curves over 25° require treatment. If a curve would naturally correct without treatment, it will merely correct quicker with treatment. Therefore, treating all curves at 25° appears to improve chances of intervening at the best possible moment to help a curve resolve. Indications for starting spine casting is a curve greater than 25° in a child over sitting age and usually younger than 3 years of age; we have initiated spinal casting on the occasional child at nearly 5 years of age. In the rare case when a child has a large curve before they begin sitting independently, a semi-rigid spine brace is used to temporize until they are suitably developed physically to start casting. There are three possible outcomes from cast treatment. The best outcome ("cured") is the curve that can be reduced to either <15° out-of-cast, or 3 successive out-of-cast measurements of <25°, in which case the patient is transitioned to a brace, then weaned out of the brace after one year (Figure 3). More moderate curves, once they plateau in casting, are also transitioned to a brace, with the expectation that the brace will be long-term treatment. Severe curves are casted until the child is old enough to undergo surgery for an expandable spine implant (5–8 years of age) (Figure 4).

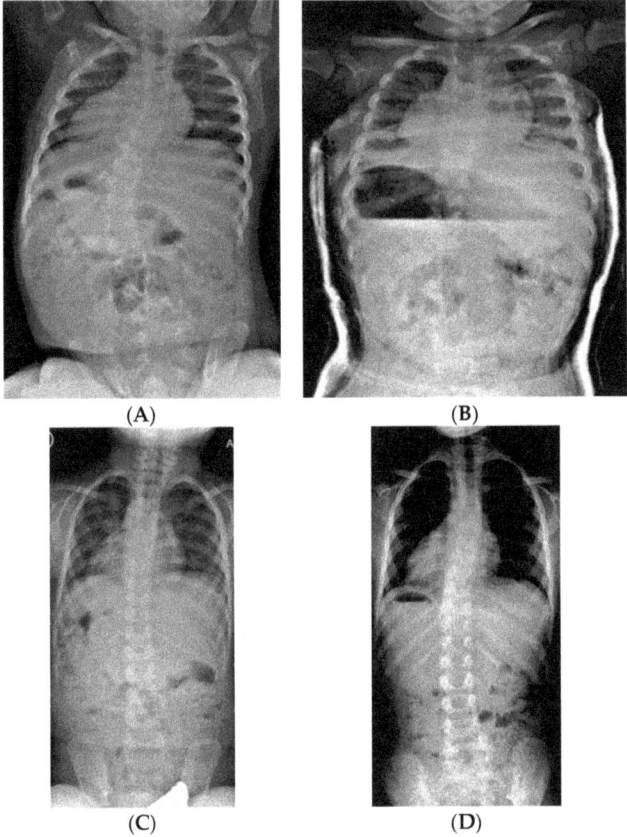

Figure 3. (**A**) 19-month-old male with PWS deletion type with 52° curve. (**B**) Same patient at 20 months old, sitting in his first spinal cast, 10° curve in cast. (**C**) Same patient at 35 months old, after completing 8 casts, 11° curve. (**D**) Same patient at 6 years old, 3 years out of cast and 2 years out of brace, with an 18° curve.

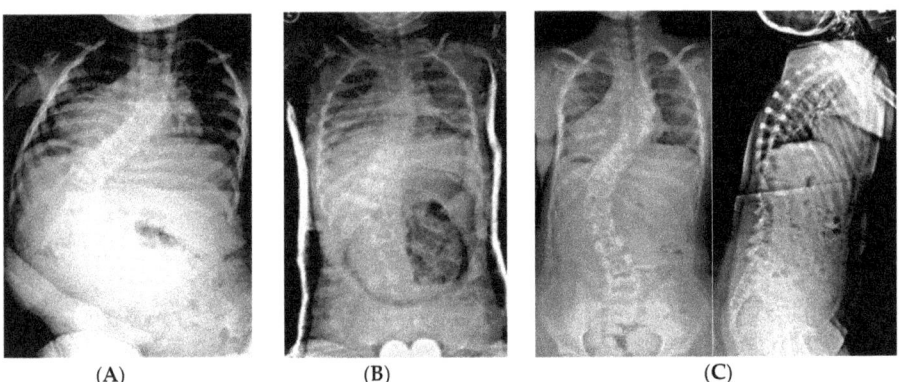

Figure 4. *Cont.*

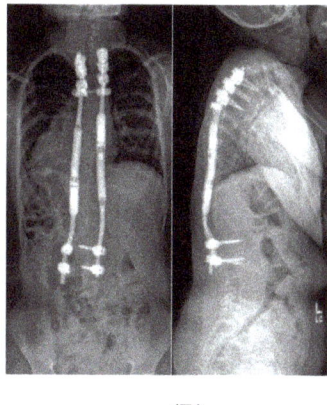 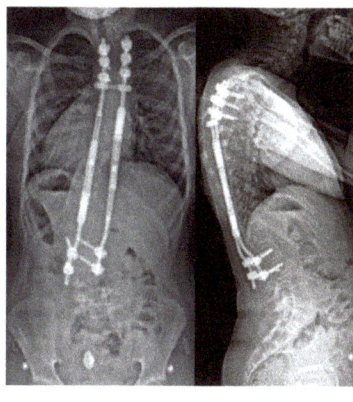

(D)   (E)

Figure 4. (**A**) 18-month-old female with PWS deletion type with 106° curve. (**B**) Same patient at 18 months old, sitting in first cast, 54° curve. (**C**) AP and lateral views of spine at 6 years old, after 18 casts, 61° curve, just prior to surgery. (**D**) AP and lateral views of spine 4 months after placing magnetically actuated spine rods T3–L3. Curve was corrected to 30°, maintaining her pre-operative kyphosis. (**E**) AP and lateral views of spine at 10 years old, just prior replacement with new expandable rods. Due to adding on, curve measures 50°, which was addressed by including L4 in the construct.

Oore et al. reported the only published series of serial casting for children with PWS, noting a reduction of curve size in their ten patients, from 45° to 37° [40]. We reviewed our results from 34 children with PWS with more than 24 months' follow-up after their initial spine cast. The average age at initial casting was 32 months (range 14–64 months) with an average of 8 casts (range 3–18). Twelve children (35%) were in the "cured" group; all were weaned out of brace at one year after completion of casting. Seven of these patients had maternal disomy 15, five had the 15q11-q13 deletion, and the average initial curve was 44° (range 27°–80°). Another 18 patients transitioned to long-term brace wear (10 with deletion, 7 with maternal disomy 15, and one having an imprinting defect). Their average initial curve of 55° (range 27°–84°) became 35° (16°–64°) at the end of casting and was 46° (27°–84°) at two years' follow-up. Four patients with severe initial curves (54°, 84°, 95°, and 106°) were controlled in casts until they reached a sufficient age for surgery (average 56 months old). Overall, the odds ratio for "curing" an initial curve of <50° was nine times that of a curve >50° in this cohort.

2.1.4. Bracing

Bracing is most appropriate for children who have spinal curves over 20°–25° but too old for casting. The goal of bracing is to prevent curve progression, but in very large curves, braces may be used to control the curve until the patient reaches a desired age for surgery. In general, curves smaller than 30° are treated with a nighttime only Providence style brace. This brace is designed to obtain maximal curve stretching, maintaining its flexibility. The brace is not appropriate for ambulation. If the curve exceeds 30°, a standard thoracic-lumbar-sacral orthosis (TLSO) is added for daytime use. Our preference is an anterior opening, custom molded brace, with a goal of achieving 40–50% diminution of the curve based on an in-brace spinal radiograph. The use of two braces together may seem excessive, but unanticipated curve improvement has occurred with this strategy (Figure 5). If a curve progresses past 50°, and future surgery is likely, then brace treatment is continued so long as in-brace radiographs show the curve below 50°, allowing the child the opportunity for further growth.

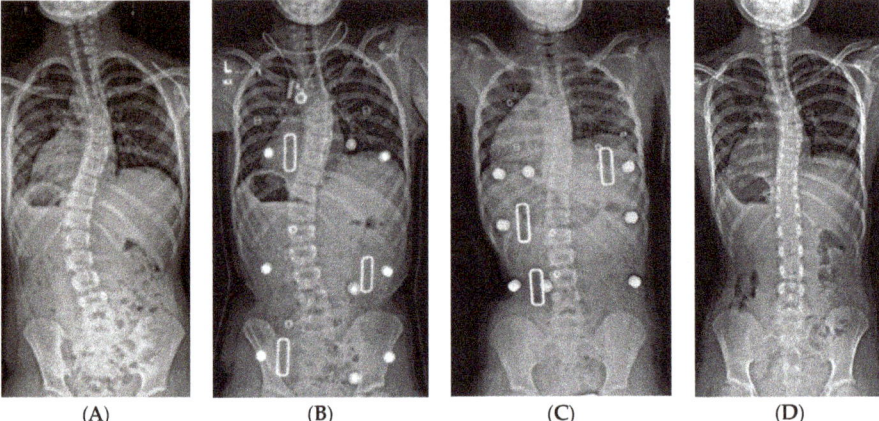

(A)   (B)   (C)   (D)

Figure 5. (**A**) 10-year-old female with PWS deletion type and 41° curve. (**B**) Standing in her daytime thoracic-lumbar-sacral orthosis (TLSO). (**C**) Supine in her nighttime Providence brace. (**D**) At 13 years, with curve improved to 25°.

2.1.5. Spine Surgery

2.1.5.1. Complications

Prior to discussing the different surgical options for children with PWS and severe scoliosis, it is important to understand why their scoliosis is different from idiopathic spine deformities, as well as what makes the child with PWS different from the typical child with regards to major surgery. It is important to think of the patient as a child with PWS who has scoliosis, and not as just a child with scoliosis who also has a rare and obscure diagnosis.

The most common complication affecting outcomes of spinal instrumentation is adding-on of the curve above or below the construct, usually as proximal or distal junctional kyphosis (PJK and DJK, respectively); PJK being the most frequent problem (Figures 6 and 7). Patients with PWS characteristically have a "head forward" posture with their C7 vertebral plumb line falling much farther anterior to the sacrum than would be seen in a typically developed person [11,13]. This occurs by a combination of flattened cervical lordosis and/or thoracic hyperkyphosis. In fact, most PWS curves are kyphoscoliotic rather than the lordoscoloisis seen in idiopathic scoliosis cases. If the sagittal alignment is "anatomically" corrected surgically, patients often will compensate by increasing kyphosis, leading to hypolordosis or even kyphosis in the cervical spine, PJK and DJK [9,41]. In addition, up to 62% of patients with PWS have low bone mineral density and other musculoskeletal manifestations [11,42–46]. The combination of the PJK/DJK and bone weakness leads to a rate of hardware pull out/failure/rod fracture between 17% and 31% [9,40,41,47,48]. The consequences can be catastrophic [49].

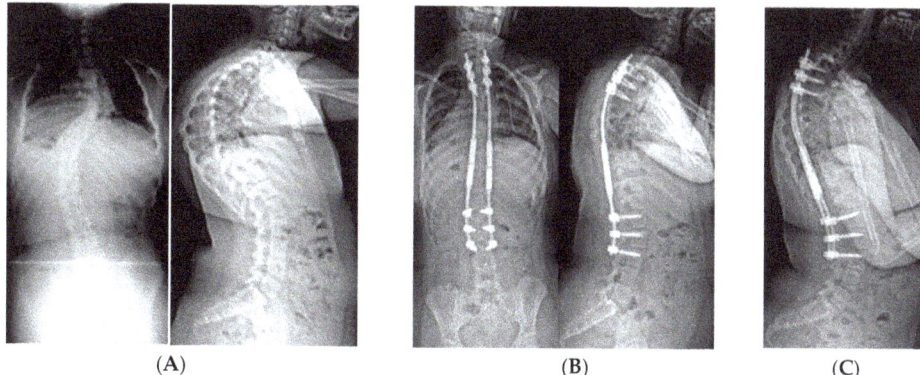

(A) **(B)** **(C)**

Figure 6. (**A**) 10-year-old female with PWS UPD type with 85° kyphosis, a 66° right thoracic and 61° left thoracolumbar curve. (**B**) Expandable, magnetically actuated rods are implanted from T2–L3, reducing her scoliotic curves to 25° or less, and her kyphosis to 48°. (**C**) 6 months post-operatively with developing proximal junctional kyphosis. Kyphosis now measures 81°.

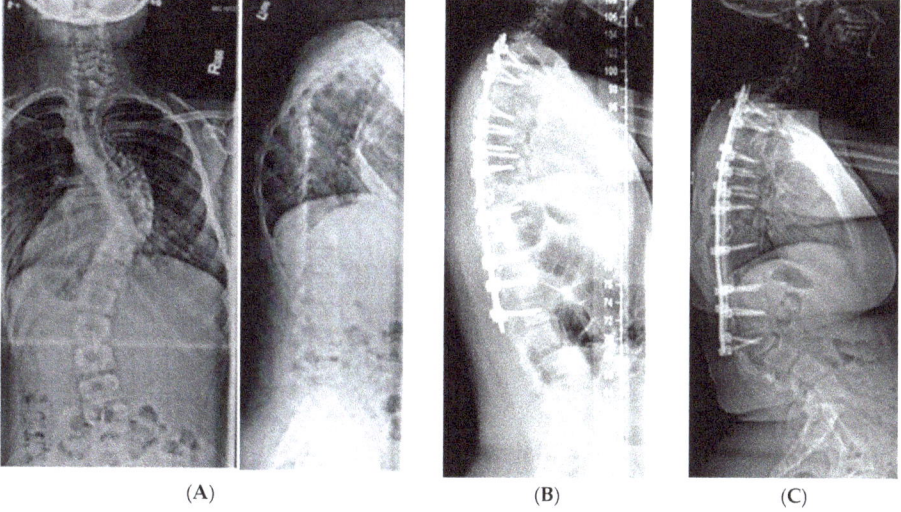

(A) **(B)** **(C)**

Figure 7. (**A**) 11-year-old female with PWS UPD type with 70° scoliosis, and 60° kyphosis. (**B**) Same patient at 12 years of age, after T2–L2 posterior spinal fusion. Overall kyphosis measures 50°. (**C**) Same patient at 3 years post-operatively with 60° distal junctional kyphosis.

In surgical planning, positioning and density of anchoring hardware (primarily pedicle screws) should be chosen with osteoporosis/osteopenia in mind. Thoracic kyphosis should be addressed judiciously – patients with kyphosis or kyphoscoliosis should not have their sagittal profile corrected to values appropriate for typical patients. In most kyphotic deformities, we strive for a resulting kyphosis of 50° to 60°, depending on the initial measurement and sagittal balance. We will select T3 or lower as our upper instrumented vertebra, to allow enough room for the patient to adjust their kyphosis across the cervical-thoracic junction.

Patients with PWS exhibit "skin picking", which can lead to invasion or injury of their incisions. Combined with potential poor quality of the soft tissues, the rate of wound dehiscence and related deep infections are reported between 19% and 38% of cases [40,41,48]. To avoid these issues, a negative pressure wound therapy bandage is placed over the incision for the first five days, both to help with any seepage and to act as an "early warning" system, as the pump will alarm if the patient breaks the pressure seal by scratching their incision. Afterwards, they are outfitted with a light brace to be worn at all times except bathing, primarily to protect the incision for 2–3 months.

Patients with PWS often have gastrointestinal problems and are nearly universally constipated. They also experience a protracted ileus post-operatively which can substantially delay recovery. Their interest in food reemerges soon after waking from surgery. If not monitored, they can easily overeat, hyperextending their stomach, and developing gastroparesis and stomach rupture, a life-threatening complication of PWS. Our protocol is for a slow bowel clean out with stool softeners and laxatives for one to two weeks prior to surgery. Post-operatively, limited clear fluids (2-4 ounces per 4 hours) are allowed until stomach sounds return. Erythromycin is used to increase gastric motility while methylnaltrexone blunts the effect of opioids on the gastrointestinal system and lactulose stimulates bowel movements. The diet is advanced slowly, relative to bowel sounds, and abdominal radiographs are obtained usually daily to monitor for signs of gastric stasis until regular bowel movements are established.

Intravenous access can be difficult in children with PWS. Since there may be a prolonged need for intravenous hydration, a central venous line is placed in the operating room, to prevent having to search for venous access in the post-operative period.

As noted in the introduction, children with PWS often have sleep apnea or other respiratory conditions; sleep apnea occurs in 80% of children, and narcolepsy in 36% [16]. Pre-operatively, a sleep study is needed along with a pulmonology evaluation to assess for the possible post-operative needs such as the use of BiPAP or CPAP. Occasionally, if they are slow to awake after surgery, they will remain intubated until they demonstrate a strong respiratory response.

2.1.5.2. Non-Fusion Spinal Instrumentation with Expandable Implants

Young children with severe infantile curves may need stabilization of the spine to allow for more symmetric chest development with growth. Typically, these are child too old for spinal casting but have substantial remaining growth with curves >50° and minimal flexibility/improvement in brace. If they cannot be maintained in brace, then an expandable implant serves to internally splint the spine. Early implant versions required manual distraction, typically performed every six months as an open procedure in the operating room (Figure 8). This strategy worked well for controlling the curve and maintaining spine growth, but with the potential complications related to surgical procedures. In 2014, expandable spinal rods became available that were magnetically actuated through the skin. The rods are lengthened every three months, using an external spinning magnet, which causes the magnet within the rod to rotate thereby lengthening the rod (Figure 4). Oore et al found that the average initial curve was reduced from 76° to 42° at time of implant surgery with no change in curve size over the subsequent two years of rod elongation [40].

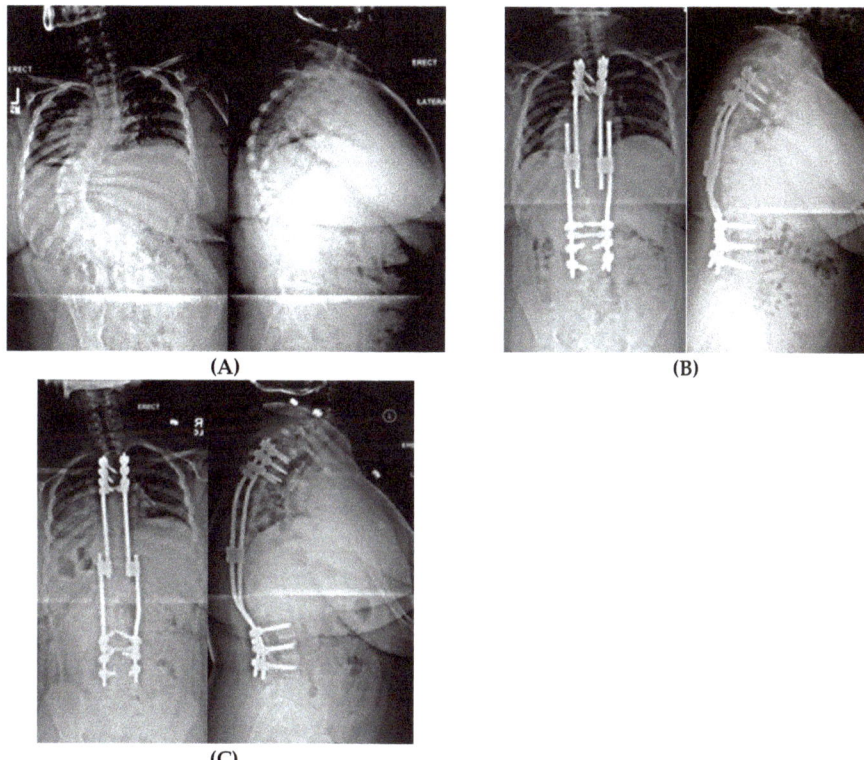

Figure 8. (A) AP and lateral radiographs of a 10-year-old female with PWS deletion type with 103° curve. **(B)** AP and lateral radiographs 1 month later, after placement of non-fusion spinal instrumentation. Curve is 57°. **(C)** 18 months later, after 50mm of lengthening, curve is 25°.

Expandable implants, as a technique, have a life span of approximately five years, after which the ongoing process of spontaneous fusion along the section of the instrumented spine leads to stiffness and an inability to lengthen further [50,51]. Therefore, the goal is to manage the curve non-operatively until the child is 5–8 years of age, in order to "grow" the spine until at least 10 years of age. Unfortunately, the magnetically actuated rods only generate 42 pounds of axial force and may fail to generate enough force to elongate after several lengthening procedures. There are also issues related to titanium wear debris noted at the time of device removal [52]. Generally, these devices have made important improvements in the treatment of severe curves seen in young children with PWS. Usually, the construct is anchored with two vertebral levels above and below, but when there is any question of bone strength, three levels are fixated.

2.1.5.3. Spinal Fusion

Spinal curves over 50° have a high propensity towards progression, even in skeletally mature patients; curves over 40° need to be closely monitored for progression. Timing of surgery can be tricky, adolescents with PWS experience delayed puberty, and females may not reach menarche or begin menses until in their 20s. PWS specific growth charts do indicate that boys and girls reach skeletal maturity essentially at the same age as their typically developing peers [53]. It is, therefore, preferable to delay spinal fusion until or after 12 years of age for females and 14 years for males. In general, teenagers with PWS have some concept of body image, but seem less perturbed by residual shoulder asymmetry or waist clefts. Achieving appropriate sagittal alignment is much more important in avoiding late deformity and assuring patient satisfaction. We try to limit our upper end vertebra to T3 or lower, even if still within the region of kyphosis; the rods are bent to accentuate kyphosis. Distally, the end vertebra is chosen much as it is for idiopathic scoliosis cases with a predisposition to fuse a level longer rather than shorter to prevent adding-on of the curve. The rods are bent to match or accentuate the pre-operative lumbar lordosis. Due to concerns of bone strength, nearly all included vertebrae are instrumented with pedicle screws bilaterally for better fixation (Figure 9).

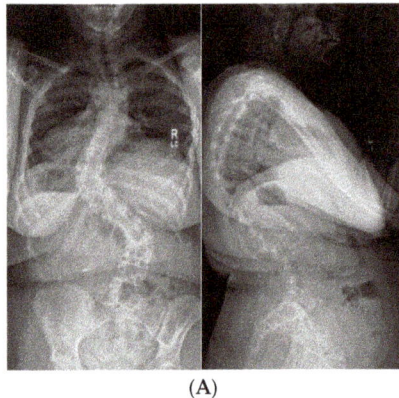 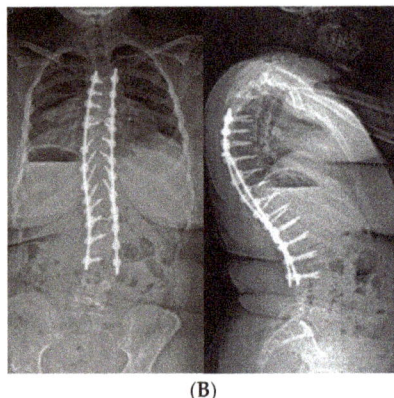

(A)   (B)

Figure 9. (**A**) 15-year-old female with PWS UPD type with 67° left thoracic and 60° right lumbar curve. She had thoracic kyphosis of 79° and lumbar lordosis of 84°. (**B**) Same patient at 4 years after T4–L3 posterior spinal fusion. The thoracic curve measures 12°, the lumbar 25° with 75° kyphosis.

3. Discussion

Growth hormone (GH) therapy was approved by the FDA in 2000 for treating genetically confirmed individuals with PWS with short stature. Growth hormone acts as a ligand for the growth hormone receptor (GHR). Approximately 50% of Caucasians with or without PWS and regardless of PWS genetic subtype have a *GHR* gene (exon-3 deletion) polymorphism which is associated with an increased response to growth hormone therapy with growth acceleration [54–56]. A significant increase in growth rate (1.7 times) is observed in both PWS and the general population when the *GHR* gene polymorphism is present. In a case-controlled study of 73 patients with genetically confirmed PWS matched for levels of scoliosis (moderate or severe) and those without scoliosis, no differences were found between the two groups in terms of gender, PWS genetic subtype or GHR gene exon-3 deletion distributions [56]. Therefore, the growth rate stimulation by the *GHR* gene polymorphism did not appear to influence the development of spine deformities in PWS.

When treated with GH, individuals with PWS respond favorably in stature, lean body mass and physical activity [1,4]. A frequent concern of parents of patients with scoliosis is whether the growth hormone could be contributing to their child's curve progression, and therefore whether the hormone supplementation should be stopped. This concern stems from similar apprehension related to the treatment of Turner syndrome, where a higher prevalence of scoliosis in patients treated with GH was suggested in some studies, but refuted by others [57,58]. Studies of children with PWS have been less equivocal. For example, de Lind van Wijngaarden et al. conducted a prospective randomized, controlled GH study of infants, prepubertal and pubertal children [59]. They found a similar onset and progression of scoliosis between those treated with GH and those not, across all three age groups. Nakamura et al. had similar findings in a retrospective study, but also noted that the GH-treated patients had improved bone mineral density as measured by dual-energy x-ray absorptiometry [60]. Other studies of children with PWS and scoliosis have noted significant impacts of GH on metabolism, lean body mass, brain development and energy level, supporting their recommendations to not discontinue treatment [4,42,60]. Data analysis of the 2007 PWSA (USA) survey found that for every month delay in beginning GH treatment, the risk of needing scoliosis surgery increased by 0.7%. Our protocol is to continue GH treatment in all cases, unless contraindicated by the patient's endocrinologist. At the time of surgery, we will only skip the dose the day of the procedure, resuming on the first post-operative day.

Other than the similarity of age of onset of the adolescent form and the overall coronal plane curve appearance, there are a number of important differences between idiopathic scoliosis and the PWS type. The most obvious is that idiopathic deformity is a lordoscoliosis of the thoracic region, while in PWS most curves are kyphoscoliotic. The exaggerated kyphosis seems to be requisite for proper overall center of balance, as correcting it surgically leads to the greatest post-surgical complications – proximal and distal junction kyphosis. Studies are needed of skeletally mature individuals with PWS, without scoliosis, to determine their natural sagittal posture, which can then inform the goals of the post-surgical alignment. Although neurological and genetic factors do play a role in scoliosis [28], no genes as yet are identified or associated with scoliosis in children with PWS, but future research is needed. For example, expression patterns for both coding and non-coding genes from tissue (e.g., skeletal muscle, bone, connective tissue) and related gene variants may prove as useful markers for development of scoliosis at a young age requiring careful surveillance.

Experience has taught us that aggressive non-surgical treatment can be successful in postponing or avoiding surgery, and even reducing the actual curve. One-third of the patients that underwent spine casting for their infantile curves had their curve decreased to the point that they could be transitioned to a brace for a year, then weaned from the brace. This is a smaller proportion of "cured" patients compared to Mehta's series (69%) [38], although the average initial curve of her 136 patients was 38°, compared to 55° for our cohort. Likewise, in brace treatment, at least two older patients had significantly improved curves with separate nighttime Providence and daytime TLSO braces (Figure 5). This most likely indicated a gradual improvement of the patients' hypotonia while maintaining their spine flexibility and applying corrective external posturing. The strengthening spinal muscles over time were able to preserve the alignment. Naturally, all of these patients need to be carefully followed even after growth cessation to verify no deterioration over time.

It cannot be overemphasized that patients with PWS treated for scoliosis should have their underlying condition understood, particularly when planning surgery. By taking into account such characteristics as hyperphagia, skin picking, the occasional violent outbursts, and planning accordingly, the patient, family and hospital staff can be kept safe during the inpatient stay. Moreover, slow advancement of diet with diligent attention to gastrointestinal function will actually decrease the length of hospital stay; if the diet is advanced too quickly, the subsequent bloating and ileus resumption may take days to resolve.

Funding: This research received no external funding.

Acknowledgments: We thank Grace Graham for expert preparation of manuscript and acknowledge the National Institute of Child Health and Human Development grant number HD02528.

Conflicts of Interest: The authors declare no conflict of interest.

References

1. Butler, M.G.; Hanchett, J.M.; Thompson, T. Clinical findings and natural history of Prader-Willi syndrome. In *Management of Prader-Willi Syndrome*, 3rd ed.; Butler, M.G., Lee, P.D.K., Whitman, Y.W., Eds.; Springer: New York, NY, USA, 2006; pp. 3–48.
2. Butler, M.G.; Thompson, T. Prader-Willi syndrome: Clinical and genetic findings. *Endocrinologist* **2000**, *10*, 3S–16S. [CrossRef]
3. Butler, M.G. Prader-Willi Syndrome: Current understanding of cause and diagnosis. *Am. J. Med. Genet.* **1990**, *35*, 319–332. [CrossRef]

4. Cassidy, S.B.; Schwartz, S.; Miller, J.L.; Driscoll, D.J. Prader-Willi syndrome. *Genet. Med.* **2012**, *14*, 10–26. [CrossRef]

5. Butler, M.G.; Hartin, S.N.; Hossain, W.A.; Manzardo, A.M.; Kimonis, V.; Dykens, E.; Gold, J.A.; Kim, S.J.; Weisensel, N.; Tamura, R.; et al. Molecular genetic classification in Prader-Willi syndrome: A multisite cohort study. *J. Med. Genet.* **2019**, *56*, 149–153. [CrossRef]

6. Butler, M.G.; Bittel, D.C.; Kibiryeva, N.; Talebizadeh, Z.; Thompson, T. Behavioral differences among subjects with Prader-Willi syndrome and type I or type II deletion and maternal disomy. *Pediatrics* **2004**, *113*, 565–573. [CrossRef]

7. Butler, M.G.; Matthews, N.A.; Patel, N.; Surampalli, A.; Gold, J.A.; Khare, M.; Thompson, T.; Cassidy, S.B.; Kimonis, V.E. Impact of genetic subtypes of Prader-Willi syndrome with growth hormone therapy on intelligence and body mass index. *Am. J. Med. Genet. A* **2019**, *179*, 1826–1835. [CrossRef]

8. de Lind van Wijngaarden, R.F.; de Klerk, L.W.; Festen, D.A.; Hokken-Koelega, A.C. Scoliosis in Prader-Willi syndrome: Prevalence, effects of age, gender, body mass index, lean body mass and genotype. *Arch. Dis. Child.* **2008**, *93*, 1012–1016. [CrossRef]

9. Greggi, T.; Martikos, K.; Lolli, F.; Bakaloudis, G.; Di Silvestre, M.; Cioni, A.; Brodano, G.B.; Giacomini, S. Treatment of scoliosis in patients affected with Prader-Willi syndrome using various techniques. *Scoliosis* **2010**, *5*, 11. [CrossRef]

10. Holm, V.A.; Laurnen, E.L. Prader-Willi syndrome and scoliosis. *Dev. Med. Child. Neurol.* **1981**, *23*, 192–201. [CrossRef]

11. Kroonen, L.T.; Herman, M.; Pizzutillo, P.D.; Macewen, G.D. Prader-Willi syndrome: Clinical concerns for the orthopaedic surgeon. *J. Pediatr. Orthop.* **2006**, *26*, 673–679. [CrossRef]

12. Nagai, T.; Obata, K.; Ogata, T.; Murakami, N.; Katada, Y.; Yoshino, A.; Sakazume, S.; Tomita, Y.; Sakuta, R.; Niikawa, N. Growth hormone therapy and scoliosis in patients with Prader-Willi syndrome. *Am. J. Med. Genet. A* **2006**, *140*, 1623–1627. [CrossRef] [PubMed]

13. Nakamura, Y.; Murakami, N.; Iida, T.; Ozeki, S.; Asano, S.; Nohara, Y.; Nagai, T. The characteristics of scoliosis in Prader-Willi syndrome (PWS): Analysis of 58 scoliosis patients with PWS. *J. Orthop. Sci.* **2015**, *20*, 17–22. [CrossRef] [PubMed]

14. Odent, T.; Accadbled, F.; Koureas, G.; Cournot, M.; Moine, A.; Diene, G.; Molinas, C.; Pinto, G.; Tauber, M.; Gomes, B.; et al. Scoliosis in patients with Prader-Willi syndrome. *Pediatrics* **2008**, *122*, e499–e503. [CrossRef] [PubMed]

15. Ghergan, A.; Coupaye, M.; Leu-Semenescu, S.; Attali, V.; Oppert, J.M.; Arnulf, I.; Poitou, C.; Redolfi, S. Prevalence and phenotype of sleep disorders in 60 adults with Prader-Willi syndrome. *Sleep* **2017**, *40*. [CrossRef]

16. Sedky, K.; Bennett, D.S.; Pumariega, A. Prader-Willi syndrome and obstructive sleep apnea: Co-occurrence in the pediatric population. *J. Clin. Sleep Med.* **2014**, *10*, 403–409. [CrossRef]

17. Tan, H.L.; Urquhart, D.S. Respiratory complications in children with Prader Willi syndrome. *Paediatr. Respir. Rev.* **2017**, *22*, 52–59. [CrossRef]

18. Gurd, A.R.; Thompson, T.R. Scoliosis in Prader-Willi syndrome. *J. Pediatr. Orthop.* **1981**, *1*, 317–320. [CrossRef]

19. Hakonarson, H.; Moskovitz, J.; Daigle, K.L.; Cassidy, S.B.; Cloutier, M.M. Pulmonary function abnormalities in Prader-Willi syndrome. *J. Pediatr.* **1995**, *126*, 565–570. [CrossRef]

20. Pacoricona Alfaro, D.L.; Lemoine, P.; Ehlinger, V.; Molinas, C.; Diene, G.; Valette, M.; Pinto, G.; Coupaye, M.; Poitou-Bernert, C.; Thuilleaux, D.; et al. Causes of death in Prader-Willi syndrome: Lessons from 11 years' experience of a national reference center. *Orphanet J. Rare Dis.* **2019**, *14*, 238. [CrossRef]

21. Proffitt, J.; Osann, K.; McManus, B.; Kimonis, V.E.; Heinemann, J.; Butler, M.G.; Stevenson, D.A.; Gold, J.A. Contributing factors of mortality in Prader-Willi syndrome. *Am. J. Med. Genet. A* **2019**, *179*, 196–205. [CrossRef]

22. Rees, D.; Jones, M.W.; Owen, R.; Dorgan, J.C. Scoliosis surgery in the Prader-Willi syndrome. *J. Bone Jt. Surg. Br.* **1989**, *71*, 685–688. [CrossRef]

23. Tokutomi, T.; Chida, A.; Asano, Y.; Ishiwata, T.; Koike, Y.; Motegi, A.; Asazuma, T.; Nonoyama, S. A non-obese boy with Prader-Willi syndrome shows cardiopulmonary impairment due to severe kyphoscoliosis. *Am. J. Med. Genet. A* **2006**, *140*, 1978–1980. [CrossRef] [PubMed]

24. Butler, M.G.; Manzardo, A.M.; Heinemann, J.; Loker, C.; Loker, J. Causes of death in Prader-Willi syndrome: Prader-Willi syndrome association (USA) 40-year mortality survey. *Genet. Med.* **2017**, *19*, 635–642. [CrossRef] [PubMed]

25. Grugni, G.; Crino, A.; Bosio, L.; Corrias, A.; Cuttini, M.; De Toni, T.; Di Battista, E.; Franzese, A.; Gargantini, L.; Greggio, N.; et al. The italian national survey for Prader-Willi syndrome: An epidemiologic study. *Am. J. Med. Genet. A* **2008**, *146A*, 861–872. [CrossRef] [PubMed]

26. Lionti, T.; Reid, S.M.; Rowell, M.M. Prader-Willi syndrome in victoria: Mortality and causes of death. *J. Paediatr. Child. Health* **2012**, *48*, 506–511. [CrossRef]

27. Laurance, B.M.; Brito, A.; Wilkinson, J. Prader-Willi syndrome after age 15 years. *Arch. Dis. Child.* **1981**, *56*, 181–186. [CrossRef]

28. Wajchenberg, M.; Astur, N.; Kanas, M.; Martins, D.E. Adolescent idiopathic scoliosis: Current concepts on neurological and muscular etiologies. *Scoliosis Spinal Disord.* **2016**, *11*, 4. [CrossRef]

29. Fendri, K.; Patten, S.A.; Kaufman, G.N.; Zaouter, C.; Parent, S.; Grimard, G.; Edery, P.; Moldovan, F. Microarray expression profiling identifies genes with altered expression in adolescent idiopathic scoliosis. *Eur. Spine J.* **2013**, *22*, 1300–1311. [CrossRef]

30. Baschal, E.E.; Wethey, C.I.; Swindle, K.; Baschal, R.M.; Gowan, K.; Tang, N.L.S.; Avarado, D.M.; Haller, G.E.; Dobbs, M.B.; Taylor, M.R.G.; et al. Exome sequencing identifies rare *HSPG2* variant associated with familial idiopathic scoliosis. *G3 (Bethesda)* **2014**, *5*, 167–174. [CrossRef]

31. Baschal, E.E.; Swindle, K.; Justice, C.J.; Baschal, R.M.; Perera, A.; Wethey, C.I.; Poole, A.; Pourquie, O.; Tassy, O.; Miller, N.H. Sequencing of the *TBX6* gene in families with familial idiopathic scoliosis. *Spine Deform.* **2015**, *3*, 288–296. [CrossRef] [PubMed]

32. Grauers, A.; Wang, J.; Einarsdottir, E.; Simony, A.; Danielsson, A.; Åkesson, K.; Ohlin, A.; Halldin, K.; Grabowski, P.; Tenne, M.; et al. Candidate gene analysis and exome sequencing confirm *LBX1* as a susceptibility gene for idiopathic scoliosis. *Spine J.* **2015**, *15*, 2239–2246. [CrossRef] [PubMed]

33. Ogura, Y.; Kou, I.; Miura, S.; Takahashi, A.; Xu, L.; Takeda, K.; Takahashi, Y.; Kono, K.; Kawakami, N.; Uno, K.; et al. A functional SNP in *BNC2* is associated with adolescent idiopathic scoliosis. *Am. J. Hum. Genet.* **2015**, *97*, 337–342. [CrossRef] [PubMed]

34. Gao, W.; Chen, C.; Zhou, T.; Yang, S.; Gao, B.; Zhou, H.; Lian, C.; Wu, Z.; Qiu, X.; Yang, X.; et al. Rare coding variants in *MAPK7* predispose to adolescent idiopathic scoliosis. *Hum. Mutat.* **2017**, *38*, 1500–1510. [CrossRef] [PubMed]

35. Butler, M.G. Magnesium supplement and the 15q11.2 BP1-BP2 microdeletion (Burnside-Butler) syndrome: A potential treatment? *Int. J. Mol. Sci.* **2019**, *20*, 2914. [CrossRef] [PubMed]

36. Cassidy, S.B.; Driscoll, D.J. Prader-Willi syndrome. *Eur. J. Hum. Genet.* **2009**, *17*, 3–13. [CrossRef] [PubMed]

37. Soriano, R.M.; Weisz, I.; Houghton, G.R. Scoliosis in the Prader-Willi syndrome. *Spine (Phila PA 1976)* **1988**, *13*, 209–211. [CrossRef] [PubMed]

38. Mehta, M.H. Growth as a corrective force in the early treatment of progressive infantile scoliosis. *J. Bone Joint Surg. Br.* **2005**, *87*, 1237–1247. [CrossRef]

39. Sanders, J.O.; D'Astous, J.; Fitzgerald, M.; Khoury, J.G.; Kishan, S.; Sturm, P.F. Derotational casting for progressive infantile scoliosis. *Pediatr. Orthop.* **2009**, *29*, 581–587. [CrossRef]

40. Oore, J.; Connell, B.; Yaszay, B.; Samdani, A.; Hilaire, T.S.; Flynn, T.; El-Hawary, R.; Children's Spine Study, G.; Growing Spine Study, G. Growth friendly surgery and serial cast correction in the treatment of early-onset scoliosis for patients with Prader-Willi syndrome. *J. Pediatr. Orthop.* **2019**, *39*, e597–e601. [CrossRef]

41. Accadbled, F.; Odent, T.; Moine, A.; Chau, E.; Glorion, C.; Diene, G.; de Gauzy, J.S. Complications of scoliosis surgery in Prader-Willi syndrome. *Spine (Phila PA 1976)* **2008**, *33*, 394–401. [CrossRef]

42. Nakamura, Y.; Nagai, T.; Iida, T.; Ozeki, S.; Nohara, Y. Growth hormone supplement treatment reduces the surgical risk for Prader-Willi syndrome patients. *Eur. Spine J.* **2012**, *21* (Suppl. 4), S483–S491. [CrossRef] [PubMed]

43. Shim, J.S.; Lee, S.H.; Seo, S.W.; Koo, K.H.; Jin, D.K. The musculoskeletal manifestations of Prader-Willi syndrome. *J. Pediatr. Orthop.* **2010**, *30*, 390–395. [CrossRef] [PubMed]

44. Sinnema, M.; Maaskant, M.A.; van Schrojenstein Lantman-de Valk, H.M.; van Nieuwpoort, I.C.; Drent, M.L.; Curfs, L.M.; Schrander-Stumpel, C.T. Physical health problems in adults with Prader-Willi syndrome. *Am. J. Med. Genet. A* **2011**, *155A*, 2112–2124. [CrossRef] [PubMed]

45. West, L.A.; Ballock, R.T. High incidence of hip dysplasia but not slipped capital femoral epiphysis in patients with Prader-Willi syndrome. *J. Pediatr. Orthop.* **2004**, *24*, 565–567. [CrossRef] [PubMed]

46. Brunetti, G.; Grugni, G.; Piacente, L.; Delvecchio, M.; Ventura, A.; Giordano, P.; Grano, M.; D'Amato, G.; Laforgia, D.; Crino, A.; et al. Analysis of circulating mediators of bone remodeling in Prader-Willi syndrome. *Calcif. Tissue Int.* **2018**, *102*, 635–643. [CrossRef] [PubMed]

47. Chung, A.S.; Renfree, S.; Lockwood, D.B.; Karlen, J.; Belthur, M. Syndromic scoliosis: National trends in surgical management and inpatient hospital outcomes: A 12-year analysis. *Spine (Phila PA 1976)* **2019**, *44*, 1564–1570. [CrossRef] [PubMed]

48. Levy, B.J.; Schulz, J.F.; Fornari, E.D.; Wollowick, A.L. Complications associated with surgical repair of syndromic scoliosis. *Scoliosis* **2015**, *10*, 14. [CrossRef]

49. de Baat, P.; van Tankeren, E.; de Lind van Wijngaarden, R.F.; de Klerk, L.W. Sudden proximal spinal dislocation with complete spinal cord injury 1 week after spinal fusion in a child with Prader-Willi syndrome: A case report. *Spine (Phila PA 1976)* **2011**, *36*, E1765–E1768. [CrossRef]

50. Cahill, P.J.; Marvil, S.; Cuddihy, L.; Schutt, C.; Idema, J.; Clements, D.H.; Antonacci, M.D.; Asghar, J.; Samdani, A.F.; Betz, R.R. Autofusion in the immature spine treated with growing rods. *Spine (Phila PA 1976)* **2010**, *35*, E1199–E1203. [CrossRef]

51. Sankar, W.N.; Skaggs, D.L.; Yazici, M.; Johnston, C.E., 2nd; Shah, S.A.; Javidan, P.; Kadakia, R.V.; Day, T.F.; Akbarnia, B.A. Lengthening of dual growing rods and the law of diminishing returns. *Spine (Phila PA 1976)* **2011**, *36*, 806–809. [CrossRef]

52. Joyce, T.J.; Smith, S.L.; Rushton, P.R.P.; Bowey, A.J.; Gibson, M.J. Analysis of explanted magnetically controlled growing rods from seven UK spinal centers. *Spine (Phila PA 1976)* **2018**, *43*, E16–E22. [CrossRef] [PubMed]

53. Butler, M.G.; Lee, J.; Cox, D.M.; Manzardo, A.M.; Gold, J.A.; Miller, J.L.; Roof, E.; Dykens, E.; Kimonis, V.; Driscoll, D.J. Growth charts for Prader-Willi syndrome during growth hormone treatment. *Clin. Pediatr. (Phila)* **2016**, *55*, 957–974. [CrossRef] [PubMed]

54. Dos Santos, C.; Essioux, L.; Teinturier, C.; Tauber, M.; Goffin, V.; Bougneres, P. A common polymorphism of the growth hormone receptor is associated with increased responsiveness to growth hormone. *Nat. Genet.* **2004**, *36*, 720–724. [CrossRef] [PubMed]

55. Butler, M.G.; Roberts, J.; Hayes, J.; Tan, X.; Manzardo, A.M. Growth hormone receptor (GHR) gene polymorphism and Prader-Willi syndrome. *Am. J. Med. Genet. A* **2013**, *161A*, 1647–1653. [CrossRef] [PubMed]

56. Butler, M.G.; Hossain, W.; Hassan, M.; Manzardo, A.M. Growth hormone receptor (GHR) gene polymorphism and scoliosis in Prader-Willi syndrome. *Growth Horm. IGF Res.* **2018**, *39*, 29–33. [CrossRef] [PubMed]

57. Cowell, C.T.; Dietsch, S. Adverse events during growth hormone therapy. *J. Pediatr. Endocrinol. Metab.* **1995**, *8*, 243–252. [CrossRef]

58. Kim, J.Y.; Rosenfeld, S.R.; Keyak, J.H. Increased prevalence of scoliosis in Turner syndrome. *J. Pediatr. Orthop.* **2001**, *21*, 765–766. [CrossRef]

59. de Lind van Wijngaarden, R.F.; de Klerk, L.W.; Festen, D.A.; Duivenvoorden, H.J.; Otten, B.J.; Hokken-Koelega, A.C. Randomized controlled trial to investigate the effects of growth hormone treatment on scoliosis in children with Prader-Willi syndrome. *J. Clin. Endocrinol. Metab.* **2009**, *94*, 1274–1280. [CrossRef]

60. Nakamura, Y.; Murakami, N.; Iida, T.; Asano, S.; Ozeki, S.; Nagai, T. Growth hormone treatment for osteoporosis in patients with scoliosis of Prader-Willi syndrome. *J. Orthop. Sci.* **2014**, *19*, 877–882. [CrossRef]

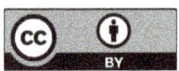

© 2020 by the authors. Licensee MDPI, Basel, Switzerland. This article is an open access article distributed under the terms and conditions of the Creative Commons Attribution (CC BY) license (http://creativecommons.org/licenses/by/4.0/).

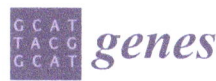

Review

The Potential Role of Activating the ATP-Sensitive Potassium Channel in the Treatment of Hyperphagic Obesity

Neil Cowen * and Anish Bhatnagar

Soleno Therapeutics, Redwood City, CA 94065, USA; anish@soleno.life
* Correspondence: neil@soleno.life

Received: 23 March 2020; Accepted: 16 April 2020; Published: 21 April 2020

Abstract: To evaluate the potential role of ATP-sensitive potassium (K_{ATP}) channel activation in the treatment of hyperphagic obesity, a PubMed search was conducted focused on the expression of genes encoding the K_{ATP} channel, the response to activating the K_{ATP} channel in tissues regulating appetite and the establishment and maintenance of obesity, the evaluation of K_{ATP} activators in obese hyperphagic animal models, and clinical studies on syndromic obesity. K_{ATP} channel activation is mechanistically involved in the regulation of appetite in the arcuate nucleus; the regulation of hyperinsulinemia, glycemic control, appetite and satiety in the dorsal motor nucleus of vagus; insulin secretion by β-cells; and the synthesis and β-oxidation of fatty acids in adipocytes. K_{ATP} channel activators have been evaluated in hyperphagic obese animal models and were shown to reduce hyperphagia, induce fat loss and weight loss in older animals, reduce the accumulation of excess body fat in growing animals, reduce circulating and hepatic lipids, and improve glycemic control. Recent experience with a K_{ATP} channel activator in Prader–Willi syndrome is consistent with the therapeutic responses observed in animal models. K_{ATP} channel activation, given the breadth of impact and animal model and clinical results, is a viable target in hyperphagic obesity.

Keywords: K_{ATP} channel activation; hyperphagic obesity; animal models; Prader–Willi syndrome

1. Introduction

Hyperphagic obesity is characterized by a markedly increased appetite and aggressive food-seeking behavior, often associated with a lack of satiety, and the accumulation of excess body fat, frequently resulting in morbid obesity and obesity-associated comorbidities. The underlying basis for hyperphagic obesity is frequently genetic, involving biallelic-inactivating mutations in known genes, as is the case of leptin receptor deficiency [1], or the deletion or lack of expression of a chromosomal segment containing a number of genes, which is characteristic of Prader–Willi syndrome [2]. Alternatively, hyperphagic obesity may follow from damage to the hypothalamus, resulting in hypothalamic obesity [3]. Hyperphagic obesity is frequently associated with both elevated morbidity and mortality and reduced quality of life [2,3]. There are very few approved treatments for any form of hyperphagic obesity and, therefore, there is a need to identify effective therapeutic targets to address the unmet medical need in these conditions. This review focuses on a single potential therapeutic target, the ATP-sensitive potassium (K_{ATP}) channel, which may have utility in various forms of hyperphagic obesity.

2. Methods

A PubMed search was conducted focused on the expression of genes encoding the K_{ATP} channel in tissues involved in the regulation of appetite and satiety, and in tissues involved in the establishment and persistence of the obese state, the role of activating the K_{ATP} channel in those tissues, studies involving pharmacological activators of the channel in obese hyperphagic animal models, and clinical studies of

K_{ATP} channel activators in obese hyperphagic syndromes. Search terms used included K_{ATP}, SUR1, SUR2b, Kir6.1, Kir6.2, ABCC8, ABCC9, KCNJ8, KCNJ11, agonist, hypothalamus, motor neuron of vagus, adipocyte, β-cell, hyperphagia, appetite, neuropeptide, obesity, obese, animal model, leptin, insulin, α-MSH, insulin-resistance, and hyperinsulinemia. Terms were combined to generate searches which identified tissues in which the genes encoding the K_{ATP} channel might be expressed that have a known role in appetite and obesity, hormones with known roles in appetite and the K_{ATP} channel, and obese or hyperphagic obese animal models in which a K_{ATP} channel agonist might have been evaluated. Prior to conducting the searches, the authors already possessed extensive knowledge of the K_{ATP} channel and its role in the regulation of appetite, having studied the channel for more than 15 years. The searches were conducted to supplement that understanding, rather than as the sole source of information summarized in this publication.

3. Results

3.1. The Structure of and Genes Encoding the K_{ATP} Channel

The K_{ATP} channel is an octomeric structure consisting of four copies of the sulfonylurea receptor (SURx) and four copies of an inwardly rectifying potassium channel (Kir6.x) [4]. The isotype of the channel is a function of the specific forms of each of the two components that are expressed in the tissue at any developmental stage. SUR1 is encoded by ABCC8; SUR2A and SUR2B are splice variants of the same gene product which is encoded by ABCC9 [4]. Kir6.2 is encoded by KCNJ11, while Kir6.1 is encoded by KCNJ8 [4]. ABCC8 and KCNJ11 both reside on chromosome 11p15.1, while ABCC9 and KCNJ8 both reside on chromosome 12p12.1 [4]. SUR1-containing forms of the channel are typically found in pancreatic β-cells, certain CNS cell types [5], adipocytes [6] and certain skeletal muscle cells but exist in other tissues as well. SUR2B-containing forms of the channel are typically found in cardiovascular smooth muscle [4] and certain skeletal muscle cells, whereas SUR2A-containing forms of the channel are found almost exclusively in cardiac tissues [4]. The channel resides in the cell membrane, and a unique isotype resides in the mitochondrial inner membrane [4].

3.2. The Role of the K_{ATP} Channel in the Central Regulation of Appetite by the Arcuate Nucleus

In mature animals or humans, the arcuate nucleus of the hypothalamus (ARC) integrates peripheral circulating hormonal signals, including leptin, insulin and ghrelin, which communicate environmental nutrient availability, into the homeostatic regulation of appetite and energy expenditure. The ARC, in the mature animal, includes two populations of neurons that respond to these hormonal signals and project into other appetite-regulatory regions. One population of neurons (NAG neurons) co-expresses neuropeptide Y (NPY), the most potent endogenous appetite-stimulatory neuropeptide, agouti-related protein (AgRP), an antagonist/inverse agonist of melanocortin 4 receptors (MC4R) [7], and γ-aminobutyric acid (GABA). NAG neurons are orexigenic and sufficient to regulate food intake [5]. A separate population of ARC neurons (POMC neurons) expresses the proopiomelanocortin (POMC) peptide and are anorexigenic. Within the ARC, POMC neurons are inhibited by NAG neurons [8], mediated primarily by GABA. Additionally, NPY has been shown to downregulate prohormone convertase 2 [9], which is a key enzyme involved in the conversion of POMC to α-melanocyte-stimulating hormone (α-MSH) which, through its interaction with MC4R, mediates the anorexigenic effects of POMC neurons. Thus, NAG neurons serve a modulatory function, through direct inhibition of POMC neurons, reduced conversion of POMC to α-MSH, and antagonism of MC4R, thereby counter-regulating the melanocortin pathway to reduce satiety and promote food intake. During early postnatal development, projections from these two populations of neurons extend to other key appetite-regulatory regions including the paraventricular nucleus (PVH), the dorsomedial nucleus (DMH), and lateral hypothalamic area (LHA), exerting opposing effects on appetite and energy expenditure [10].

NPY injected into the brain either in the ventricles or in different hypothalamic nuclei induces a robust feeding response, even in sated animals [11]. NPY achieves this effect by reducing the latency to eat, delaying satiety and thereby augmenting meal size and meal duration [11]. NPY also causes treated animals to be more motivated to obtain food [11]. Specifically activating neurons pharmacologically with AgRP induces a robust hyperphagic response in rodents with a distinct temporal dynamic from that of NPY [7], NPY results in immediate feeding while AgRP increases food intake, but the effect is delayed and occurs over a longer time scale. In adult animals, NAG neuron ablation results in rapid starvation [12].

Leptin inhibits the excitability of NAG neurons, reducing their firing rate and hyperpolarizing their resting membrane potential [13]. This inhibition is mediated through leptin's activation of ATP-sensitive potassium channels (K_{ATP}) via phosphoinositide-3-kinase (PI3-K) [5,14,15]. Activation of K_{ATP} channels (i.e., keeping them open) serves to hyperpolarize the resting membrane potential. While it is unclear whether hyperpolarizing the resting membrane potential affects intra-cellular proNPY mRNA or NPY protein levels, it clearly results in limiting the release of NPY by these neurons (Figure 1). Since NPY and AgRP are co-localized in the same secretory vesicles, factors that affect NPY secretion affect AgRP secretion to the same degree [16]. Depolarizing the NAG neuron resting membrane potential results in a doubling of the NPY release rate, which returned to normal values when the resting membrane potential returned to a neutral condition [17]. In adult animals, K_{ATP} channels in the NAG neurons appear to include only SUR1, but not SUR2 [5,18]. At this stage, exposure to diazoxide free base (DFB), a potent K_{ATP} channel activator, resulted in significant hyperpolarization of the resting membrane potential in 100% of NAG neurons, and DFB more extensively hyperpolarized the resting energy potential of NAG neurons than leptin [5].

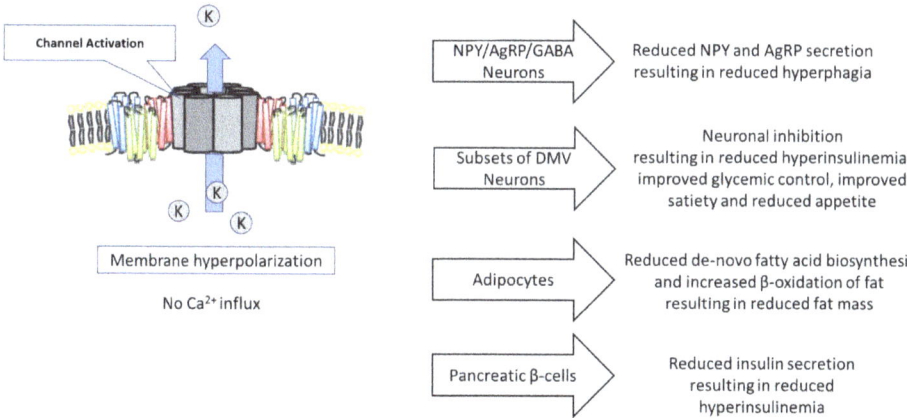

Figure 1. The Potential Role of the K_{ATP} Channel in the Regulation of Cellular and Physiological Processes Associated with Establishing and Maintaining the Obese Hyperphagic State.

3.3. The Role of the K_{ATP} Channel in the Regulation of Neuronal Function in the Dorsal Motor Nucleus of the Vagus

The dorsal vagal complex (DVC) is an autonomic regulatory center located in the caudal medulla. Primary viscerosensory information is processed within the nucleus tractus solitarii (NTS) and subsequently relayed to the dorsal motor nucleus of vagus (DMV). Neurons within the DMV are parasympathetic motor neurons as they project to the periphery and regulate the tone of most of the subdiaphragmatic organs and, thus, regulate feeding, digestion, and energy and glucose homeostasis [19,20]. The activity of DMV neurons is largely controlled by local circuits and by inputs from other brain regions including the hypothalamus [21–23]. Hormones, metabolic signals, gastrointestinal signals, or pharmacological agents have the potential to alter the activity of DMV neurons and thereby modulate the parasympathetic outflow to the organs.

Deletion of the melanocortin 4 receptor (MC4R) in the DMV results in hyperinsulinemia and modest insulin resistance in a weight-independent manner and without changes in glucose tolerance or blood glucose levels [24]. Sohn et al. [25] examined the role of melanocortin 4 receptors (MC4R) in the regulation of cholinergic neurons of the DMV which have been hypothesized to regulate insulin secretion. In these studies, MTII (a MC3R/MC4R agonist) hyperpolarized the membrane potential of cholinergic neurons within the DMV, but failed to hyperpolarize the membrane potential of cholinergic neurons in mice which were deficient for MC4R. The MTII-induced hyperpolarization of DMV cholinergic neurons was accompanied by a decrease in input resistance characteristic of the activation of a K^+ channel which was reversed by tolbutamide, a K_{ATP} antagonist, leading to the conclusion that the K^+ channel mediating MC4R-induced membrane hyperpolarization in these neurons is the K_{ATP} channel. The results of this study show that activation of MC4Rs decreases parasympathetic tone following the activation of K_{ATP} channels, which may result in decreased insulin secretion.

Insulin-induced hypoglycemia enhances vagal activity [26], while hyperglycemia depresses vagal tone [27]. Eliminating or blocking components of the insulin receptor pathway centrally, such as phosphatidylinositol 3 kinase (PI3K) or the K_{ATP} channel, disrupts vagal control of energy homeostasis [28,29], and insulin applied centrally improves hepatic gluconeogenesis in a vagally mediated manner in models of diabetes [30–32]. Moreover, insulin applied to the dorsal vagal complex affects the function of peripheral targets [33,34]. Thus, insulin may alter neural activity in the dorsal vagal complex to affect visceral function. Blake et al. [35] evaluated the effect of insulin on excitation of gastric-related neurons in the DMVand showed that insulin acts on insulin receptors located on glutamatergic afferent terminals synapsing on DMV neurons. They also showed that insulin did not affect inhibitory transmission in DMV neurons, and that there are direct effects of insulin on action potential (AP) frequency in DMV neurons, independent of fast synaptic transmission. They showed that the decrease in AP frequency was consistent with a PI3K-dependent activation of the K_{ATP} channel. Pocai et al. [36] showed that mice lacking the SUR1 subunit of the K_{ATP} channel are resistant to the inhibitory effect of insulin on gluconeogenesis, suggesting that SUR1 containing K_{ATP} channels are responsible for insulin-mediated actions within the dorsal motor nucleus of vagus.

Grill et al. [37] have reported leptin receptor gene expression in the dorsal vagal complex, including the DMV. In addition, fourth ventricle administration of leptin reduces food ingestion and weight gain, and these appetite effects are mimicked by microinjection of leptin into the DVC. Williams et al. [38] studied the effects of leptin on membrane potential in DMV neurons. They showed that leptin hyperpolarizes the majority of DMV neurons, which was consistent with the opening of a K^+ channel. Using tolbutamide and a PI3K inhibitor, the authors showed that leptin failed to hyperpolarize DMV neurons pre-exposed to tolbutamide and the application of tolbutamide depolarized neurons that had been hyperpolarized by leptin, implicating the K_{ATP} channel in the hyperpolarization. Leptin receptors are expressed widely in autonomic centers implicated in regulating ingestive behaviors, including the vagal complex and several hypothalamic sites. DMV motor neuron activity has been linked with behaviors related to feeding and satiety [38]. Enhancement of feeding behavior is directly associated with increases in DMV motor activity, whereas satiety is directly correlated with decreases in DMV motor activity [39,40]. Leptin suppression of DMV motor activity may result in satiety [38]. Additionally, leptin suppression of activity within the DVC may be closely related to the autonomic effects of leptin on blood pressure, glucose production, and/or insulin sensitivity [41–43].

Leptin, insulin and α-MSH interacting with their respective receptors, LepR, InsR, and MC4R, each achieve some or all of their respective effects in the DMV via a PI3K-mediated opening of the K_{ATP} channel, resulting in membrane hyperpolarization which leads to inhibition of neuronal signaling. The use of a K_{ATP} channel activator which is capable of penetrating the DVC has the potential to recapitulate the effects of leptin, insulin and α-MSH, with the likely result being reductions in hyperinsulinemia, reductions in hepatic gluconeogenesis, reductions in appetite and improved satiety (Figure 1).

3.4. The Role of The K_{ATP} Channel in the Regulation of Adipocyte Metabolism and Fat Mass

There is also evidence that activation of K_{ATP} channels in peripheral tissues, including adipose tissue, may be important for body weight regulation. Shi et al. [6] detected the expression of SUR1 in human adipocytes using RT-PCR. Shi [6] evaluated lipogenesis in human adipocytes treated with a K_{ATP} channel activator or an antagonist, using fatty acid synthase (FAS), which catalyzes the synthesis of palmitate from acetyl-CoA and malonyl-CoA, and glycerol-3-phosphate dehydrogenase (GPDH) activities as lipogenic markers. Glibenclamide, a K_{ATP} channel antagonist, caused a significant increase in FAS and GPDH activity, which were completely blocked by DFB. Forty eight-hour treatment with glibenclamide caused a significant inhibition in lipolysis, which was substantially recovered by DFB exposure. Thus, closing the K_{ATP} channel in human adipocytes increased the de novo synthesis of fatty acids and downregulated lipolysis, while activating the channel substantially reversed these effects.

Alemzadeh et al. [44] evaluated the effect of activating the K_{ATP} channel on fat oxidation rate in obese Zucker rats. The Zucker rat has defective leptin signaling due to a mutation in the leptin receptor which results in hyperphagic obesity, in which reduced lipid oxidation contributes to the obese state. Obese Zucker rats were treated either with vehicle or DFB. Treated animals had significantly higher fat oxidation without a significant change in glucose oxidation, as well as lower fat mass compared to vehicle-treated animals. Alemzadeh and Tushaus [45] evaluated the effect of activating the K_{ATP} channel on the expression of genes involved in hepatic fatty acid biosynthesis in Zucker diabetic fatty (ZDF) rats. ZDF rats carry the same defect in leptin signaling as Zucker fatty rats and also have a genetic predisposition to diabetes. ZDF rats were randomized to DFB or vehicle control. Treatment was associated with mRNA reductions of hepatic sterol regulatory element-binding protein-1c, FAS, acetyl CoA carboxylase, hormone-sensitive lipase, and peroxisome proliferator agonist receptor-γ, without altering acyl-CoA oxidase, peroxisome proliferator receptor-α, or carnitine palmitoyl transferase-1. ACC and FAS are the enzymes primarily responsible for the synthesis of medium- and long-chain fatty acids, where ACC catalyzes the first synthetic step and FAS catalyzes a series of 2-carbon additions.

The K_{ATP} channel appears to be a key regulator of both fatty acid biosynthesis and β-oxidation of fat. One of the peripheral effects of treatment of obese individuals with a K_{ATP} channel activator should be loss of body fat (Figure 1). Similarly, K_{ATP} channel activators, by this mechanism, should prevent the accumulation of excess body fat in individuals who are prone or genetically predisposed to such accumulation.

3.5. The Role of the K_{ATP} Channel in Reducing Hyperinsulinemia

The K_{ATP} channel has a crucial role in insulin secretion which was summarized in the following way by Komatsu et al. [46]. On elevation of plasma glucose concentration, glucose enters the pancreatic β-cells through the glucose transporter on the plasma membrane. Glucose is then phosphorylated by glucokinase and subjected to glycolysis, by which pyruvate is generated in the cytoplasm. Pyruvate is metabolized equally by pyruvate dehydrogenase and pyruvate carboxylase (PC) in the β-cells and passes into the mitochondria. The former reaction leads to generation of adenosine triphosphate (ATP) in the respiratory chain and the latter is accompanied by efflux of tricarboxylic acid (TCA) cycle intermediates as anaplerosis. ATP is a signaling molecule for insulin secretion in β-cells, because the cell is equipped with ATP-sensitive K^+ channels (K_{ATP} channels), which close on elevation of cytoplasmic ATP or ATP/adenosine diphosphate ratio. As the K_{ATP} channel is the primary determinant of the membrane potential of the β-cells, closure of these channels causes membrane depolarization. The membrane depolarization opens L-type voltage-dependent Ca^{2+} channels (VDCC), followed by Ca^{2+} influx and elevation of cytosolic free Ca^{2+} concentration ($[Ca^{2+}]_i$). The elevation of $[Ca^{2+}]_i$ rapidly increases the rate of insulin exocytosis.

Insulin is a powerful anabolic hormone secreted from pancreatic β-cells that acts on multiple tissues to stimulate the synthesis and storage of carbohydrates, lipids, and proteins [47]. Adipose tissue remodeling can occur via lipid hypertrophy and/or hyperplasia, and there is evidence that insulin has direct effects on cellular lipid metabolism [48] and adipocyte differentiation [49]. Insulin acts to inhibit lipolysis in adipocytes in the postprandial state [50], while promoting lipid storage through stimulating the uptake, synthesis, and storage of triglycerides in adipocytes [51]. Insulin stimulates adipogenesis via multiple mechanisms [52].

Hyperinsulinemia is a very early pathobiological event in the cascade of homeostatic dysfunction leading to obesity, insulin resistance, and type 2 diabetes [53]. For example, preclinical evidence from male C57BL/6 mice shows that insulin levels are elevated several weeks prior to the onset of obesity [54]. Similarly, hyperinsulinemia precedes insulin resistance, obesity, and enhanced lipogenesis in Lep ob/ob mice [55–57]. Onset of hyperinsulinemia is a primary causal factor in animal models of obesity and in some human populations [47]. Induction of VMH lesions in animal models results in hyperinsulinemia, obesity and hyperphagia [58]. The use of streptozotocin in these models results in the partial destruction of pancreatic β-cells, which reverses the hyperphagia and weight gain observed in the model [59]. This suggests that both hyperphagia and weight gain follow from hyperinsulinemia in lesioned animals. On the other hand, if there is strict control of energy intake in lesioned animals, there is no hyperphagia, but hyperinsulinemia and weight gain occur nonetheless [60,61].

K_{ATP} channel activators can partially suppress insulin secretion, are approved for the treatment of hyperinsulinemia, and would be useful to reduce the contribution of hyperinsulinemia to hyperphagia and obesity (Figure 1).

3.6. Insulin Resistance and Hyperinsulinemia

While it is clear that increases in insulin resistance can result in hyperinsulinemia, it is equally true that persistent hyperinsulinemia contributes to the development of insulin resistance both by reductions in the numbers of receptors and by postreceptor effects. Kobayashi and Olefsky [62] studied the effect of experimental hyperinsulinemia on insulin resistance in rat adipocytes. Hyperinsulinemia was induced using a gradually increasing dose of insulin, which led to a significant reduction in insulin receptors and a rightward shift in the insulin-glucose transport dose–response curve. The decrease in insulin sensitivity is the predicted functional consequence of these observed changes. When the insulin injections were stopped, insulin receptors and insulin sensitivity rapidly returned to normal. Hyperinsulinemia also increased insulin resistance in humans over 2 day treatment with exogenous insulin [63], and in patients with insulinomas [64].

Obici et al. [31] investigated the effect of downregulation of hypothalamic insulin receptor, as is characteristic of insulin resistance, on hyperphagia and fat mass and showed that the selective decrease in hypothalamic insulin receptor protein was accompanied by a rapid onset of hyperphagia and increased fat mass. Thus, central insulin resistance likely also contributes to hyperphagia and obesity.

Improvements in insulin sensitivity can be achieved using a K_{ATP} channel activator. Ratzmann et al. [65] studied the impact of K_{ATP} channel activator treatment on insulin sensitivity in obese subjects. Insulin sensitivity was studied on two separate days before and after 4 days of treatment with DFB. The authors concluded that treatment resulted in a 50% increase in insulin sensitivity in comparison to the pretreatment value. Wigand and Blackard [66] showed that 7 days of treatment with a K_{ATP} channel activator resulted in increased expression of both high and low affinity insulin receptors in treated subjects. In animal models, K_{ATP} channel activator-mediated improvements in insulin sensitivity were conditioned by increased mRNA and protein levels for glucose transporter 4 and increased protein expression for insulin receptor substrate-1 [67], and hepatic tissue levels of activated PKB/Akt (p-Akt, phosphorylated Akt), expressed as a ratio of p-Akt to Akt protein (p-Akt/Akt), were increased by treatment. DFB treatment of Zucker diabetic fatty rats resulted in improved insulin resistance compared to controls [68].

Škrha et al. [69] studied the effect of K_{ATP} channel activator treatment on insulin resistance in insulinoma and control subjects. A euglycemic clamp procedure was applied to subjects before and after 3 days of DFB administration. At baseline, the insulinoma patients were more insulin resistant than the controls, as measured by glucose disposal rate and metabolic clearance rate of insulin. Three days of treatment with DFB resulted in reduced basal insulin levels, increased tissue sensitivity to insulin and improved metabolic clearance rate of insulin. After treatment, the insulin sensitivity of insulinoma subjects was not significantly different from healthy control subjects.

3.7. The Use of K_{ATP} Channel Activators in Animal Models of Hyperphagic Obesity

The following animal models have been shown to be hyperphagic: Zucker fatty rat [70], Zucker diabetic fatty rat [70], db/db mouse [70], Otsuka Long Evans Tokushima Fatty rat [70], ventromedial hypothalamus lesioned animal models [70], and streptozotocin-induced diabetic rat [71]. The Magel2 mouse can be rendered obese with some elevation of appetite by ad libitum access to a high-fat diet [72]. The high-fat diet-induced obese (DIO) mouse also appears to have elevated appetite, while the DIO rat is clearly hyperphagic [70]. The experience with K_{ATP} channel activators in these nine models is discussed below. In animal models, changes in hyperphagia are typically assessed in the context of ad libitum access to food and measured directly by assessing either changes in energy intake or indirectly by the evaluation of the impact of changes in hyperphagia on weight and fat mass.

3.7.1. Magel2 Knockout Mice—A Model of Prader–Willi Syndrome

Magel2, encoding a MAGE-like protein, resides within the Prader–Willi syndrome (PWS) critical region of chromosome 15 in humans and its loss or lack of expression may account for several of the observed characteristics of the disease. When administered a high-fat diet, Magel2 null mice display several features of PWS, including elevated appetite and obesity [73]. In a study by Bischof and Wevrick [72], wild-type and Magel-2 null mice were rendered obese after being fed a high-fat diet. Both sets of mice received DFB with continued ad libitum access to a high-fat diet. With treatment, both groups of mice showed significant weight loss, and fat mass loss. Fasting glucose measurements of both strains after 12 weeks of HFD were in the high normal range. Four weeks of treatment significantly lowered fasting glucose measurements of both strains. The Magel2 null mice were better able to sustain energy expenditure in treadmill tests following treatment compared to their pretreatment performance.

3.7.2. Zucker Fatty Rat—A Model of LepR Deficiency

The Zucker fatty rat has a mutation in the leptin receptor which renders NAG neurons and other tissues non-responsive to leptin regulation. NPY messenger RNA levels are elevated 2- to 3-fold in Zucker fatty rats compared to their lean littermates [74]. This results in hyperphagia and obesity.

There are multiple publications covering the use of K_{ATP} channel activators in Zucker fatty rats [44,75–79]. The results of Alemzadeh and Holshouser [77] are provided by way of example. Eleven-week-old animals were randomized to receive DFB or vehicle control. Treatment was associated with a significant reduction in energy consumed per day per 100 gm body weight, reductions in plasma glucose and reductions in fasting insulin and leptin compared to vehicle-treated animals. Alemzadeh et al. [44] showed that relative to vehicle-treated controls, DFB treatment significantly reduced energy intake, weight gain, and circulating triglycerides and showed increased β-oxidation of fat and basal metabolic rate (BMR).

3.7.3. Zucker Diabetic Fatty Rat—A Model of LepR Deficiency

The Zucker diabetic fatty rat includes a further mutation, which, in the context of the LepR mutation in this strain, accelerates the development of diabetes.

Alemzadeh and Tushaus [45,68] conducted two studies of the effect of activating the K_{ATP} channel in the Zucker diabetic fatty rat. In each study, six-week-old animals were subdivided into three groups, DFB treated, pair-fed and control animals, with the latter two receiving vehicle treatment.

Treated animals gained significantly less weight than the pair-fed or control animals, even though the pair-fed animals consumed the same energy per day. Treated animals consumed significantly less energy per day compared to controls. Compared to either pair-fed or control animals, treated animals also had significantly lower glucose, higher insulin, lower triglycerides, lower HbA1c, and lower hepatic triglyceride and cholesterol content.

3.7.4. db/db Mouse—A Model of LepR Deficiency

Both NPY and AgRP levels are elevated in db/db diabetic mice [80], contributing to hyperphagia. Lee [81] evaluated the effect of K_{ATP} channel activator treatment on food intake in (db/db) diabetic mice. Diabetic (db/db) mice consume nearly twice the amount of food as do control heterozygous mice. Treatment with DFB resulted in dose dependent reductions in food intake. At the highest dose, food intake was reduced by 50% compared to control diabetic animals.

3.7.5. Otsuka Long Evans Tokushima Fatty Rat—A Model of CCK1 Receptor Deficiency

Hyperphagia in the Otsuka Long Evans Tokushima fatty (OLETF) rat is due to the absence of cholecystokinin (CCK)-1 receptors in both the gastrointestinal track and the brain. OLETF rats have a deficit in their ability to limit the size of meals and in contrast to CCK-1 receptor knockout mice, do not compensate for this increase in the size of their spontaneous meals, resulting in hyperphagia. Prior to becoming obese and in response to pair feeding, OLETF rats have increased expression of NPY in the compact region of the dorsomedial hypothalamus (DMH), and this overexpression contributes to their overall hyperphagia [82].

Guo et al. [83] evaluated the effects of treatment with a K_{ATP} channel activator in the OLETF rat. DFB or vehicle control was administered starting at 8 through 30 weeks of age. Long Evans Tokushima Otsuka (LETO) rats also served as controls. LETO rats are not genetically predisposed to obesity or diabetes. Weight gain over the 22 weeks in the treated OLETF animals was less than in the LETO controls and significantly less than in the OLETF vehicle-treated animals. Compared to controls, treated animals had significantly lower circulating triglyceride and less intra-abdominal fat, and markedly lower accumulation of fat in the liver and pancreas. Fasting glucose and insulin in treated animals were comparable to the non-diabetic LETO animals and significantly lower than controls.

3.7.6. Hypothalamic Injured Rat—A Model of Hyperinsulinemia Driven Hyperphagic Obesity

In animals, ventromedial hypothalamic (VMH) lesions cause hyperphagia and obesity [61]. In these animals, there is central dysregulation of insulin secretion resulting in hyperinsulinemia, obesity and hyperphagia. Both hyperphagia and weight gain follow from hyperinsulinemia in this model. If there is restriction of energy intake in lesioned animals, there is no hyperphagia, but hyperinsulinemia and weight gain occur nonetheless.

Larue-Achagiotis and Le Magnen [84] evaluated the effect of K_{ATP} channel activator treatment on feeding behaviour in normal and VMH lesioned Wistar rats. DFB was administered as an intra-venous dose. Rats are typically nocturnal feeders. Meal size during the night is approximately 2x the average daytime meal size. Rats also eat more meals per night than during the day. Lesioned animals increased their food intake by more than 50% at night and by approximately 300% during the day, and tend to consume similar meal sizes in both daytime and night-time. Treatment reduced food intake in a dose dependent manner. At lower doses, treatment induced a latent period without a change in meal size. At higher doses, treatment was associated with a longer latency period followed by reduced meal size.

3.7.7. Hypothalamic Injured Chicken—A Model of Hyperinsulinemia Driven Hyperphagic Obesity

The effect of activating the K_{ATP} channel on hyperphagia associated with hypothalamic injury in a white leghorn chicken model was evaluated by Sonoda [85]. Controls underwent a sham operation. Lesioned animals showed a 2-fold increase in food consumption. DFB was administered for 4 days.

Treatment resulted in a statistically significant reduction in food consumption. Average daily food consumption increased once treatment was withdrawn.

3.7.8. Streptozotocin Induced Diabetic Rat

NPY expression is also elevated in rats made diabetic by streptozotocin treatment, contributing to hyperphagia and weight gain in these models [71]. Matsuda et al. [86] evaluated the effects of activating the K_{ATP} channel in a streptozotocin-induced diabetic Wistar rat model. Male Wistar rats were either treated with a 30 mg injection of streptozotocin (to induce diabetes) or vehicle injection. One week following streptozotocin treatment, animals were randomized to either DFB or vehicle. The authors did not evaluate food consumption, but they did examine rate of weight gain at 2, 4 and 6 weeks. At each time point, treated animals showed significantly lower rates of weight gain than vehicle control animals.

3.7.9. High-Fat Diet-Induced Obese Mouse

The effect of activating the K_{ATP} channel in high-fat diet-induced obese mice was evaluated by Bischof and Wevrick [72] and described above in relation to the Magel2 mouse model of PWS. Surwit [87] also evaluated the effect of activating the K_{ATP} channel on high-fat diet-induced obese mice. After 4 weeks on the high-fat diet (HFD), mice were randomized to control or DFB treatment groups and continued HFD. Compared to HFD controls, treated HFD animals showed a significantly lower rate of weight gain, lower leptin, lower circulating non-esterified fatty acids and triglycerides, lower epididymal and retroperitoneal fat pad weights, lower plasma insulin, and lower plasma glucose. Glucose and insulin levels in treated HFD animals were markedly lower than LFD controls.

3.7.10. Tabular Summary of Animal Model Results

A tabular summary of responses to activating the K_{ATP} channel in nine animal models of hyperphagic obesity is presented in Table 1.

Table 1. Tabular summary of responses to K_{ATP} channel activator treatment in nine animal models of hyperphagic obesity.

Model	Energy Intake	Weight	Body Fat	Glycemic Control	Circulating Lipids	Hepatic Lipids
Magel2 mouse	NM	Weight loss	Loss of body fat	Improved	NM	NM
ZF rat	Reduced	Reduced rate of gain	NM	Improved	Improved	NM
ZDF rat	Reduced	Reduced rate of gain	NM	Improved	Improved	Improved
db/db mouse	Reduced	NM	NM	NM	NM	NM
OTLEF rat	Reduced	Reduced rate of gain	NM	Improved	Improved	Improved
Hypothalamic injury rat	Reduced	NM	NM	NM	NM	NM
Hypothalamic injury chicken	Reduced	NM	NM	NM	NM	NM
Streptozotocin diabetic rat	NM	Reduced rate of gain	NM	NM	NM	NM
HFD obese mouse	Reduced	Weight loss or reduced rate of gain	Loss of body fat	Improved	Improved	NM

NM—parameter was not measured.

3.8. Experience with the Diazoxide Choline Controlled-Release Tablet (DCCR) in Prader–Willi Syndrome

Prader–Willi syndrome (PWS) is a complex genetic neurobehavioral/metabolic disorder with an estimated birth incidence of 1:15,000 to 1:25,000 males and females [88]. Clinical features of

PWS include hypotonia and poor feeding in infancy; low muscle mass is present throughout life; the accumulation of excess body fat typically begins at approximately age 2 and continues into adulthood [89]. Ultimately, the central neurological defect of the disease results in an obsession with food, aggressive food seeking, and reduced satiety. This results in hyperphagia, and a progression to morbid obesity if the energy intake is not carefully managed [89]. Intellectual disability, growth hormone deficiency, behavioral problems, including aggressive and threatening behaviors, and neuroendocrine abnormalities are also characteristic of PWS [88]. The death rate among PWS patients is markedly elevated [90]. According to a 2014 survey of parents and caregivers of PWS patients, reducing hunger and improving food-related behaviors were the most important unmet needs in PWS that could be addressed in the development of a new therapeutic [91]. There are no approved therapeutics for the treatment of hyperphagia in PWS. DCCR is a novel, patent-protected, extended-release, crystalline salt tablet formulation of diazoxide which is administered once daily.

The effect of DCCR in PWS was tested in clinical study PC025, a single-center pilot study which enrolled 13 overweight or obese male and female subjects between the ages of 10 and 22 years old, with genetically confirmed PWS [92]. Treatment with DCCR resulted in greater improvements in hyperphagia at higher doses and in subjects with more marked baseline hyperphagia. DCCR treatment also resulted in statistically significant, dose dependent reductions in fat mass, increases in lean body mass, with a corresponding reduction in waist circumference. Treatment also resulted in the reduction of aggressive and threatening behaviors. There were trends for the improvement of lipids and insulin resistance.

4. Discussion

The K_{ATP} channel plays a central role in the regulation of a number of physiological processes, which, in the context of the underlying genetic or structural defects in many forms of syndromic hyperphagic obesity, cumulatively contribute to elevations in appetite and aggressive food seeking, lack of satiety, accumulation of excess body fat and the establishment and perpetuation of the obese state.

Hyperphagia, in most forms of hyperphagic obesity, is due to both enhanced orexigenic drive and diminished anorectic signaling. Activation of the K_{ATP} channel in NAG neurons should replicate the effects of leptin and insulin, hyperpolarizing the resting membrane potential of the cell and, thereby, reducing secretion of NPY and AgRP and also likely GABA. The net effect of this downregulation of secretion should be reductions in hyperphagia and more generally in appetite. These are anticipated to occur because reductions in NPY should directly and instantaneously reduce appetite. It should also result in reduced NPY-mediated suppression of the activity of prohormone convertase 2, leading to more extensive processing of POMC to αMSH and thereby enhancing anorectic signaling through the interaction of αMSH with MC4R. Reductions in AgRP, since it is an inverse agonist of MC4R, should also enhance anorectic signaling. Finally, reductions in GABA secretion by the NAG neurons should reduce the inhibitory action of GABA on POMC neurons and thereby enhance anorectic signaling. Even in the context of leptin or insulin resistance, it is possible to activate the K_{ATP} channel, resulting in the hyperpolarization of the resting membrane potential thereby reducing secretion of NPY and AgRP and, as a consequence, this approach can effectively reduce hyperphagia and appetite without a need to first restore either leptin sensitivity or insulin sensitivity. This effect on appetite would be further enhanced by improvements in satiety mediated through activation of the K_{ATP} channel in the DMV.

The accumulation of excess body fat is a fundamental characteristic of hyperphagic obesity and can be driven by excess energy intake which results in the preferential directing of excess energy to fat, or by hyperinsulinemia and/or insulin resistance. Directly activating the K_{ATP} channel in adipocytes should result in increases in β-oxidation of fat and reduced de novo synthesis of fatty acids and triglyceride accumulation. This direct effect alone should result in reduced fat deposition and/or reductions in fat mass. These effect would be complemented by the effects of K_{ATP} channel activators on hyperinsulinemia and insulin resistance. Insulin resistance tends to cause a preferential deposition of consumed energy as fat. Hyperinsulinemia has a similar effect on energy storage in fat. It also suppresses lipolysis and thereby contributes to the persistent accumulation of fat. Reductions in hyperinsulinemia result directly from the effect of activation of the K_{ATP} channel in the pancreatic β-cell, and indirectly from activating the channel in the DMV. Insulin resistance can be reduced via reductions in hyperinsulinemia and by direct effects resulting from activating the channel in the DMV. The net effect of these responses to K_{ATP} channel activation should be reduced fat mass and reduced accumulation of fat.

Beyond the effect of K_{ATP} channel activation-mediated improvements in insulin resistance on adipocytes, more generally, these improvements in insulin resistance should result in improved glycemic control.

Dyslipidemia is frequently observed in hyperphagic obesity, particularly when the individual is insulin resistant. Activating the K_{ATP} channel in the DMV has the potential to reduce hepatic synthesis and secretion of triglyceride-rich lipoprotein particles by the liver, correcting or improving dyslipidemia. Given that there is reduced triglyceride synthesis by the liver, there should, as a consequence, be reduced hepatic lipid content.

Treatment with K_{ATP} channel activators in nine animal models of hyperphagic obesity resulted in a range of therapeutic responses that are completely consistent with the predicted ressponses that follow from activating the channel in NAG neurons, the DMV, adipocytes and the pancreatic β-cell. These included reductions in hyperphagia, weight loss and body fat loss in mature animals, reductions in the rate of weight gain and body fat accumulation in growing animals, improved circulating and hepatic lipids, and improved glycemic control. These nine animal models included both genetic and induced models of hyperphagic obesity. The underlying basis for hyperphagia and excess weight gain in these models included disrupted leptin responsiveness, hyperinsulinemia, insulin resistance, and reduced satiety resulting in increased meal size.

The extant experience with DCCR in a small pilot study of patients with PWS was consistent with the animal model results, increasing the likelihood of effective translation of animal model results to clinical efficacy. In the published study, treated PWS subjects showed reductions in hyperphagia, loss of body fat, reductions in circulating lipids and improvements in insulin resistance, each anticipated from the activation of the K_{ATP} channel and consistent with the results observed in animal models of hyperphagic obesity. These results provide motivation to the more extensive evaluation of the efficacy of K_{ATP} channel activators in PWS.

Based on the animal model results, treatment of subjects who are genetically predisposed to hyperphagic obesity, but do not yet present with either hyperphagia or marked obesity, could result in preventing or delaying the transition to hyperphagia, to limiting the accumulation of excess body fat and to delaying or preventing glycemic dysregulation, which consistently follows obesity. Similarly, treatment of subjects who are obese and hyperphagic could result in the reduction of elimination of hyperphagia, reduction in body fat, improved lipid profiles and, potentially, improvements in glycemic control.

5. Conclusions

Given this range of relevant therapeutic responses that follow from activating the K_{ATP} channel, pharmacological activators of the channel could be a useful treatment option in syndromic hyperphagic obesity and may have utility in delaying the progression of these conditions, where obesity and hyperphagia are not evident from birth.

Author Contributions: Conceptualization, N.C. and A.B.; methodology, N.C.; investigation, N.C.; writing—original draft preparation, N.C.; writing—review and editing, N.C. and A.B.; visualization, N.C. All authors have read and agreed to the published version of the manuscript.

Funding: This research received no external funding.

Acknowledgments: The authors would like to thank Jack Yanovski for his feedback on early drafts of the manuscript.

Conflicts of Interest: The authors declare no conflict of interest.

References

1. Dubern, B.; Clément, K. Leptin and leptin receptor-related monogenic obesity. *Biochimie* **2012**, *94*, 2111–2115. [CrossRef]
2. Butler, M.G.; Miller, J.L.; Forster, J.L. Prader-Willi Syndrome—Clinical Genetics, Diagnosis and Treatment Approaches: An Update. *Curr. Pediatr. Rev.* **2019**, *15*, 207–244. [CrossRef]
3. Lustig, R.H. Hypothalamic obesity: Causes, consequences, treatment. *Pediatr. Endocrinol. Rev.* **2008**, *6*, 220–227.
4. Foster, M.N.; Coetzee, W. KATP Channels in the Cardiovascular System. *Physiol. Rev.* **2016**, *96*, 177–252. [CrossRef]
5. Baquero, A.F.; De Solis, A.J.; Lindsley, S.R.; Kirigiti, M.A.; Smith, M.S.; Cowley, M.; Zeltser, L.; Grove, K.L. Developmental switch of leptin signaling in arcuate nucleus neurons. *J. Neurosci.* **2014**, *34*, 9982–9994. [CrossRef] [PubMed]
6. Shi, H.; Moustaid-Moussa, N.; Wilkison, W.O.; Zemel, M. Role of the sulfonylurea receptor in regulating human adipocyte metabolism. *FASEB J.* **1999**, *13*, 1833–1838. [CrossRef] [PubMed]
7. Krashes, M.J.; Shah, B.P.; Koda, S.; Lowell, B.B. Rapid versus delayed stimulation of feeding by the endogenously released AgRP neuron mediators GABA, NPY, and AgRP. *Cell Metab.* **2013**, *18*, 588–595. [CrossRef] [PubMed]
8. Cansell, C.; Denis, R.; Joly-Amado, A.; Castel, J.; Luquet, S.H. Arcuate AgRP neurons and the regulation of energy balance. *Front. Endocrinol.* **2012**, *3*. [CrossRef] [PubMed]
9. Cyr, N.E.; Toorie, A.M.; Steger, J.S.; Sochat, M.M.; Hyner, S.; Perelló, M.; Stuart, R.; Nillni, E.A. Mechanisms by which the orexigen NPY regulates anorexigenic α-MSH and TRH. *Am. J. Physiol. Metab.* **2013**, *304*, E640–E650. [CrossRef]
10. Bouret, S.G. Organizational actions of metabolic hormones. *Front. Neuroendocr.* **2013**, *34*, 18–26. [CrossRef]
11. Beck, B. Neuropeptide Y in normal eating and in genetic and dietary-induced obesity. *Philos. Trans. R. Soc. B Boil. Sci.* **2006**, *361*, 1159–1185. [CrossRef] [PubMed]
12. Luquet, S.H.; Perez, F.A.; Hnasko, T.S.; Palmiter, R.D. NPY/AgRP Neurons Are Essential for Feeding in Adult Mice but Can Be Ablated in Neonates. *Science* **2005**, *310*, 683–685. [CrossRef] [PubMed]
13. Baver, S.B.; Hope, K.; Guyot, S.; Bjørbaek, C.; Kaczorowski, C.; O'Connell, K.M.S. Leptin modulates the intrinsic excitability of AgRP/NPY neurons in the arcuate nucleus of the hypothalamus. *J. Neurosci.* **2014**, *34*, 5486–5496. [CrossRef]
14. Spanswick, D.; Smith, M.A.; Groppi, V.E.; Logan, S.D.; Ashford, M. Leptin inhibits hypothalamic neurons by activation of ATP-sensitive potassium channels. *Nature* **1997**, *390*, 521–525. [CrossRef] [PubMed]
15. Top, M.V.D.; Lee, K.; Whyment, A.D.; Blanks, A.M.; Spanswick, D.C. Orexigen-sensitive NPY/AgRP pacemaker neurons in the hypothalamic arcuate nucleus. *Nat. Neurosci.* **2004**, *7*, 493–494. [CrossRef] [PubMed]
16. Ramamoorthy, P.; Wang, Q.; Whim, M.D. Cell Type-Dependent Trafficking of Neuropeptide Y-Containing Dense Core Granules in CNS Neurons. *J. Neurosci.* **2011**, *31*, 14783–14788. [CrossRef]
17. Stricker-Krongrad, A.; Barbanel, G.; Beck, B.; Burlet, A.; Nicolas, J.; Burlet, C. K+-stimulated neuropeptide Y release into the paraventricular nucleus and relation to feeding behavior in free-moving rats. *Neuropeptides* **1993**, *24*, 307–312. [CrossRef]
18. Top, M.V.D.; Lyons, D.; Lee, K.; Coderre, E.; Renaud, L.; Spanswick, D.C. Pharmacological and molecular characterization of ATP-sensitive K+ conductances in CART and NPY/AgRP expressing neurons of the hypothalamic arcuate nucleus. *Neuroscience* **2007**, *144*, 815–824. [CrossRef]
19. Laughton, W.B.; Powley, T.L. Localization of efferent function in the dorsal motor nucleus of the vagus. *Am. J. Physiol. Integr. Comp. Physiol.* **1987**, *252*, R13–R25. [CrossRef]
20. Berthoud, H.-R. The vagus nerve, food intake and obesity. *Regul. Pept.* **2008**, *149*, 15–25. [CrossRef]
21. Saper, C.B.; Loewy, A.; Swanson, L.; Cowan, W. Direct hypothalamo-autonomic connections. *Brain Res.* **1976**, *117*, 305–312. [CrossRef]
22. Swanson, L.W.; Sawchenko, P.E. Parventricular nucleus: A site for the integration of neuroendocrine and autonomic mechanisms. *Neuroendocrinology* **1980**, *31*, 410–417. [CrossRef] [PubMed]

23. Zsombok, A.; Smith, B. Plasticity of central autonomic neural circuits in diabetes. *Biochim. Biophys. Acta* **2008**, *1792*, 423–431. [CrossRef] [PubMed]

24. Berglund, E.D.; Liu, T.; Kong, X.; Sohn, J.-W.; Vong, L.; Deng, Z.; Lee, C.E.; Lee, S.; Williams, K.W.; Olson, D.P.; et al. Melanocortin 4 receptors in autonomic neurons regulate thermogenesis and glycemia. *Nat. Neurosci.* **2014**, *17*, 911–913. [CrossRef] [PubMed]

25. Sohn, J.-W.; Harris, L.E.; Berglund, E.D.; Liu, T.; Vong, L.; Lowell, B.B.; Balthasar, N.; Williams, K.W.; Elmquist, J.K. Melanocortin 4 receptors reciprocally regulate sympathetic and parasympathetic—Preganglionic neurons. *Cell* **2013**, *152*, 612–619. [CrossRef]

26. Hjelland, I.; Oveland, N.P.; Leversen, K.; Berstad, A.; Hausken, T. Insulin-Induced Hypoglycemia Stimulates Gastric Vagal Activity and Motor Function without Increasing Cardiac Vagal Activity. *Digestion* **2005**, *72*, 43–48. [CrossRef]

27. Maeda, C.Y.; Fernandes, T.G.; Lulhier, F.; Irigoyen, M.C.C. Streptozotocin diabetes modifies arterial pressure and baroreflex sensitivity in rats. *Braz. J. Med. Biol. Res.* **1995**, *28*, 497–501.

28. Plum, L.; Schubert, M.; Brüning, J.C. The role of insulin receptor signaling in the brain. *Trends Endocrinol. Metab.* **2005**, *16*, 59–65. [CrossRef]

29. Plum, L.; Belgardt, B.F.; Brüning, J.C. Central insulin action in energy and glucose homeostasis. *J. Clin. Investig.* **2006**, *116*, 1761–1766. [CrossRef]

30. Lam, T.K.T.; Pocai, A.; Gutierrez-Juarez, R.; Obici, S.; Bryan, J.; Aguilar-Bryan, L.; Schwartz, G.J.; Rossetti, L. Hypothalamic sensing of circulating fatty acids is required for glucose homeostasis. *Nat. Med.* **2005**, *11*, 320–327. [CrossRef]

31. Obici, S.; Feng, Z.; Karkanias, G.; Baskin, D.G.; Rossetti, L. Decreasing hypothalamic insulin receptors causes hyperphagia and insulin resistance in rats. *Nat. Neurosci.* **2002**, *5*, 566–572. [CrossRef] [PubMed]

32. Obici, S.; Zhang, B.B.; Karkanias, G.; Rossetti, L. Hypothalamic insulin signaling is required for inhibition of glucose production. *Nat. Med.* **2002**, *8*, 1376–1382. [CrossRef]

33. Huang, H.-N.; Lu, P.-J.; Lo, W.-C.; Lin, C.-H.; Hsiao, M.; Tseng, C.J. In Situ Akt Phosphorylation in the Nucleus Tractus Solitarii Is Involved in Central Control of Blood Pressure and Heart Rate. *Circulation* **2004**, *110*, 2476–2483. [CrossRef] [PubMed]

34. Krowicki, Z.; Nathan, N.A.; Hornby, P.J. Gastric motor and cardiovascular effects of insulin in dorsal vagal complex of the rat. *Am. J. Physiol. Content* **1998**, *275*, G964–G972. [CrossRef] [PubMed]

35. Blake, C.B.; Smith, B. Insulin reduces excitation in gastric-related neurons of the dorsal motor nucleus of the vagus. *Am. J. Physiol. Integr. Comp. Physiol.* **2012**, *303*, R807–R814. [CrossRef] [PubMed]

36. Pocai, A.; Lam, T.K.T.; Gutierrez-Juarez, R.; Obici, S.; Schwartz, G.J.; Bryan, J.; Aguilar-Bryan, L.; Rossetti, L. Hypothalamic KATP channels control hepatic glucose production. *Nature* **2005**, *434*, 1026–1031. [CrossRef] [PubMed]

37. Grill, H.J.; Schwartz, M.W.; Kaplan, J.M.; Foxhall, J.S.; Breininger, J.; Baskin, D.G. Evidence that the caudal brainstem is a target for the inhibitory effect of leptin on food intake. *Endocrinology* **2002**, *143*, 239–246. [CrossRef]

38. Williams, K.W.; Zsombok, A.; Smith, B. Rapid inhibition of neurons in the dorsal motor nucleus of the vagus by leptin. *Endocrinology* **2006**, *148*, 1868–1881. [CrossRef]

39. Rogers, R.C.; Hermann, G.E. Oxytocin, oxytocin antagonist, TRH, and hypothalamic paraventricular nucleus stimulation effects on gastric motility. *Peptides* **1987**, *8*, 505–513. [CrossRef]

40. Abrahamsson, H.; Jansson, G. Elicitation of Reflex Vagal Relaxation of the Stomach from Pharynx and Esophagus in the Cat. *Acta Physiol. Scand.* **1969**, *77*, 172–178. [CrossRef]

41. Ferreira, M.; Browning, K.N.; Sahibzada, N.; Verbalis, J.G.; Gillis, R.A.; Travagli, R.A. Glucose effects on gastric motility and tone evoked from the rat dorsal vagal complex. *J. Physiol.* **2001**, *536*, 141–152. [CrossRef] [PubMed]

42. Schwartz, M.W.; Porte, D. Diabetes, Obesity, and the Brain. *Science* **2005**, *307*, 375–379. [CrossRef] [PubMed]

43. Bogacka, I.; Roane, D.S.; Xi, X.; Zhou, J.; Li, B.; Ryan, D.; Martin, R.J. Expression Levels of Genes Likely Involved in Glucose-sensing in the Obese Zucker Rat Brain. *Nutr. Neurosci.* **2004**, *7*, 67–74. [CrossRef] [PubMed]

44. Alemzadeh, R.; Karlstad, M.; Tushaus, K.; Buchholz, M. Diazoxide enhances basal metabolic rate and fat oxidation in obese Zucker rats. *Metabolism* **2008**, *57*, 1597–1607. [CrossRef] [PubMed]

45. Alemzadeh, R.; Tushaus, K. Diazoxide attenuates insulin secretion and hepatic lipogenesis in zucker diabetic fatty rats. *Med. Sci. Monit.* **2005**, *11*, BR439–BR448.
46. Komatsu, M.; Takei, M.; Ishii, H.; Sato, Y. Glucose-stimulated insulin secretion: A newer perspective. *J. Diabetes Investig.* **2013**, *4*, 511–516. [CrossRef]
47. Page, M.M.; Johnson, J.D. Mild Suppression of Hyperinsulinemia to Treat Obesity and Insulin Resistance. *Trends Endocrinol. Metab.* **2018**, *29*, 389–399. [CrossRef]
48. Templeman, N.M.; Skovsø, S.; Page, M.M.; E Lim, G.; Johnson, J.D. A causal role for hyperinsulinemia in obesity. *J. Endocrinol.* **2017**, *232*, R173–R183. [CrossRef]
49. Gagnon, A.; Sorisky, A. The effect of glucose concentration on insulin-induced 3T3-L1 adipose cell differentiation. *Obes. Res.* **1998**, *6*, 157–163. [CrossRef]
50. Nielsen, T.S.; Jessen, N.; Jørgensen, J.O.L.; Moller, N.; Lund, S. Dissecting adipose tissue lipolysis: Molecular regulation and implications for metabolic disease. *J. Mol. Endocrinol.* **2014**, *52*, R199–R222. [CrossRef]
51. Czech, M.P.; Tencerova, M.; Pedersen, D.J.; Aouadi, M. Insulin signalling mechanisms for triacylglycerol storage. *Diabetologia* **2013**, *56*, 949–964. [CrossRef] [PubMed]
52. Cristancho, A.G.; Lazar, M.A. Forming functional fat: A growing understanding of adipocyte differentiation. *Nat. Rev. Mol. Cell Boil.* **2011**, *12*, 722–734. [CrossRef] [PubMed]
53. Corkey, B. Banting Lecture 2011: Hyperinsulinemia: Cause or Consequence? *Diabetes* **2011**, *61*, 4–13. [CrossRef] [PubMed]
54. Mehran, A.E.; Templeman, N.M.; Brigidi, G.S.; Lim, G.E.; Chu, K.-Y.; Hu, X.; Botezelli, J.D.; Asadi, A.; Hoffman, B.; Kieffer, T.J.; et al. Hyperinsulinemia Drives Diet-Induced Obesity Independently of Brain Insulin Production. *Cell Metab.* **2012**, *16*, 723–737. [CrossRef]
55. D'Souza, A.M.; Johnson, J.D.; Clee, S.M.; Kieffer, T.J. Suppressing hyperinsulinemia prevents obesity but causes rapid onset of diabetes in leptin-deficient Lepob/ob mice. *Mol. Metab.* **2016**, *5*, 1103–1112. [CrossRef] [PubMed]
56. Wang, B.; Charukeshi, C.P.; Pippin, J.J. Leptin- and Leptin Receptor-Deficient Rodent Models: Relevance for Human Type 2 Diabetes. *Curr. Diabetes Rev.* **2014**, *10*, 131–145. [CrossRef]
57. Gray, S.L.; Donald, C.; Jetha, A.; Covey, S.D.; Kieffer, T.J. Hyperinsulinemia Precedes Insulin Resistance in Mice Lacking Pancreatic β-Cell Leptin Signaling. *Endocrinology* **2010**, *151*, 4178–4186. [CrossRef]
58. Hales, C.; Kennedy, G.; Byrne, C.D.; Brindle, N.P.J.; Wang, T.W.M.; Zorzano, A.; Balon, T.W.; Brady, L.J.; Rivera, P.; Garetto, L.P.; et al. Plasma glucose, non-esterified fatty acid and insulin concentrations in hypothalamic-hyperphagic rats. *Biochem. J.* **1964**, *90*, 620–624. [CrossRef]
59. York, D.A.; Bray, G.A. Dependence of Hypothalamic Obesity on Insulin, the Pituitary and the Adrenal Gland11. *Endocrinology* **1972**, *90*, 885–894. [CrossRef]
60. Han, P.; Frohman, L. Hyperinsulinemia in tube-fed hypophysectomized rats bearing hypothalamic lesions. *Am. J. Physiol. Content* **1970**, *219*, 1632–1636. [CrossRef]
61. Goldman, J.; Bernardis, L.; Frohman, L. Food intake in hypothalamic obesity. *Am. J. Physiol. Content* **1974**, *227*, 88–91. [CrossRef] [PubMed]
62. Kobayashi, M.; Olefsky, J.M. Effect of experimental hyperinsulinemia on insulin binding and glucose transport in isolated rat adipocytes. *Am. J. Physiol. Metab.* **1978**, *235*, E53. [CrossRef]
63. Rizza, R.A.; Mandarino, L.J.; Genest, J.; Baker, B.A.; Gerich, J.E. Production of insulin resistance by hyperinsulinemia in man. *Diabetologia* **1985**, *28*, 70–75. [CrossRef] [PubMed]
64. Shanik, M.H.; Xu, Y.; Škrha, J.; Dankner, R.; Zick, Y.; Roth, J. Insulin Resistance and Hyperinsulinemia: Is hyperinsulinemia the cart or the horse? *Diabetes Care* **2008**, *31*, S262–S268. [CrossRef] [PubMed]
65. Ratzmann, K.P.; Ruhnke, R.; Kohnert, K.D. Effect of pharmacological suppression of insulin secretion on tissue sensitivity to insulin in subjects with moderate obesity. *Int. J. Obes.* **1983**, *7*, 453–458.
66. Wigand, J.; Blackard, W. Downregulation of insulin receptors in obese men. *Diabetes* **1979**, *28*, 287–291. [CrossRef]
67. Alemzadeh, R.; Zhang, J.; Tushaus, K.; Koontz, J. Diazoxide enhances adipose tissue protein kinase B activation and glucose transporter-4 expression in obese Zucker rats. *Med. Sci. Monit.* **2004**, *10*, BR53–BR60.
68. Alemzadeh, R.; Tushaus, K.M. Modulation of Adipoinsular Axis in Prediabetic Zucker Diabetic Fatty Rats by Diazoxide. *Endocrinology* **2004**, *145*, 5476–5484. [CrossRef]
69. Škrha, J.; Svacina, S.; Šrámková, J.; Páv, J. Use of euglycaemic clamping in evaluation of diazoxide treatment of insulinoma. *Eur. J. Clin. Pharmacol.* **1989**, *36*, 199–201. [CrossRef]

70.   Lutz, T.A.; Woods, S.C. Overview of animal models of obesity. *Curr. Protoc. Pharmacol.* **2012**, *58*, 5–61. [CrossRef]

71.   Dube, M.G.; Kalra, S.P.; Kalra, P.S. Low abundance of NPY in the hypothalamus can produce hyperphagia and obesity. *Peptides* **2007**, *28*, 475–479. [CrossRef] [PubMed]

72.   Bischof, J.M.; Wevrick, R. Chronic diazoxide treatment decreases fat mass and improves endurance capacity in an obese mouse model of Prader-Willi syndrome. *Mol. Genet. Metab.* **2018**, *123*, 511–517. [CrossRef] [PubMed]

73.   Knani, I.; Earley, B.J.; Udi, S.; Nemirovski, A.; Hadar, R.; Gammal, A.; Cinar, R.; Hirsch, H.J.; Pollak, Y.; Gross, I.; et al. Targeting the endocannabinoid/CB1 receptor system for treating obesity in Prader-Willi syndrome. *Mol. Metab.* **2016**, *5*, 1187–1199. [CrossRef] [PubMed]

74.   Dryden, S.; Pickavance, L.; Frankish, H.M.; Williams, G. Increased neuropeptide Y secretion in the hypothalamic paraventricular nucleus of obese (fa/fa) Zucker rats. *Brain Res.* **1995**, *690*, 185–188. [CrossRef]

75.   Alemzadeh, R.; Slonim, A.E.; Zdanowicz, M.M.; Maturo, J. Modification of insulin resistance by diazoxide in obese Zucker rats. *Endocrinology* **1993**, *133*, 705–712. [CrossRef] [PubMed]

76.   Alemzadeh, R.; Jacobs, W.; Pitukcheewanont, P. Antiobesity effect of diazoxide in obese zucker rats. *Metabolism* **1996**, *45*, 334–341. [CrossRef]

77.   Alemzadeh, R.; Holshouser, S. Effect of diazoxide on brain capillary insulin receptor binding and food intake in hyperphagic obese Zucker rats. *Endocrinology* **1999**, *140*, 3197–3202. [CrossRef]

78.   Standridge, M.; Alemzadeh, R.; Zemel, M.; Koontz, J.; Moustaid-Moussa, N. Diazoxide down-regulates leptin and lipid metabolizing enzymes in adipose tissue of Zucker rats. *FASEB J.* **2000**, *14*, 455–460. [CrossRef]

79.   Hensley, I.; E Lawler, J.; Alemzadeh, R.; Holshouser, S.J. Diazoxide effects on hypothalamic and extra-hypothalamic NPY content in Zucker rats. *Peptides* **2001**, *22*, 899–908. [CrossRef]

80.   De Luca, C.; Kowalski, T.J.; Zhang, Y.; Elmquist, J.K.; Lee, C.; Kilimann, M.W.; Ludwig, T.; Liu, S.-M.; Chua, S.C. Complete rescue of obesity, diabetes, and infertility in db/db mice by neuron-specific LEPR-B transgenes. *J. Clin. Investig.* **2005**, *115*, 3484–3493. [CrossRef]

81.   Lee, S. Effects of diazoxide on insulin secretion and metabolic efficiency in the db/db mouse. *Life Sci.* **1981**, *28*, 1829–1840. [CrossRef]

82.   Bi, S.; Moran, T.H. Obesity in the Otsuka Long Evans Tokushima Fatty Rat: Mechanisms and Discoveries. *Front. Nutr.* **2016**, *3*. [CrossRef] [PubMed]

83.   Guo, Z.; Bu, S.; Yu, Y.; Ghatnekar, G.; Wang, M.; Chen, L.; Bu, M.; Yang, L.; Zhu, B.; Feng, Z.; et al. Diazoxide prevents abdominal adiposity and fatty liver in obese OLETF rats at prediabetic stage. *J. Diabetes Complicat.* **2008**, *22*, 46–55. [CrossRef] [PubMed]

84.   Larue-Achagiotis, C.; Le Magnen, J. Effects of a Diazoxide inhibition of insulin release on food intake of normal and hyperphagic hypothalamic rats. *Pharmacol. Biochem. Behav.* **1978**, *9*, 717–720. [CrossRef]

85.   Sonoda, T. Hyperinsulinemia and its role in maintaining the hypothalamic hyperphagia in chickens. *Physiol. Behav.* **1983**, *30*, 325–329. [CrossRef]

86.   Matsuda, M.; Kawasaki, F.; Mikami, Y.; Takeuchi, Y.; Saito, M.; Eto, M.; Kaku, K. Rescue of beta-cell exhaustion by diazoxide after the development of diabetes mellitus in rats with streptozotocin-induced diabetes. *Eur. J. Pharmacol.* **2002**, *453*, 141–148. [CrossRef]

87.   Surwit, R.S.; Dixon, T.M.; Petro, A.E.; Daniel, K.W.; Collins, S. Diazoxide restores β3-adrenergic receptor function in diet-induced obesity and diabetes. *Endocrinology* **2000**, *141*, 3630–3637. [CrossRef]

88.   McCandless, S.E.; Committee on Genetics American Academy of Pediatrics. Clinical Report-Health supervision for children with Prader-Willi syndrome. *Pediatrics* **2011**, *127*, 195–204. [CrossRef]

89.   Miller, J.L.; Lynn, C.H.; Driscoll, D.C.; Goldstone, A.P.; Gold, J.-A.; Kimonis, V.; Dykens, E.; Butler, M.G.; Shuster, J.J.; Driscoll, D.J. Nutritional phases in Prader-Willi syndrome. *Am. J. Med. Genet. Part. A* **2011**, *155*, 1040–1049. [CrossRef]

90.   Hedgeman, E.; Ulrichsen, S.P.; Carter, S.; Kreher, N.C.; Malobisky, K.P.; Braun, M.M.; Fryzek, J.; Olsen, M.S. Long-term health outcomes in patients with Prader–Willi Syndrome: A nationwide cohort study in Denmark. *Int. J. Obes.* **2017**, *41*, 1531–1538. [CrossRef]

91. Summary of the Impact of PWS on Individuals and Their Families and Views on Treatments: Results of an International Online Survey. Available online: https://www.fpwr.org/pws-patient-voices (accessed on 19 April 2020).

92. Kimonis, V.E.; Surampalli, A.; Wencel, M.; Gold, J.-A.; Cowen, N.M. A randomized pilot efficacy and safety trial of diazoxide choline controlled-release in patients with Prader-Willi syndrome. *PLoS ONE* **2019**, *14*, e0221615. [CrossRef] [PubMed]

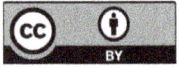 © 2020 by the authors. Licensee MDPI, Basel, Switzerland. This article is an open access article distributed under the terms and conditions of the Creative Commons Attribution (CC BY) license (http://creativecommons.org/licenses/by/4.0/).

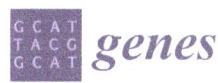

Article

Growth Trajectories in Genetic Subtypes of Prader–Willi Syndrome

Daisy A. Shepherd [1,2], Niels Vos [1,3], Susan M. Reid [1,2], David E. Godler [1,2], Angela Guzys [1], Margarita Moreno-Betancur [1,2] and David J. Amor [1,2,*]

[1] Murdoch Children's Research Institute, Royal Children's Hospital, Parkville 3052, Australia; daisy.shepherd@mcri.edu.au (D.A.S.); niels_vos132@msn.com (N.V.); sue.reid@mcri.edu.au (S.M.R.); david.godler@mcri.edu.au (D.E.G.); angela.guzys@mcri.edu.au (A.G.); margarita.moreno@mcri.edu.au (M.M.-B.)
[2] Department of Paediatrics, University of Melbourne, Parkville 3052, Australia
[3] Department of Clinical Genetics, Amsterdam UMC, University of Amsterdam, Amsterdam Reproduction & Development Research Institute, 1105 AZ Amsterdam, The Netherlands
* Correspondence: david.amor@mcri.edu.au

Received: 26 May 2020; Accepted: 30 June 2020; Published: 2 July 2020

Abstract: Prader–Willi syndrome (PWS) is a rare disorder caused by the loss of expression of genes on the paternal copy of chromosome 15q11-13. The main molecular subtypes of PWS are the deletion of 15q11-13 and non-deletion, and differences in neurobehavioral phenotype are recognized between the subtypes. This study aimed to investigate growth trajectories in PWS and associations between PWS subtype (deletion vs. non-deletion) and height, weight and body mass index (BMI). Growth data were available for 125 individuals with PWS (63 males, 62 females), of which 72 (57.6%) had the deletion subtype. There was a median of 28 observations per individual (range 2–85), producing 3565 data points distributed from birth to 18 years of age. Linear mixed models with cubic splines, subject-specific random effects and an autoregressive correlation structure were used to model the longitudinal growth data whilst accounting for the nature of repeated measures. Height was similar for males in both PWS subtypes, with non-deletion females being shorter than deletion females for older ages. Weight and BMI were estimated to be higher in the deletion subtype compared to the non-deletion subtype, with the size of difference increasing with advancing age for weight. These results suggest that individuals with deletion PWS are more prone to obesity.

Keywords: Prader–Willi syndrome; weight; obesity; BMI; pediatric; linear mixed models

1. Introduction

Prader–Willi syndrome (PWS) is a rare multisystem disorder caused by the loss of transcription of several genes and RNA transcripts on the paternally inherited copy of chromosome 15 [1]. Key early clinical features are infantile hypotonia and poor sucking with failure to thrive, followed in childhood by food seeking and hyperphagia that may lead to morbid obesity [2,3] and early mortality [4] if not externally controlled. Other features are hypogonadism, short stature and small hands and feet. The neurodevelopmental phenotype includes intellectual disability that is usually mild and behavior problems including compulsions, tantrums and skin picking [5].

There are two main molecular classes of PWS. In approximately 65% of cases, PWS is caused by a deletion which removes either 5.0 Mb (class I deletion) or 5.9 Mb (class II deletion) of the paternal chromosome within 15q11-13 [5,6]. In the remaining cases, there is no alteration to the copy number at 15q11-13, and instead the loss of expression from a paternal allele is due either to maternal uniparental disomy of chromosome 15 (matUPD15) or, less commonly, an imprinting center defect (ICD).

Although there is considerable overlap in the clinical phenotypes between deleted and non-deleted subtypes of PWS, several genotype–phenotype correlations have emerged. Individuals with the typical 15q11-q13 deletions have been reported to have lower cognitive ability, including IQ scores, than those with matUPD [7–12], whereas the risk for autistic-like behaviors [8,13,14] and the development of mental health issues (e.g., psychosis) [12,15] is elevated in those with the matUPD subtype. These differences all relate to central nervous system function and suggest that there are differences in brain gene expression between the subtypes [10]. The most likely biological explanation for such differences is that the 15q11-13 region contains both imprinted and non-imprinted genes that contribute to the PWS phenotype, with the contribution of non-imprinted genes being limited to deletion cases [16]. For example, the characteristic fair skin in deletion PWS is attributed to haploinsufficiency for the non-imprinted gene *OCA2* at 15q12-13 [17]. Another potential source of phenotypic heterogeneity between deletion and matUPD subtypes is that matUPD15 typically arises from a trisomy 15 conceptus with subsequent trisomy rescue; therefore, the phenotype in some cases of matUPD15 may be influenced by the presence of residual trisomy cells in the placenta and/or the individuals, or by the unmasking of an autosomal recessive gene located on chromosome 15 [18].

Comparisons between the deletion and non-deletion subtypes of PWS provide a means of separating the effects of maternally imprinted genes (which should apply to both subtypes) from those resulting from a single copy loss of non-imprinted genes (which should only apply to deletion cases) [16]. Although growth parameters have been studied extensively in PWS, including the publication of standardized growth charts for children with [19] and without [20] growth hormone treatment, there is limited evidence linking growth to the genetic subtype of PWS. This study aimed to investigate the associations between a PWS individual's genetic subtype (deletion vs. non-deletion) and their anthropometric measure (height, weight, BMI).

2. Materials and Methods

2.1. Victorian Prader–Willi Syndrome Register

This study draws data from the Victorian Prader–Willi Syndrome Register (VPWSR). The VPWSR collects and stores information about individuals with PWS who were born, living and/or receiving services in Victoria, Australia [6]. Ethics approval (RCH HREC ID number 20851) covers the collection of demographic and diagnostic information from medical records for the public good and fulfils state and federal privacy legislation requirements. Families are also provided with the opportunity to consent to receiving questionnaires every 3 years until the age of 18. These questionnaires ask about health, medication use, hyperphagia and other behaviors relevant to PWS. Additional longitudinal data on height and weight are collected for patients of the PWS multidisciplinary clinic of the Royal Children's Hospital, Melbourne. At the time of this study, the register contained information for 212 individuals with PWS (born in years 1971–2018), with 82 individuals consenting to receive the additional three-yearly questionnaires.

2.2. Study Cohort

From the VPWSR, we identified a retrospective cohort of individuals with a known molecular mechanism and at least one recorded height and weight measurement. For each growth measurement, the individual's age (recorded in years as an unrounded decimal) was calculated based on the patient's date of birth and the date of measurement as recorded in the register. The study cohort focused on measurements taken from 0 to 18 years of age only, due to the majority of data points falling in this interval. The body mass index (BMI) was calculated from the recorded height and weight measurements (weight (kg) / height (m^2)). The final data set of interest contained information about: (i) each individual's genetic subtype (categorized as deletion or non-deletion), (ii) measurements of height, weight and BMI, (iii) each individual's date of birth, (iv) gender and (v) age at the time of each measurement.

2.3. Statistical Analysis

The primary aim of this analysis was to investigate the associations between genetic subtype and anthropometric measures in our cohort of PWS individuals. During the analysis, two different modeling approaches were considered for addressing different questions, as described below. In addition, growth is known to follow different trajectories in males versus females with PWS [20], therefore, analyses were performed for each of the genders separately.

2.3.1. Modeling Longitudinal Growth of Anthropometric Measures

Longitudinal growth models were fitted to estimate the mean growth over time in the observed data and to provide comparison to the normal growth trajectories. An exploratory analysis highlighted a number of characteristics in the data which needed to be addressed when modeling the growth of each anthropometric measure: the non-linear growth over age, the heterogeneity among individuals and the correlation of repeated measures on the same individual. To model the non-linear relationship between age and each outcome, natural cubic B-splines were fitted separately for each genetic subgroup and gender [21]. The spline approach essentially fits separate models to each specified age interval, with the age range divided into intervals through the placement of knots, and provides flexibility in modeling non-linear growth over time. Due to the limited number of observations at older ages, natural cubic B-splines were chosen over unmodified cubic B-splines to improve the stability of the results, particularly beyond the boundary knots [22]. Using natural cubic B-splines allowed for potential non-linear growth over age intervals and generated smooth growth curves for each anthropometric measure by genetic subtype. Age was included as a predictor in the fitted models, with the number and placement of knots (in relation to age) considered during model selection. A combination of the Akaike information criterion (AIC), the Bayesian information criterion (BIC) and visualizations of the raw data and residuals were used to determine the preferred knot placement in the final growth models. In addition, visualizations of the estimated growth curves were used to assess and avoid potential overfitting by ensuring the curves were smooth whilst explaining the signal in the data in comparison to the raw data (i.e., not driven by noise).

To account for the heterogeneity in growth between PWS individuals, linear mixed models (LMMs) with natural cubic B-splines were fitted to include individual-specific random effects in the model. LMMs are a popular choice when modeling repeated measures, due to their ability to account for the imbalance in the distribution of repeated measures for different individuals in the sample [21]. When building the growth models, the inclusion of random intercepts and random slopes were both considered. Random intercepts were fitted to account for the variation in intercept (i.e., height/weight/BMI at birth) for each individual, with random slopes fitted to account for the individual variability in growth over age. When fitting the growth models, we considered both an unstructured correlation structure (assuming each variance and covariance is unique) and a first-order continuous autoregressive correlation structure (assuming measures closer in age are more correlated than measures more distant). The visual inspection of residuals against age alongside variograms were used to determine the most appropriate correlation structure to include in the final growth models.

In addition to point estimates, approximate 95% confidence intervals were estimated to be around the predicted mean growth for each outcome for each subtype, using model-based bootstrap methods for mixed models. Model parameters from the cubic spline models are complex to interpret directly, and therefore these models were used to provide age-specific estimates of anthropometric measures and graphically depict the association between genetic subtype and anthropometric growth in our observed data (without any adjustment), whilst comparing them to the normal growth trajectories. Normal growth information from the Centers for Disease Control and Prevention (CDC) were used in the comparison [23]. These data provided percentiles for the growth of anthropometric measures in children between the ages of 2 and 20 years and were included on the growth charts alongside the growth of the PWS individuals.

For each genetic subgroup (deletion/non-deletion) and gender, the final longitudinal growth models fitted an LMM with individual-specific random effects (random intercept and slope) with natural cubic B-splines (knots at ages 2, 5, 10 and 15 years) and an autoregressive (AR(1)) correlation structure.

2.3.2. Estimating Average Rate of Growth over Age

The previously fitted cubic spline models provided estimates of the differences between mean outcomes for the deletion and non-deletion subgroups across a range of ages in our data (unadjusted). After the visual inspection of the estimated growth curves, we observed the average rate of growth appeared to vary between the genetic subgroups over age. Therefore, we aimed to compare and quantify the average rate of growth over age between the genetic subgroups for each anthropometric measure.

The parameters of the previously fitted spline models do not allow a direct interpretation of the average rate of growth. Therefore, in a second set of analyses, a separate LMM with linear splines was fitted for each outcome. Linear spline models assume a linear relationship between knots, enabling a direct interpretation of fitted model parameters as representing the average growth rate over the interval. The fitted linear spline models included age and genetic subtype as predictors, with an interaction term between age and genetic subtype to allow for different rates of growth between the two subtypes within each age interval. The interpretation of estimated interaction terms provided an estimate of the average difference in the average rate of growth between the genetic subgroups in each age interval.

In addition, each model was explored in two forms: unadjusted and adjusted for the individual's year of birth (grouped by decade and included as a linear predictor in the model). This adjustment was explored to account for the fact that, compared to the deletion group, data from the non-deletion group were obtained more recently, when different management options were available (e.g., growth hormone availability, the early implementation of food intake restraint). The earliest two decades (1970–1979 and 1980–1989) were grouped together for the adjusted analysis due to no non-deletion individuals being born before 1981 in this cohort. The same model fitting procedure was applied as outlined in Section 2.3.1.

The final models fitted an LMM with individual-specific random effects (random intercept and slope) with linear splines (knots at ages 2, 5, 10 and 15 years) and an autoregressive (AR(1)) correlation structure. Models with fewer knots also provided an adequate fit for the data, with this knot placement was selected to enable the interpretation of the average rate of growth between smaller age intervals and to align them with the previously estimated growth curves.

All of the statistical analyses were performed in R 3.6.1 [24], with the additional packages lme4 [25], nlme [26] and splines [24] used to fit the models, and the ggplot2 package [27] used to produce the growth charts.

3. Results

3.1. Description of the Study Cohort

The study cohort included 125 people with PWS (63 males, 62 females) with available growth data (Table 1). Of these, 72 (57.6%) had a paternal 15q11.2-q13 deletion, with the remaining 53 (42.4%) categorized as non-deletion (37 had matUPD15; five had an imprinting defect; 11 with other non-deletion). Individuals in the deletion group were born fairly consistently over all decades; however, a large proportion of the non-deletion cohort were born from the year 2000 onwards (83.0%). Of the 125 individuals, 119 (95.2%) had repeated measurements for weight and height over the age range of interest, with an average of 29 observations per individual (range 2–85, median 28). This produced a total of 3565 data points distributed from birth to 18 years of age across the 125 individuals.

Table 1. Characteristics of the study cohort.

			Genetic Subtype	
			Deletion (*n* = 72)	Non-Deletion (*n* = 53)
Females	*n* (%)		31 (50)	31 (50)
	Number of measurements		915	723
	Age at time of measurement, years–median (IQR)		7.0 (3.2–12.0)	4.7 (2.0–8.9)
	Year of birth–*n* (%)			
		1970–1989	4 (12.9)	1 (3.2)
		1990–1999	13 (41.9)	3 (9.7)
		2000–2009	9 (29.0)	14 (45.2)
		2010–2019	5 (16.1)	13 (41.9)
	Participants with ≥ 1 measurement in each age interval–*n* (%)			
		Birth–2 years	26 (83.9)	26 (83.9)
		> 2–5 years	23 (74.2)	21 (67.7)
		> 5–10 years	24 (77.4)	21 (67.7)
		> 10–15 years	18 (58.1)	10 (32.3)
		> 15 years	15 (48.4)	8 (25.8)
Males	*n* (%)		41 (65.1)	22 (34.9)
	Number of measurements		1225	702
	Age at time of measurement, years–median (IQR)		7.6 (3.7–12.3)	4.8 (2.0–8.6)
	Year of birth–*n* (%)			
		1970–1989	11 (26.8)	2 (9.1)
		1990–1999	12 (29.3)	3 (13.6)
		2000–2009	7 (17.1)	6 (27.3)
		2010–2018	11 (26.8)	11 (50.0)
	Participants with ≥ 1 measurement in each age interval–*n* (%)			
		Birth–2 years	27 (65.9)	20 (90.9)
		> 2–5 years	28 (68.3)	19 (86.4)
		> 5–10 years	32 (78.0)	16 (72.7)
		> 10–15 years	26 (63.4)	9 (40.9)
		> 15 years	21 (51.2)	6 (27.3)

IQR, interquartile range.

3.2. Growth in PWS Individuals and Comparison to Expected Growth in the Population

Exploratory data analysis provided insight into the structure and nature of the data and directed the model building process. Spaghetti plots provided visualization of the raw data (Figure 1) with a combination of metrics used to determine the most appropriate growth model. LMMs with the AR(1) correlation structure were the preferred fitted model, with the four-knot model improving the AIC and BIC (see Table S1 and Figure S1 for an example of the model fitting metrics). A higher number of knots in the model made a small improvement in the AIC and BIC but appeared to be overfitting the observed data in visualizations of the estimated growth curves, and thus the four-knot model was preferred.

The final cubic spline models were used to generate estimated growth charts, as presented in Figures 2–4, with each figure including the comparative quantiles of normal growth range obtained from the CDC. To align with the available growth information from the CDC, the growth charts presented here are restricted to individuals aged two years to eighteen years. Estimates of each outcome (without adjustment) were generated at specific age points (age 2, 5, 10, 15 and 18 years) using the fitted models to provide comparison between the genetic subgroups for each gender (Table 2). It is important to note that there were fewer observations obtained for the oldest age group in both subtypes and genders (18 years of age), and therefore interpretations for the older age group were made considering this.

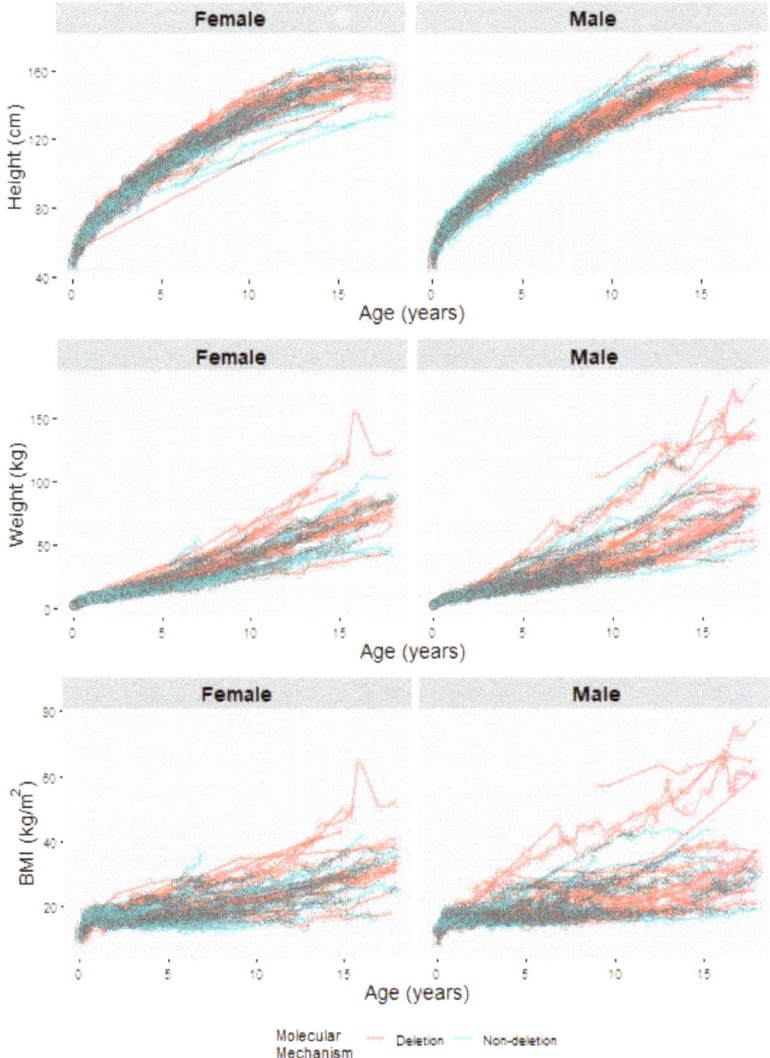

Figure 1. Spaghetti plot of the raw data for each outcome measure from the 125 participants in the study cohort.

Table 2. Estimates of mean outcome measure by age for individuals with the deletion or non-deletion mechanism of Prader–Willi syndrome (PWS) in the observed data (without adjustment), estimated using linear mixed models with cubic splines.

Gender	Outcome	Age (Years)	Deletion		Non-Deletion		Difference (Deletion – Non-Deletion)	
			Mean	(SE)	Mean	(SE)	Mean	[95% CI]
Female	Height (cm)	2	81.23	(0.81)	82.61	(1.19)	−1.38	[−4.32, 1.56]
		5	104.63	(0.78)	104.62	(1.20)	0.01	[−2.91, 2.93]
		10	137.58	(0.83)	133.00	(1.37)	4.58	[1.31, 7.85]
		15	152.36	(0.87)	144.49	(1.46)	7.87	[4.40, 11.34]
		18	153.11	(1.12)	141.71	(2.04)	11.40	[6.65, 16.15]
Female	Weight (kg)	2	10.46	(1.99)	10.33	(0.63)	0.13	[−4.13, 4.39]
		5	23.25	(1.97)	19.81	(1.15)	3.44	[−1.22, 8.10]
		10	49.26	(2.05)	38.73	(2.62)	10.53	[3.74, 17.32]
		15	73.22	(2.08)	65.21	(4.27)	8.01	[−1.69, 17.71]
		18	80.26	(2.32)	80.73	(5.38)	−0.47	[−12.44, 11.50]
Female	BMI (kg/m^2)	2	16.88	(0.95)	17.41	(0.80)	−0.53	[−3.07, 2.01]
		5	20.76	(0.94)	18.73	(0.81)	2.03	[−0.50, 4.56]
		10	26.22	(0.98)	22.37	(0.90)	3.85	[1.13, 6.57]
		15	31.80	(1.00)	27.05	(0.94)	4.75	[1.95, 7.55]
		18	34.00	(1.14)	32.18	(1.26)	1.82	[−1.65, 5.29]
Male	Height (cm)	2	81.85	(0.83)	81.41	(1.37)	0.44	[−2.89, 3.77]
		5	106.70	(0.78)	103.78	(1.32)	2.92	[−0.27, 6.11]
		10	136.17	(0.80)	138.58	(1.49)	−2.41	[−5.93, 1.11]
		15	153.60	(0.88)	155.23	(1.96)	−1.63	[−6.10, 2.84]
		18	157.01	(1.05)	159.16	(2.74)	−2.15	[−8.25, 3.95]
Male	Weight (kg)	2	8.75	(5.27)	11.27	(0.66)	−2.52	[−13.57, 8.53]
		5	19.75	(3.89)	19.30	(1.43)	0.45	[−8.17, 9.07]
		10	47.92	(3.51)	44.72	(3.35)	3.20	[−6.89, 13.29]
		15	82.62	(5.73)	66.94	(5.45)	15.68	[−0.77, 32.13]
		18	101.11	(7.54)	81.50	(6.80)	29.61	[−1.51, 40.73]
Male	BMI (kg/m^2)	2	18.35	(1.28)	15.93	(1.11)	2.42	[−1.10, 5.94]
		5	20.89	(1.16)	16.02	(1.09)	4.87	[1.56, 8.18]
		10	26.49	(1.72)	23.14	(1.17)	3.35	[−0.98, 7.68]
		15	34.53	(2.78)	31.22	(1.45)	3.31	[−3.10, 9.72]
		18	39.95	(3.39)	35.02	(1.90)	4.93	[−3.15, 13.01]

3.2.1. Height

For females with PWS, individuals with each genetic subtype tended to have a similar growth trajectory until the age of 10 years, after which the rate of growth appeared slower for the non-deletion subtype (Figure 2). At the ages of 10 and 15 years, the difference in height between the genetic subgroups is more pronounced, with the deletion individuals being, on average, 4.6 cm (95% CI: 1.3, 7.9) and 7.9 cm (95% CI: 4.4, 11.3) taller than the non-deletion individuals, respectively. By the age of 18, there appears to be a slight decline in the average height. However, there is high uncertainty here due to measurements obtained from fewer individuals at this time point (three individuals > 17 years of age in the non-deletion group), with two of these specific individuals being the shortest in the cohort and therefore driving the estimations. For males, the growth trajectory was similar between the genetic subgroups, with the estimated difference in mean height being relatively small over different ages (the size of mean difference ranging from 0.4 cm to 2.9 cm; Table 3). Between the ages of 5 and 10 years, there appeared to be a quicker rate of growth for non-deletion individuals. When compared to the normative growth range, the predicted height by age appeared to be lower than the CDC 50th percentile curve for both males and females and both genetic subtypes. For individuals aged 15 years and above, the predicted mean height was even lower than the CDC 10th percentile for both genders and subtypes.

Table 3. Mean difference in the rate of growth across age intervals, between individuals with the deletion or non-deletion mechanism of PWS, estimated using linear mixed models with linear splines (unadjusted), with an interaction term between age and genetic subtype.

Outcome	Age (Years)	Average Difference in Mean Rate of Growth (*Deletion – Non-Deletion*)					
		Females			Males		
		Estimate	[95% CI]	*p*-Value	Estimate	[95% CI]	*p*-Value
Height (cm/year)	< 2	0.10	[−1.09, 1.29]	0.87	1.35	[−0.20, 2.91]	0.09
	2–5	0.37	[−1.23, 1.98]	0.65	−1.30	[−3.14, 0.5]	0.17
	5–10	0.14	[−0.92, 1.20]	0.80	−1.41	[−2.55, −0.28]	0.01
	10–15	−0.75	[−1.75, 0.25]	0.14	2.76	[1.64, 3.89]	<0.01
	> 15	1.09	[−0.76, 2.93]	0.25	1.82	[−0.29, 3.93]	0.09
Weight (kg/year)	< 2	0.73	[−0.71, 2.16]	0.32	−0.15	[−2.56, 2.26]	0.90
	2–5	−0.36	[−2.14, 1.41]	0.69	0.19	[−2.08, 2.46]	0.87
	5–10	1.03	[−0.14, 2.20]	0.08	−0.23	[−1.67, 1.21]	0.75
	10–15	−1.56	[−2.66, −0.46]	0.01	3.71	[2.30, 5.12]	<0.01
	> 15	−1.87	[−3.90, 0.16]	0.07	1.36	[−1.30, 4.02]	0.32
BMI ((kg/m²)/year)	< 2	1.36	[0.58, 2.15]	<0.01	1.07	[−0.11, 2.25]	0.07
	2–5	−1.06	[−2.08, −0.05]	0.04	−0.57	[−1.85, 0.70]	0.38
	5–10	−0.12	[−0.76, 0.54]	0.73	−0.42	[−1.22, 0.38]	0.31
	10–15	−0.38	[−0.99, 0.24]	0.23	0.40	[−0.39, 1.19]	0.32
	> 15	−0.94	[−2.10, 0.22]	0.11	0.20	[−1.27, 1.67]	0.79

3.2.2. Weight

When looking at weight over age, individuals in the deletion subgroup generally had a higher average weight than those in the non-deletion group for both genders, with the size of the difference varying with age (Figure 2). For females with PWS, the mean weight between subtypes was similar in younger ages (mean difference of 0.1 kg at age two, 95% CI: −4.1, 4.4). However, from ages 7 to 15 years, the difference in mean weight was more substantial, with deletion individuals estimated to be, on average, 10.5 kg heavier than the non-deletion individuals at age 10 (95% CI: 3.7, 17.3) and 8 kg heavier at age 15 (95% CI: −1.7, 17.7). For females with PWS in this cohort, individuals in the non-deletion subgroup had an average predicted weight higher than the CDC 75th percentile, with the predicted weight for individuals in the deletion subgroup even exceeding the CDC 90th percentile for ages of 5 years and above.

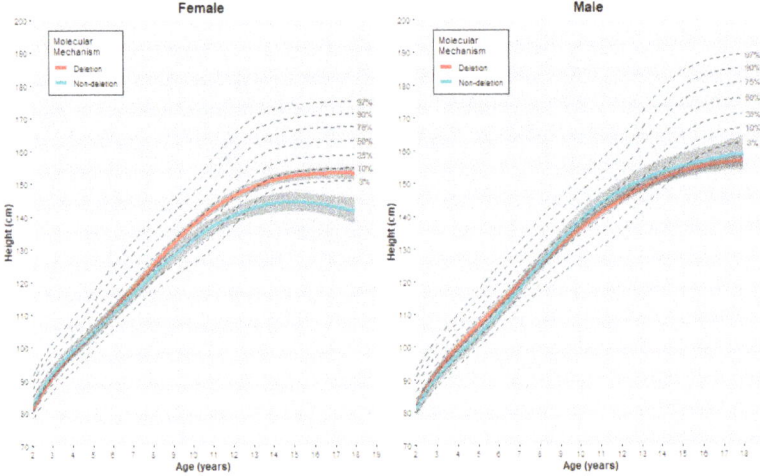

Figure 2. Estimated growth curves for the height of individuals with the deletion and non-deletion mechanism causing PWS in our study cohort (colored lines), alongside the normative percentile ranges of height growth (dashed gray lines).

The difference in mean weight between the genetic subgroups was less pronounced for males aged 10 years or younger. However, for individuals aged 10 years or above, the mean weight was estimated to be higher for the deletion subgroup. By age 15, the mean weight was estimated to be, on average, 15.7 kg heavier for males with the deletion subtype than the non-deletion subtype (95% CI: −0.8, 32.3). In comparison to the normative growth range, the non-deletion subgroup had an average predicted weight higher than the CDC 75th percentile for males aged 7 years and above, with the average predicted weight in the deletion subgroup being higher than the CDC 90th percentile.

3.2.3. Body Mass Index (BMI)

For BMI, individuals with the deletion mechanism tended to have a higher BMI than those in the non-deletion subgroup, with the size and impact of difference varying with age (Figure 3). For females, the difference was more pronounced in individuals aged 5 to 15 years. At ages 10 and 15 years, females with the deletion mechanism were estimated to have a mean BMI 3.9 units (95% CI: 1.1, 6.6) and 4.8 units (95% CI: 2.0, 7.6) higher than the non-deletion individuals in the cohort, respectively. When comparing to the normative growth range for age four and above, the predicted mean BMI for non-deletion females was higher than the CDC 90th percentile, and even higher than the CDC 97th percentile for deletion females.

This relationship was similar for males with PWS, with the mean predicted BMI being higher in the deletion individuals across all ages. At age five, the mean BMI was estimated to be, on average, 4.9 units higher in the deletion individuals than in the non-deletion individuals (95% CI: 1.6, 8.2). When compared to the normative growth range, the predicted mean BMI for the non-deletion subgroup was higher than the 90th percentile for males aged 7 years and above. For deletion males in the study cohort, the estimated mean BMI in the deletion subgroup exceeded the 97th percentile limit for ages 3 years and above.

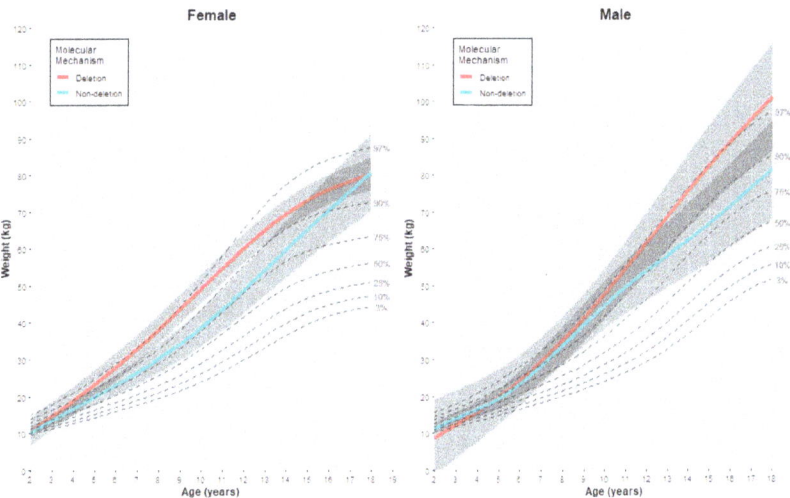

Figure 3. Estimated growth curves for the weight of individuals with the deletion or non-deletion mechanism causing PWS in our study cohort (colored lines), alongside the normative percentile ranges of weight growth (dashed gray lines).

Given that the BMI is based on the height and weight of an individual, observations in the growth patterns in BMI can be linked to the other growth charts. For males with PWS, the substantially higher BMI in older ages appears to be driven by a combination of extremes: short stature and high weight in comparison to the normative growth ranges at this age range. For females with PWS, the BMI still exceeds the CDC 90th percentiles but has a less substantial increase in older ages in comparison to the males.

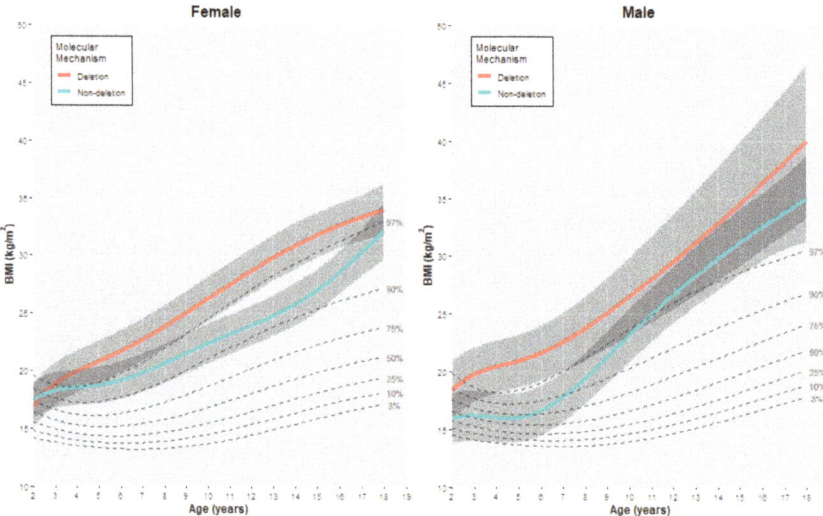

Figure 4. Estimated growth curves for the BMI of individuals with the deletion or non-deletion mechanism causing PWS in our study cohort (colored lines), alongside the normative percentile ranges of BMI growth (dashed gray lines).

3.3. Comparing the Average Rate of Growth between Genetic Subgroups

After exploring the average differences in measures between the genetic subgroups, LMMs with linear splines were used to estimate and compare the average rate of growth between the deletion and non-deletion individuals. Adjustment for year of birth had little to no impact on effect estimates and therefore the unadjusted results are presented here, to allow comparison with the previously estimated growth curves in Section 3.2. Estimates of the unadjusted difference in the average rate of growth are provided in Table 3 (see Table S2 for the adjusted estimates).

3.3.1. Height

The average rate of growth in height was similar for females less than 10 years of age, with the average difference in the rate of growth being relatively small across all ages (Table 3). For males with PWS, the non-deletion subgroup grew at a faster average rate than the deletion subgroup over the ages of 5 to 10 years (unadjusted difference in mean rate of growth = 1.4 cm/year, 95% CI: 0.3, −2.6, $p = 0.01$), aligning with visual observations from the estimated growth curves. However, for males older than 10 years, the deletion subgroup had a slightly quicker average rate of growth (age 10–15: 2.8 cm/year, 95% CI: 1.6, 3.9, $p < 0.01$; and age > 15: 1.8 cm/year, 95% CI: −0.3, 3.9, $p = 0.09$), contributing to similar estimates in mean height between the subgroups.

3.3.2. Weight

For younger females (less than 5 years old), the average rate of growth in weight was similar between the genetic subgroups. During the ages 5 to 10 years, the deletion individuals were growing at a faster rate than the non-deletion individuals, by an additional mean growth of 1.0 kg per year (95% CI: −0.1, 2.2, $p = 0.08$). However, after the age of 10, the non-deletion individuals had a substantially quicker mean rate of weight growth (1.6 kg/year for ages 10–15, and 1.9 kg/year for ages 15 and older).

This contributed to the difference in mean weight between the subtypes, reducing in older ages as observed from the estimated growth curve.

For males aged 10 years and younger, the average mean rate of weight growth was similar between the genetic subgroups. However, between the ages of 10 and 15 years, there was a substantially larger rate of growth for the deletion individuals, contributing to the larger mean weight in ages 10 years and above. During this age range, the weight for the deletion individuals was increasing, on average, 3.7 kg per year faster than the non-deletion individuals (95% CI: 2.3, 5.1, $p < 0.01$).

3.3.3. Body Mass Index (BMI)

The average rate of growth in BMI was relatively similar between the genetic subgroups (Table 3). This observation was consistent for both genders. There were some differences in the rate of growth from birth to age two, with the deletion individuals tending to grow at a faster rate than the non-deletion individuals (difference in mean rate of growth in females of 1.4 units/year and 1.1 units/year in males). These estimates were consistent with the growth trajectories observed in Figure 4, with the rate of growth in BMI being fairly consistent, particularly in older individuals.

4. Discussion

In this large longitudinal study of 125 individuals with PWS, with analysis using linear mixed models, has shown and described differences in growth patterns between deletion and non-deletion subtypes. The mean weight and BMI were estimated to be higher in the deletion subtype in both genders in this cohort, particularly over the age of 5 years. The mean height was similar in both subtypes for males, with the mean height in deletion females being higher than for non-deletion females over the age of 10 years. For females with PWS, the size of difference in mean weight and mean BMI was more pronounced over the age range of 5 to 15 years, while the difference in mean weight for males was more pronounced over the age of 10 years and fairly consistent over age for BMI. Furthermore, the rate of growth in weight was faster for the deletion subtype in males, particularly in the aforementioned age range (10 years and older). Consistent with published PWS growth charts [19,20], our results show that, compared to the general population, the heights of Australian PWS patients are mostly below the CDC 50th percentile, and weights and BMI are mostly above the CDC 75th percentile.

Our results are comparable to two previous studies of large PWS cohorts aged 16 years and older. Laurier et al. [28] studied 154 PWS adults aged 16–54 years and found a higher mean BMI in the deletion group compared to the non-deletion group (44 vs. 38.9 kg/m^2). Similarly, Coupaye et al. [29] studied 73 PWS adults aged 16–58 years and found that, compared to UPD patients, deletion patients had a higher mean weight (99.4 vs. 81.0 kg) and BMI (40.9 vs. 34.6 kg/m^2), but little difference in height. Two earlier studies did not observe a substantial difference in mean BMI between genetic subtypes [30,31]. Studies of neonates [32] and children and adolescents [33] with PWS have also not observed a substantial difference in anthropometric measures between genetic subgroups, suggesting that the differences may emerge with increasing age.

Collectively, these results suggest that deletion PWS patients are more prone to obesity with advancing age, although the underlying mechanisms are not clear. A detailed study of body composition and metabolic profile compared deletion and UPD subgroups but did not observe substantial differences in body fat, adipocyte size, insulin resistance, fasting total ghrelin level or resting energy expenditure, as measured by indirect calorimetry [29]. The examination of endocrine parameters also detected no difference between the two subgroups in GF-1 levels, cortisol levels or the frequency of hypogonadism, but hypothyroidism was more common in the deletion subgroup [29]. Two studies have also examined hyperphagia scores but did not observe a substantial difference in hyperphagia between the two subtypes [29,34]. Yet, it is possible that small differences in hyperphagia or metabolic measures could still lead to a substantial difference in BMI when acting over a timescale of many years. We hypothesize that the observed differences in BMI between the subtypes are most likely central in origin, and may be mediated through differences in gene expression in the brain and associated neurobehavioral phenotypes.

In comparison to the large cross-sectional studies of Laurier et al. [28] and Coupaye et al. [29], a strength of our study was the use of longitudinal growth data obtained from the VPWSR. As a result, a large proportion of individuals in our study cohort (95.2%) had multiple measures for each anthropometric outcome at varying ages, especially up to age 15. The repeated measures enabled us to control for the variability in the outcome measures of the specific individual, and explore the mean growth over a continuous range of ages. As discussed in the methods section, linear mixed models (LMMs) are a popular choice for modeling repeated measures, due to their ability to handle multiple measures on the same individual and robustness to an imbalance in repeated measures for different individuals in the sample. In addition, the use of a first-order continuous autoregressive correlation structure accommodated the within-subject correlations, assuming an individual's measures at closer ages were more correlated than measures at distant ages. The natural cubic B-spline models provided estimates of growth at varying ages for each genetic subgroup to generate growth curves, with the linear spline models providing estimates of differences in the average rate of growth across subtypes within age intervals. While the assumption of a linear trend under the linear spline model may be slightly simplistic, given that growth is rarely completely linear, the use of such models enabled an efficient estimate of a parameter with a clear and direct interpretation as the average difference between the mean rate of growth across genetic subtypes; an interpretation that is difficult to extract from the cubic B-spline model. Both modeling approaches were useful in addressing different aims, and providing a more detailed insight into the association between genetic subtype and anthropometric measure.

A limitation of this study is that we did not have data about potential confounders or mediators, including potential differences in diet, endocrine factors that are common in PWS [35], physical activity or the use of psychotropic medications. It is also possible that the use of growth hormones may differ between the subtypes, however, it is notable that in Australia, all children with genetically diagnosed PWS receive subsidized growth hormone treatment under the Pharmaceutical Benefit Scheme (PBS) until age 18, unless otherwise contraindicated [36], and without regard to genetic subtype. To account for the varying management of PWS over the years (e.g., growth hormones becoming publicly available in 2011 to those under 18 years of age), an adjustment for an individual's decade of birth was explored within our linear spline models, although the adjustment had little to no effect on the rate of growth estimates. However, this is essentially a proxy measure using the available data in our cohort and may be limited in completely accounting for the changing landscape of PWS management over the years, which could explain some of the differences between the subtypes observed. In addition, the cubic spline models did not include an adjustment for decade of birth and were used to solely estimate the unadjusted differences observed in our study cohort. Therefore, the estimated difference between subtypes using these models could be due to the deletion cohort being born earlier than the non-deletion cohort. However, based on the minimal effect of adjustment within the linear spline models, we suspect this adjustment would also have a minimal effect in the cubic spline models and the estimates of differences. It should also be noted that there is molecular heterogeneity within each of the subtypes, with the deletion subtype comprising class I and class 2 deletion patients and the non-deletion subtype comprising matUPD and imprinting defect patients, and there may be further differences within these categories that could only be determined by a larger study.

5. Conclusions

In summary, in this large sample, we have estimated higher mean weight and BMI in patients with the deletion subtype of PWS compared to patients with the non-deletion subtype. Height was similar for males in both PWS subtypes, with non-deletion females being shorter than deletion females for older ages. Furthermore, the average rate of growth in weight was faster for the deletion subtype in males, particularly in individuals over the age of 10 years. We hypothesize that these differences may stem from known neurobehavioral differences between the subtypes and subtype-specific differences in gene expression.

Supplementary Materials: The following are available online at http://www.mdpi.com/2073-4425/11/7/736/s1, Figure S1: Comparison of the variograms and residual plots for a LMM (random slope only), a LMM (random slope and random intercept and a LMM with AR(1) correlation structure when fitting growth models (with 4 knots) for height for the female deletion subgroup, Table S1: Comparison of the Akaike information criterion and Bayesian information criterion for a LMM (random slope only), a LMM (random slope and random intercept and a LMM with AR(1) correlation structure when fitting growth models for height for the female deletion subgroup, Table S2: Mean difference in rate of growth across age intervals between individuals with the deletion and non-deletion mechanism of PWS, estimated using linear mixed models with linear splines (adjusted for year of birth), with an interaction term between age and genetic subtype.

Author Contributions: Conceptualization, D.J.A., N.V. and D.E.G.; Data curation, S.M.R.; Formal analysis, D.A.S.; Methodology, D.AS. and M.M.-B.; Project administration, D.J.A.; Resources, S.M.R. and A.G.; Supervision, D.E.G., M.M.-B. and D.J.A.; Writing–original draft, D.A.S. and D.J.A.; Writing–review and editing, N.V., S.M.R., D.E.G., A.G., M.M.-B. and D.J.A. All authors have read and agreed to the published version of the manuscript.

Funding: This study was supported by the Victorian Government's Operational Infrastructure Support Program, with the salaries supported by the Next Generation Clinical Researchers Program – Career Development Fellowship, funded by the Medical Research Future Fund (MRF1141334 to D.E.G.). Margarita Moreno-Betancur is the recipient of an Australian Research Council Discovery Early Career Award (project number DE190101326) funded by the Australian Government. The Victorian Prader–Willi Syndrome Register is supported by the Do-Bees and Trailblazers Auxiliaries of the Royal Children's Hospital Foundation.

Conflicts of Interest: The authors declare no conflict of interest.

References

1. Cassidy, S.B.; Schwartz, S.; Miller, J.L.; Driscoll, D.J. Prader-Willi syndrome. *Genet. Med.* **2012**, *14*, 10–26. [CrossRef] [PubMed]

2. Butler, M.G. Prader-Willi syndrome: Current understanding of cause and diagnosis. *Am. J. Med. Genet.* **1990**, *35*, 319–332. [CrossRef] [PubMed]

3. Butler, M.G. Management of obesity in Prader-Willi syndrome. *Nat. Clin. Pract. Endocrinol. Metab.* **2006**, *2*, 592–593. [CrossRef] [PubMed]

4. Lionti, T.; Reid, S.M.; Rowell, M.M. Prader-Willi syndrome in Victoria: Mortality and causes of death. *J. Paediatr. Child Health* **2012**, *48*, 506–511. [CrossRef]

5. Butler, M.G.; Miller, J.L.; Forster, J.L. Prader-Willi syndrome—Clinical genetics, diagnosis and treatment approaches: An update. *Curr. Pediatr. Rev.* **2019**, *15*, 207–244. [CrossRef]

6. Lionti, T.; Reid, S.M.; White, S.M.; Rowell, M.M. A population-based profile of 160 Australians with Prader-Willi syndrome: Trends in diagnosis, birth prevalence and birth characteristics. *Am. J. Med. Genet. A* **2015**, *167A*, 371–378. [CrossRef]

7. Butler, M.G.; Bittel, D.C.; Kibiryeva, N.; Talebizadeh, Z.; Thompson, T. Behavioral differences among subjects with Prader-Willi syndrome and type I or type II deletion and maternal disomy. *Pediatrics* **2004**, *113*, 565–573. [CrossRef]

8. Milner, K.M.; Craig, E.E.; Thompson, R.J.; Veltman, M.W.; Thomas, N.S.; Roberts, S.; Bellamy, M.; Curran, S.R.; Sporikou, C.M.; Bolton, P.F. Prader-Willi syndrome: Intellectual abilities and behavioural features by genetic subtype. *J. Child Psychol. Psychiatry* **2005**, *46*, 1089–1096. [CrossRef]

9. Roof, E.; Stone, W.; MacLean, W.; Feurer, I.D.; Thompson, T.; Butler, M.G. Intellectual characteristics of Prader-Willi syndrome: Comparison of genetic subtypes. *J. Intellect. Disabil. Res.* **2000**, *44 Pt 1*, 25–30. [CrossRef]

10. Torrado, M.; Araoz, V.; Baialardo, E.; Abraldes, K.; Mazza, C.; Krochik, G.; Ozuna, B.; Leske, V.; Caino, S.; Fano, V.; et al. Clinical-etiologic correlation in children with Prader-Willi syndrome (PWS): An interdisciplinary study. *Am. J. Med. Genet. A* **2007**, *143A*, 460–468. [CrossRef]

11. Whittington, J.; Holland, A.; Webb, T.; Butler, J.; Clarke, D.; Boer, H. Cognitive abilities and genotype in a population-based sample of people with Prader-Willi syndrome. *J. Intellect. Disabil. Res.* **2004**, *48*, 172–187. [CrossRef] [PubMed]

12. Yang, L.; Zhan, G.D.; Ding, J.J.; Wang, H.J.; Ma, D.; Huang, G.Y.; Zhou, W.H. Psychiatric illness and intellectual disability in the Prader-Willi syndrome with different molecular defects—A meta analysis. *PLoS ONE* **2013**, *8*, e72640. [CrossRef] [PubMed]

13. Descheemaeker, M.J.; Govers, V.; Vermeulen, P.; Fryns, J.P. Pervasive developmental disorders in Prader-Willi syndrome: The Leuven experience in 59 subjects and controls. *Am. J. Med. Genet. A* **2006**, *140*, 1136–1142. [CrossRef] [PubMed]

14. Veltman, M.W.; Craig, E.E.; Bolton, P.F. Autism spectrum disorders in Prader-Willi and Angelman syndromes: A systematic review. *Psychiatr. Genet.* **2005**, *15*, 243–254. [CrossRef] [PubMed]

15. Soni, S.; Whittington, J.; Holland, A.J.; Webb, T.; Maina, E.; Boer, H.; Clarke, D. The course and outcome of psychiatric illness in people with Prader-Willi syndrome: Implications for management and treatment. *J. Intellect. Disabil. Res.* **2007**, *51*, 32–42. [CrossRef] [PubMed]

16. Holland, A.J.; Whittington, J.E.; Butler, J.; Webb, T.; Boer, H.; Clarke, D. Behavioural phenotypes associated with specific genetic disorders: Evidence from a population-based study of people with Prader-Willi syndrome. *Psychol. Med.* **2003**, *33*, 141–153. [CrossRef]

17. Spritz, R.A.; Bailin, T.; Nicholls, R.D.; Lee, S.T.; Park, S.K.; Mascari, M.J.; Butler, M.G. Hypopigmentation in the Prader-Willi syndrome correlates with P gene deletion but not with haplotype of the hemizygous P allele. *Am. J. Med. Genet.* **1997**, *71*, 57–62. [CrossRef]

18. Gardner, R.J.M.; Amor, D.J. *Chromosome Abnormalities and Genetic Counseling*, 5th ed.; Oxford Monographs on Medical Genetics; Oxford University Press: New York, NY, USA, 2018.

19. Butler, M.G.; Lee, J.; Cox, D.M.; Manzardo, A.M.; Gold, J.A.; Miller, J.L.; Roof, E.; Dykens, E.; Kimonis, V.; Driscoll, D.J. Growth charts for Prader-Willi syndrome during growth hormone treatment. *Clin. Pediatr.* **2016**, *55*, 957–974. [CrossRef]

20. Butler, M.G.; Lee, J.; Manzardo, A.M.; Gold, J.A.; Miller, J.L.; Kimonis, V.; Driscoll, D.J. Growth charts for non-growth hormone treated Prader-Willi syndrome. *Pediatrics* **2015**, *135*, e126–e135. [CrossRef]

21. Grajeda, L.M.; Ivanescu, A.; Saito, M.; Crainiceanu, C.; Jaganath, D.; Gilman, R.H.; Crabtree, J.E.; Kelleher, D.; Cabrera, L.; Cama, V.; et al. Modelling subject-specific childhood growth using linear mixed-effect models with cubic regression splines. *Emerg. Themes Epidemiol.* **2016**, *13*, 1. [CrossRef]

22. Hastie, T.; Tibshirani, R.; Friedman, J. *The Elements of Statistical Learning, Data Mining, Inference and Prediction*; Springer: New York, NY, USA, 2001.

23. Centres for Disease Control and Prevention. *CDC Growth Charts*; Centers for Disease Control and Prevention, National Center for Health Statistics: Atlanta, GA, USA, 2010.

24. R Core Team. *R: A Language and Environment for Statistical Computing*; R Foundation for Statistical Computing: Vienna, Austria, 2017.

25. Bates, D.; Machler, M.; Bolker, B.; Walker, S. Fitting Linear Mixed-Effects Models using lme4. *J. Stat. Softw.* **2015**, *67*, 1–48. [CrossRef]

26. Pinheiro, J.; Bates, D.; DebRoy, S.; Sarkar, D.; R Development Core Team. *nlme: Linear and Nonlinear Mixed Effects Models. R Package*; R Foundation for Statistical Computing: Vienna, Austria, 2013.

27. Wickham, H. *ggplot2: Elegant Graphics for Data Analysis*; Springer: New York, NY, USA, 2009.

28. Laurier, V.; Lapeyrade, A.; Copet, P.; Demeer, G.; Silvie, M.; Bieth, E.; Coupaye, M.; Poitou, C.; Lorenzini, F.; Labrousse, F.; et al. Medical, psychological and social features in a large cohort of adults with Prader-Willi syndrome: Experience from a dedicated centre in France. *J. Intellect. Disabil. Res.* **2015**, *59*, 411–421. [CrossRef] [PubMed]

29. Coupaye, M.; Tauber, M.; Cuisset, L.; Laurier, V.; Bieth, E.; Lacorte, J.M.; Oppert, J.M.; Clement, K.; Poitou, C. Effect of genotype and previous GH treatment on adiposity in adults with Prader-Willi syndrome. *J. Clin. Endocrinol. Metab.* **2016**, *101*, 4895–4903. [CrossRef] [PubMed]

30. Kennedy, L.; Bittel, D.C.; Kibiryeva, N.; Kalra, S.P.; Torto, R.; Butler, M.G. Circulating adiponectin levels, body composition and obesity-related variables in Prader-Willi syndrome: Comparison with obese subjects. *Int. J. Obes.* **2006**, *30*, 382–387. [CrossRef] [PubMed]

31. Theodoro, M.F.; Talebizadeh, Z.; Butler, M.G. Body composition and fatness patterns in Prader-Willi syndrome: Comparison with simple obesity. *Obesity* **2006**, *14*, 1685–1690. [CrossRef] [PubMed]

32. Butler, M.G.; Sturich, J.; Myers, S.E.; Gold, J.A.; Kimonis, V.; Driscoll, D.J. Is gestation in Prader-Willi syndrome affected by the genetic subtype? *J. Assist. Reprod. Genet.* **2009**, *26*, 461–466. [CrossRef]

33. Varela, M.C.; Kok, F.; Setian, N.; Kim, C.A.; Koiffmann, C.P. Impact of molecular mechanisms, including deletion size, on Prader-Willi syndrome phenotype: Study of 75 patients. *Clin. Genet.* **2005**, *67*, 47–52. [CrossRef]

34. Dykens, E.M.; Maxwell, M.A.; Pantino, E.; Kossler, R.; Roof, E. Assessment of hyperphagia in Prader-Willi syndrome. *Obesity* **2007**, *15*, 1816–1826. [CrossRef] [PubMed]

35. Muscogiuri, G.; Formoso, G.; Pugliese, G.; Ruggeri, R.M.; Scarano, E.; Colao, A. Prader-Willi syndrome: An uptodate on endocrine and metabolic complications. *Rev. Endocr. Metab. Disord.* **2019**, *20*, 239–250. [CrossRef]

36. Scheermeyer, E.; Hughes, I.; Harris, M.; Ambler, G.; Crock, P.; Verge, C.F.; Craig, M.E.; Bergman, P.; Werther, G.; van Driel, M.; et al. Response to growth hormone treatment in Prader-Willi syndrome: Auxological criteria versus genetic diagnosis. *J. Paediatr. Child Health* **2013**, *49*, 1045–1051. [CrossRef]

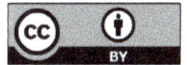 © 2020 by the authors. Licensee MDPI, Basel, Switzerland. This article is an open access article distributed under the terms and conditions of the Creative Commons Attribution (CC BY) license (http://creativecommons.org/licenses/by/4.0/).

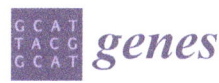

Article

The Gut Microbiota Profile in Children with Prader–Willi Syndrome

Ye Peng [1,†], Qiming Tan [2,†], Shima Afhami [3], Edward C. Deehan [3], Suisha Liang [1], Marie Gantz [4], Lucila Triador [2], Karen L. Madsen [5], Jens Walter [3,6,7], Hein M. Tun [1,*] and Andrea M. Haqq [2,3,*]

1   HKU-Pasteur Research Pole, School of Public Health, University of Hong Kong, Hong Kong 999077, China; pengye@connect.hku.hk (Y.P.); suishal@connect.hku.hk (S.L.)
2   Department of Pediatrics, University of Alberta, Edmonton, AB T6G 2R3, Canada; qtan3@ualberta.ca (Q.T.); triador@ualberta.ca (L.T.)
3   Department of Agricultural Food & Nutritional Science, University of Alberta, Edmonton, AB T6G 2R3, Canada; afhami@ualberta.ca (S.A.); deehan@ualberta.ca (E.C.D.); jwalter1@ualberta.ca (J.W.)
4   Biostatistics & Epidemiology Division, RTI International, Durham, DC 27709, USA; mgantz@rti.org
5   Department of Medicine, University of Alberta, Edmonton, AB T6G 2R3, Canada; kmadsen@ualberta.ca
6   Department of Biological Sciences, University of Alberta, Edmonton, AB T6G 2R3, Canada
7   APC Microbiome Ireland, School of Microbiology, and Department of Medicine, University College Cork–National University of Ireland, T12 YN60 Cork, Ireland
*   Correspondence: heinmtun@hku.hk (H.M.T.); haqq@ualberta.ca (A.M.H.)
†   These authors contributed equally to this work.

Received: 18 July 2020; Accepted: 5 August 2020; Published: 7 August 2020

Abstract: Although gut microbiota has been suggested to play a role in disease phenotypes of Prader–Willi syndrome (PWS), little is known about its composition in affected children and how it relates to hyperphagia. This cross-sectional study aimed to characterize the gut bacterial and fungal communities of children with PWS, and to determine associations with hyperphagia. Fecal samples were collected from 25 children with PWS and 25 age-, sex-, and body mass index-matched controls. Dietary intake data, hyperphagia scores, and relevant clinical information were also obtained. Fecal bacterial and fungal communities were characterized by 16S rRNA and ITS2 sequencing, respectively. Overall bacterial α-diversity and compositions of PWS were not different from those of the controls, but 13 bacterial genera were identified to be differentially abundant. Interestingly, the fungal community, as well as specific genera, were different between PWS and controls. The majority of the variation in the gut microbiota was not attributed to differences in dietary intake or the impact of genotype. Hyperphagia scores were associated with fungal α-diversity and relative abundance of several taxa, such as *Staphylococcus*, *Clostridium*, *SMB53*, and *Candida*. Further longitudinal studies correlating changes in the microbiome with the degree of hyperphagia and studies integrating multi-omics data are warranted.

Keywords: Prader–Willi syndrome; gut microbiota; bacteria; fungi; diet; hyperphagia; obesity; cross-sectional

---

1. Introduction

Prader–Willi syndrome (PWS) is a complex genetic disorder known as the most common syndromic cause of childhood obesity. It is caused by the lack of expression of paternal alleles in 15q11-13, with an incidence of 1 in 10,000 to 15,000 live births worldwide [1,2]. Three common forms of PWS are deletion (65–75%), maternal uniparental disomy (UPD; 20–30%), and imprinting defects (ID; 1–3%) [3]. Affected children typically experience excessive and rapid weight gain between 12 months and 6 years of age, which coincides with an onset of hyperphagia (abnormally increased appetite). Hyperphagia is a critical diagnostic feature of PWS, characterized by a deficit in satiety, food preoccupations, and problematic food-seeking behaviors [4]. Patients with PWS are at elevated risk of developing morbid obesity and associated life-threatening complications, unless eating is externally controlled. Although symptom severity varies, hyperphagia generally requires individuals to have a restricted lifestyle with constant supervision, which hinders their independence and significantly affects the quality of life of these patients, as well as their families [5].

Recent studies suggest that PWS-associated obesity is accompanied by alterations in the gut microbiota, offering new insights into the pathophysiology of obesity in patients with PWS. Zhang et al. were the first to demonstrate that children with PWS-associated obesity (n = 17) and those with idiopathic obesity (n = 21) shared similar dysbiotic gut microbiota features, characterized by a higher diversity and abundance of toxin-producing and potentially pathogenic bacteria, compared to lean controls [6]. In addition, the colonization of germ-free mice with a microbial community from a subject with PWS transferred some aspects of the obesity phenotype, such as higher inflammation and larger adipocytes. The authors concluded that the gut microbiota may play an important role in inducing and promoting obesity and metabolic complications in PWS, and hence could be a potential therapeutic target. Moreover, work from Olsson et al. recently showed that, compared to obese controls, the fecal microbiota of adults with PWS-associated obesity was characterized by higher phylogenetic diversity, and was associated with markers of insulin sensitivity [7]. In addition, the gut microbial communities in patients with PWS were more similar to their non-PWS parents than those of obese controls [7].

Characterization of the gut microbiota in individuals with PWS is an important initial step in understanding the role of the microbiome in the course and outcome of hyperphagia, obesity, and metabolic deterioration in PWS. The only two observational studies characterizing the gut microbiome in PWS have reported inconsistent findings, which may be attribuTable to the differences in age and ethnicity of their subjects and in the specific control groups included. Additionally, no studies have yet assessed the gut microbiota profile of PWS in childhood populations in North America. Although fungi have been shown to be implicated in health and diseases, including metabolic disorders [8], differences in the fungal community between individuals with and without PWS have not been assessed at all. Furthermore, little is known about whether gut microbiota in overweight or obese (OWOB) subjects are distinct from those in normal weight (NW) subjects within the PWS population. To gain insight into the potential links between the microbiome and clinical manifestations of PWS, additional investigations are needed to define the microbial signatures specific to PWS, as well as to the OWOB within PWS. In this study, we profiled the fecal microbiota in children with PWS and compared it to that of healthy matched controls, while also assessing for associations between microbial composition and hyperphagic symptoms. As hyperphagia in PWS likely results in nutrient intake differences between PWS and controls, we further investigated the relationship between diet and fecal microbial composition.

2. Materials and Methods

2.1. Subjects

This cross-sectional study was completed in Edmonton, Alberta, Canada, from February 2017 to July 2018, and was approved by the University of Alberta's Research Ethics Boards (Pro00069925). A prior written/verbal informed consent was obtained from the children and their parents or legal guardians to participate in the study. Children with genetically confirmed PWS (n = 25; aged 3–17 years) were recruited from the Pediatric Endocrine Clinic at the Stollery Children's Hospital, as well as remotely through collaboration with the Foundation for Prader–Willi Research (Canada/United States) and the PWS Association (United States). Controls (CON) (n = 25) included age-, sex-, and body mass index (BMI) z-score-matched participants, who were recruited by advertising on bulletin boards and via e-mail distribution lists at the University of Alberta. We collected a fecal sample and data on hyperphagia, dietary intake, and anthropometric measurements. Additional parent-reported information including gestational age, delivery mode, and infant feeding methods; use of probiotics and proton pump inhibitors, as well as medication was also collected. Exclusion criteria were (a) a pre-existing condition that could affect body weight; (b) use of antibiotics 30 days prior to study, or (c) administration of pre/probiotic supplements or antibiotics. Growth hormone therapy was permitted, as this treatment is commonly used in patients with PWS to counteract their endogenous deficiency of growth hormone.

2.2. Assessments

Hyperphagia was assessed using the Hyperphagia Questionnaire, a multi-item, provider-reported instrument widely used in clinical practice that has been specifically designed and validated to capture hyperphagic symptoms in PWS [9]. Each item was rated on a five-point scale (1 = not a problem to 5 = severe and/or frequent problem). The scores were calculated by summing the following items: behavior (items 2, 4, 5, 8, 10); drive (items 1, 3, 6, 9); severity (items 7, 11); and total (items 1 to 11) scores (see example questionnaire in Appendix A).

Dietary intake was assessed using a three-day dietary record; children and parents were asked to provide detailed information on the food and beverages consumed by the children over two non-consecutive weekdays and one weekend day. Analysis of dietary data was performed using Food Processor SQL (Version 11.4, ESHA Research Inc., Salem, OR, USA). Daily intake of energy and macronutrients (carbohydrates, protein, lipids, sugar, dietary fiber, sat/unsaturated fat, and cholesterol) was estimated. For correlation analyses, nutrient intakes were adjusted for total daily energy intake using the nutrient residual method [10].

Weight, height, and waist circumference (WC) were measured following standardized procedures described by the National Health and Nutrition Examination Survey Anthropometry Procedures Manual [11]. Weight was measured to the nearest 0.1 kg using an electronic weighing scale. Height was measured to the nearest 0.1 cm using a wall-mounted stadiometer. WC was recorded to the nearest 0.1 cm with a non-stretch measuring tape between the bottom of the lower rib and the iliac crest. BMI-for-age percentile (BMI %ile) and BMI z-scores were calculated and classified according to the World Health Organization BMI-for-age growth standards (for 5–19 years) [12]. Normal weight was defined as a BMI z-score ≤ 1 SD, while overweight was defined as >1 to ≤2 SD, and obesity as > 2 SD.

2.3. Fecal Sample Collection, DNA Sequencing, and Microbiome Analysis

Subjects were provided with OMNIgene·GUT kits (DNA Genotek, Inc., Ottawa, CA, USA) and instructed to collect feces at home, and send the sample through expedited mail delivery service on the day of collection. In OMNIgene·GUT kits, samples were diluted in a proprietary solution, which has been previously shown to keep microbial DNA stable [13]. Within 24 h of receipt, fecal slurries were aliquoted and immediately frozen at −80 °C until being sent to Microbiome Insights Inc. (Vancouver, BC, Canada) for sequencing. DNA was extracted from the fecal homogenates using the PowerMag Soil DNA Isolation Kit (MoBio Laboratories, Carlsbad, CA, USA) per manufacturer's protocol. PCR amplification of the bacterial 16S rRNA gene targeting the V3–V4 region and the fungal ITS2 gene was performed with dual-barcoded primers, as previously described [14]. Amplicons were sequenced with an Illumina MiSeq using the 300 bp paired-end kit (v.3). Sequences were deposited at the European Nucleotide Archive under PRJEB34398 (16S data) and PRJEB34790 (ITS2 data). Sequences were denoised and taxonomically classified, using Greengenes (v. 13_8) as the reference database. Sequences were clustered into operational taxonomic units (OTUs) using Mothur v. 1.39.5 [15], following the recommended procedure that are illustrated on the mothur website (https://mothur.org/wiki/miseq_sop/) [15].

The potential for contamination was addressed by co-sequencing DNA amplified from specimens, and from four each of template-free controls and extraction kit reagents, processed the same way as the specimens. Two positive controls consisting of cloned SUP05 DNA were also included (number of copies = 2×10^6). Operational taxonomic units were considered putative contaminants (and were removed) if their mean abundance in controls reached or exceeded 25% of their mean abundance in specimens. In addition, OTUs that had fewer than three occurrences (counts) in 10% of the samples were considered noise, and were removed prior to statistical analysis.

2.4. Statistical Analyses

The significance of differences in dietary intake and diversity between PWS and CON, as well as between the subgroups (i.e., OWOB PWS vs. NW PWS, OWOB CON vs. NW CON, OWOB PWS vs. OWOB CON, and NW PWS vs. NW CON) were tested using a two-sided Wilcoxon test, using the *wilcox.test* function in R package stats v3.5.1 and Dunn's tests in R package *dunn.test* v1.3.5 with Bonferroni correction, respectively. To assess α-diversity, the Shannon, Simpson, and Chao1 indices were calculated for the overall bacterial community, as well as for major bacterial and fungal phylum using the diversity function in R package vegan v2.5-6 and the chao1 function in R package fossil v0.3.7, respectively. Inter-subject β-diversity, represented by Bray–Curtis, distance-based dissimilarity, was calculated for both the bacterial and the fungal communities using the *vegdist* function in R package vegan v2.5-6. Permutational multivariate analysis of variance (PERMANOVA) was used to assess differences in community structure, with group as the main fixed factor and with 9999 permutations for significance testing, using the *adonis* function in R package vegan. Canonical correspondence analysis (CCA) using the *cca* function with the *envfit* function in R package vegan (999 permutations) was used to assess the association between subject characteristics and dissimilarity between the microbial communities mentioned above, using OTU-level data.

Linear discriminant analysis effect size (LEfSe; https://huttenhower.sph.harvard.edu/galaxy/) was determined, in order to identify differentially abundant bacterial and fungal genera between PWS and CON, as well as between the two subgroups within PWS and CON (i.e., OWOB PWS vs. NW PWS, and OWOB CON vs. NW CON); *p*-values < 0.05 were considered statistically significant for the first step (Wilcoxon tests), while Linear Discriminant Analysis (LDA) minimal threshold was set at 2. as previously described [16]. Additionally, the random forest algorithm provided in *RandomForestClassifier* of the Python module *sklearn.ensemble* was used to construct a classification model using genus-level relative abundance data. The original model was built by including all bacterial or fungal genera, with variance in the stratified samples. Following that, genera with a Gini importance greater than or equal to the 90% quantile in each original model were selected to construct the final model, of which performance of classification was assessed using 5-fold cross-validation.

For genera with occurrence frequency greater than 50% among all subjects, Spearman's correlations were calculated using the *cor.test* function in R package stats v3.5.1, in order to assess associations between diversity indices and taxa abundance with dietary intakes in the whole dataset, and hyperphagia scores in both the whole dataset and within the PWS group. The *p*-values were corrected for multiple testing using the Bonferroni method, and resulting *q*-values of less than 0.1 were regarded as statistically significant. Binary logistic regression models in SPSS were used to investigate the associations between adjusted dietary carbohydrate intake (adj-CHO) and hyperphagia scores, and abundances of the marker taxa were detected by random forest classifiers while adjusting for the group and its interaction. In the models, adj-CHO values, hyperphagia scores, and the microbial abundances were dichotomized into "above-the-median" and "below-the-median".

In addition, Spearman's correlations calculated using the *cor.test* function in R package *stats* v3.5.1 were also used to construct bacterial–fungal inter-kingdom networks for microbial families with occurrence frequency greater than 50% in each subgroup. All taxon pairs with Spearman's Rho ≥ 0.3 or ≤ −0.3 with *p*-values < 0.05 were visualized using Cytoscape [17].

3. Results

Next-generation sequencing of PCR-generated amplicons of the V3–V4 region of bacterial 16S rRNA gene and fungal ITS2 gene resulted in an average of 57,133 and 5732 quality-filtered reads per sample, respectively. Samples for the ITS2 gene containing fewer than 1000 sequences were excluded from downstream analyses (six from PWS, seven from CON). After quality control, a total of 2498 bacterial OTUs and 255 fungal OTUs were identified in the samples. These OTUs were annotated and assigned taxonomy ranging from phylum to species.

3.1. Gut Bacterial Communities in PWS

No significant difference was observed between PWS and CON, or between the subgroups for overall bacterial α-diversity (Supplementary Table S1). However, more targeted analyses within bacterial phyla showed higher Chao1 richness of *Actinobacteria* in PWS compared to CON, as well as in NW PWS when compared to NW CON. In addition, fecal samples from subjects with PWS displayed a lower α-diversity of *Proteobacteria* than healthy controls assessed by the Shannon and Simpson indices, which both estimate species richness and evenness with the Shannon index giving more weight on evenness and the Simpson index on richness, respectively [18]. Between OWOB subgroups, the Simpson index of *Proteobacteria* was lower in PWS OWOB than in the matched CON (Supplementary Table S1).

PERMANOVA showed no significant difference in the overall bacterial community structure between PWS and CON subjects ($p = 0.389$, Figure 1A). CCA results suggest potential association between weight ($p = 0.016$), sex ($p = 0.001$), age ($p = 0.004$), and calorie-adjusted dietary factors (fiber ($p = 0.008$), protein ($p = 0.017$), cholesterol ($p = 0.001$), and sugar ($p = 0.040$)) and bacterial community structure (Figure 1C). There were no significant differences of the overall bacterial community structure between the genetic subtypes of PWS (deletion versus UPD form ($p > 0.05$)).

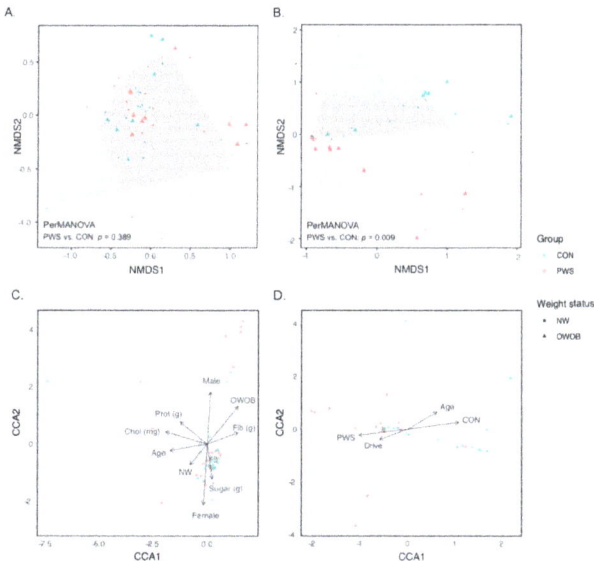

Figure 1. Phylum-level relative abundance in bacterial communities (**A**) and fungal communities (**B**). Linkages between the microbial community and environmental variables. The first two axes of the canonical correspondence analysis (CCA) display bacterial (**C**) and fungal (**D**) community (dots) and phenotypes (arrows) with significant linkage ($p < 0.05$). PWS: Prader–Willi syndrome; CON: control. Arrows show the level and direction of impact of significant factors.

3.2. Gut Fungal Communities in PWS

The α-diversity of fungal communities between PWS and CON and between the subgroups was not different. However, within the phylum *Basidiomycota*, the Shannon index suggests higher species diversity for children in the OWOB PWS group than those in the OWOB CON group (Supplementary Table S1). Interestingly, the fungal communities of PWS subjects were significantly different from those of the match CON ($p = 0.009$, PERMANOVA, Figure 1B). PWS ($p = 0.001$), age ($p = 0.002$), and hyperphagic drive score ($p = 0.012$) might be factors associated with the observed differences (CCA, Figure 1D), whereas we did not find any association between body weight and fungal community ($p > 0.05$). No significant differences of the overall fungal community structure were found between the genetic subtypes of PWS (deletion versus UPD form ($p > 0.05$)).

3.3. Abundance of Certain Taxa Is Associated with PWS

LEfSe identified differentially abundant bacterial taxa between PWS and CON, and also between the subgroups in PWS. The genus *Prevotella* showed a higher abundance in children with PWS, whereas *Oscillospira* and unclassified *Enterobacteriaceae* genera were more abundant in healthy controls (Figure 2A). Within PWS, the genera *Sutterella* and *Clostridium* were more abundant in OWOB, while higher abundance of *Turicibacter* and unclassified *Barnesiellaceae* were observed in NW subjects (Figure 2C). Among the fungal taxa, the genera *Candida*, *Mrakia*, and unclassified *Agaricomycetes* and *Basidiomycota* were in higher abundance in PWS compared with CON; whereas CON showed higher fecal abundances of *Saccharomyces* (Figure 2B). Within PWS, unclassified *Basidiomycota* was more abundant in OWOB compared to NW (Figure 2D).

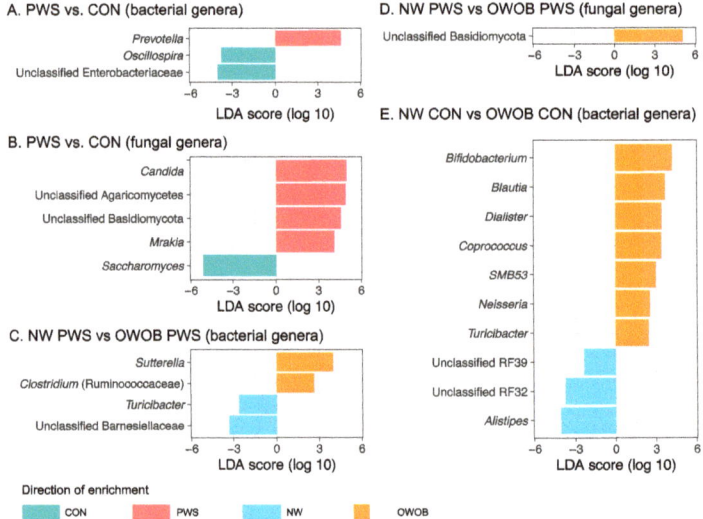

Figure 2. Discriminative features in the linear discriminant analysis effect size (LEfSe) analysis. (**A**) Discriminative bacterial genera in PWS vs. CON. (**B**) Discriminative fungal genera in PWS vs CON. (**C**) Discriminative bacterial genera in NW PWS vs. OWOB PWS groups. (**D**) Discriminative fungal genera in NW PWS vs. OWOB PWS groups. (**E**) Discriminative bacterial genera in NW CON vs. OWOB CON groups. PWS: Prader–Willi syndrome; CON: control. NW: normal weight; OWOB: overweight or obese.

We also constructed random forest classifiers to further identify taxa discriminating PWS from CON (Supplementary Figures S1–S10). All final models showed high discriminatory power, as indicated by an area under the receiver operating characteristic curve of ≥0.80 (Supplementary Figures S8–S10). The algorithm detected 13 bacterial genera, with only four of them belonging to the same genera, identified by the differential analyses above. The additional OTUs identified by this method were related to *Staphylococcus*, *Propionibacterium*, *Akkermansia*, *Haemophilus*, unclassified *RF39* and *Christensenellaceae*, *Anaerostipes*, *Dorea*, and *SMB53* (Figures 2A and 3A). Conversely, most of the selected fungal taxa (*Mrakia*, *Candida*, *Saccharomyces*, and unclassified *Agaricomycetes* and *Basidiomycota*) in the model were previously identified by LEfSe, except for the unclassified *Ascomycota* (Figures 2B and 3B). The differential abundances of both bacterial and fungal genera under the different random forest models tested are summarized in Supplementary Table S2.

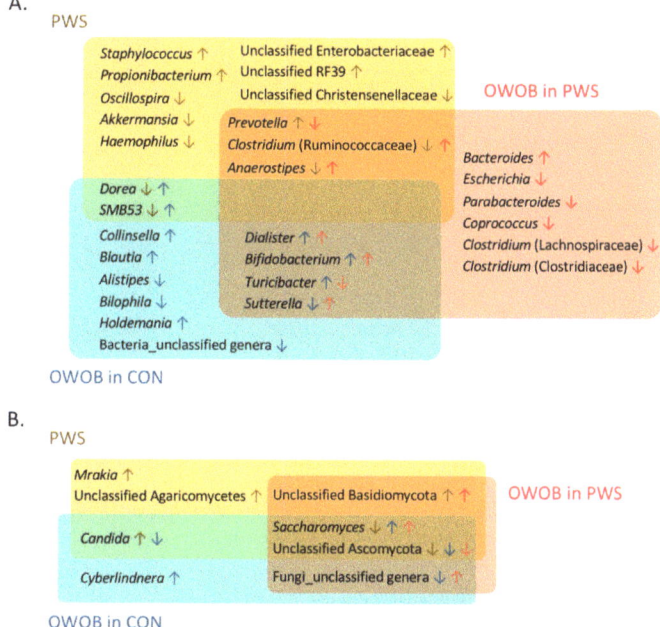

Figure 3. Overlap of differentially abundant bacterial (**A**) and fungal (**B**) taxa detected in Random Forest models for the PWS, OWOB PWS, and OWOB CON groups. PWS: Prader–Willi syndrome; CON: control; NW: normal weight; OWOB: overweight or obese. Upwards arrows indicate higher abundance, whereas downwards arrows indicate lower abundance than the reference group(s) (PWS vs. CON; OWOB in CON vs. NW in CON; OWOB in PWS vs. NW in CON).

3.4. Gut Microbiota and Dietary Carbohydrate Intake in the Whole Dataset

Sugar intake was found to be positively associated with the relative abundance of an unclassified *Christensenellaceae* (Spearman's Rho (ρ) = 0.44, *q*-value = 0.071) and bacterial α-diversity (Shannon index: ρ = 0.38, *q*-value = 0.020; and Simpson index: ρ = 0.37, *q*-value = 0.027; Supplementary Figure S11A,B). Dietary fiber intake was negatively correlated with the relative abundance of *Saccharomyces* (ρ = 0.40, *q*-value = 0.055) and fungal Shannon diversity (ρ = −0.44, *q*-value = 0.023; Supplementary Figure S11C,D). In addition, carbohydrate intake (CHO) was positively associated with the relative abundance of *Saccharomyces* (ρ = 0.45, *q*-value = 0.021; Supplementary Figure S11B), while also positively associated with bacterial Shannon diversity (ρ = 0.32, *q*-value = 0.066; Supplementary Figure S11B).

Dietary analysis showed no significant differences in dietary protein and fat intakes between PWS and CON ($p > 0.05$), whereas CHO was significantly lower in PWS compared to CON ($p = 0.002$; Table 1). We used logistic regression models to investigate whether differential abundances of the taxa between PWS and CON detected by the random forest models were associated with differences in adjusted dietary CHO (adj-CHO), while adjusting for the group and their interaction (adj-CHO * group). We found that a lower abundance of unclassified *Christensenellaceae* was significantly associated with lower adj-CHO intake (adjusted odds ratio = 0.14 (95% CI: 0.02–0.94); p = 0.043), but was not associated with the group (adjusted odds ratio = 0.61 (95% CI, 0.09–4.02); p = 0.608). In addition, there was no significant association between the interaction of adj-CHO or PWS and any taxon (Supplementary Table S4).

Table 1. Participant Characteristics.

	PWS (*n* = 25)	CON (*n* = 25)	*p*-Values
Sex (F/M)	14/11	9/16	0.256
Age (years)	6.2 (5.2, 12.9)	8.8 (6.3, 10.5)	0.455
BMI %ile	79.3 (65.5, 94.1)	76.6 (51.2, 91.5)	0.655
Weight status (OWOB/NW)	10/15	8/17	0.769
Hyperphagia scores **	19 (16, 26)	15 (14, 18)	0.014 *
Protein (g)	71 (65, 76)	64 (56, 73)	0.071
Carbohydrate (g)	189 (149, 206.3)	225 (193, 240)	0.002 *
Sugar (g)	198 (179, 212)	203 (184, 224)	0.441
Dietary fiber (g)	19 (16, 23)	17 (14, 21)	0.168
Fat (g)	204 (184, 211)	202 (196, 209)	0.848
SatFat (g)	195 (192, 203)	198 (195, 204)	0.147
UnSatFat (g)	376 (368, 390)	373 (362, 388)	0.386
Cholesterol (mg)	179 (107, 306)	163 (109, 267)	0.848

F: female; M: male; PWS: Prader–Willi syndrome; BMI %ile: body mass index-for-age percentile; OWOB: overweight or obese; NW: normal weight. Data presented as Median (25th and 75th percentiles). Comparison between the CON and PWS groups—continuous data: Wilcoxon test (two-sided); categorical data: Fisher's exact test. * $p < 0.05$. ** Score ranging from 12 to 39 for the PWS group and from 12 to 25 for the control group (minimum possible score for the hyperphagia questionnaire is 11/55).

3.5. Gut Microbiota and Hyperphagia in PWS

Since PWS is characterized by hyperphagia, we also explored associations using Spearman's correlations between hyperphagic symptoms and fecal microbiota composition. In the whole study dataset, no significant correlations were observed between hyperphagia and bacterial features ($q > 0.1$). However, severity scores were negatively correlated with unclassified *Ascomycota* ($\rho = -0.47$, q-value = 0.015), while behavior scores were correlated with an unclassified fungal taxon ($\rho = -0.45$, q-value = 0.023; Figure 4A). Furthermore, the behavior score was positively associated with fungal Simpson diversity ($\rho = 0.42$, q-value = 0.029; Figure 4B). When further investigating the correlations within the PWS group, the relative abundance of the unclassified fungi was observed again to be negatively correlated with the behavior score ($\rho = -0.65$, q-value = 0.014, Figure 4C). Strong associations were also found between behavior score and fungal α-diversity (Shannon diversity index: $\rho = 0.71$, q-value = 0.002; and Simpson diversity index: $\rho = 0.76$, q-value < 0.001; Figure 4D). In addition, the total score was positively associated with fungal α-diversity (Shannon diversity index: $\rho = 0.50$, q-value = 0.089; Simpson diversity index: $\rho = 0.57$, q-value = 0.032; Figure 4D). Using logistic regression models, we found no significant association between hyperphagia scores and microbial abundance (above vs. below median) in the whole dataset (Supplementary Table S5).

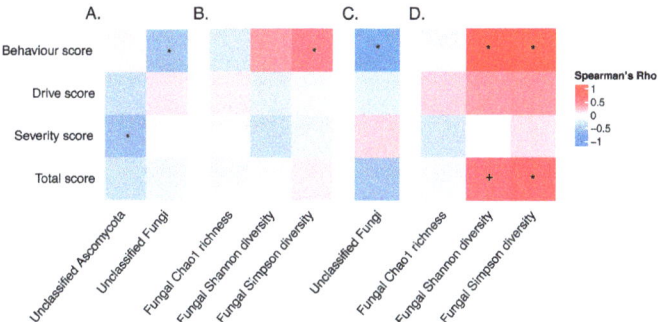

Figure 4. Correlation between hyperphagia and microbiota. (**A**) Correlation of hyperphagia score with fungal genus level in the whole dataset. (**B**) Correlation of hyperphagia scores with fungal species-level diversity in the whole dataset. (**C**) Correlation of hyperphagia score with fungal genus-level abundance within the PWS group. (**D**) Correlation of hyperphagia scores with fungal species-level diversity within the PWS group. The q-values were generated using the Bonferroni method: + indicates q-values between 0.05 and 0.1; * indicates q-values less than 0.05.

3.6. Inter-Kingdom Ecological Networks in PWS

In addition to different microbial compositions, we observed a difference within the inter-kingdom ecological networks between the PWS and CON groups (Figure 5). Specifically, at the family level, microbial communities in PWS had overall denser bacteria-fungal networks than those of the CON group, as illustrated by an increase in the number of nodes (taxa) and edges (significant interactions) in PWS. Within subgroups, microbial communities in the OWOB group appeared to have fewer bacteria-fungi network than those in the NW group, with a smaller number of nodes (NW CON: 27, OWOB: 23; NW PWS: 38, OWOB PWS: 34) and neighbors (NW CON 3.19, OWOB: 1.83; NW PWS: 3.42, OWOB PWS: 3.18). In addition, there were more positive inter-kingdom interactions than negative interactions within the four subgroups (116 positive interactions vs. 67 negative interactions in total). The ratio of positive to negative interactions was higher in the PWS subjects (2.18 in OWOB PWS, 1.71 in NW PWS) than in the CON (1.33 OWOB CON, 1.53 NW CON), suggesting that the microbial community is more cooperative in PWS than CON. Taken together, these results suggest a complex relationship between the bacteria and fungi in the gut microbiota, and that disease-specific differences are present in PWS.

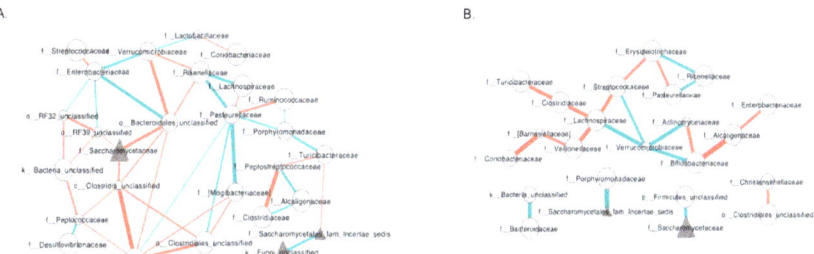

Figure 5. *Cont.*

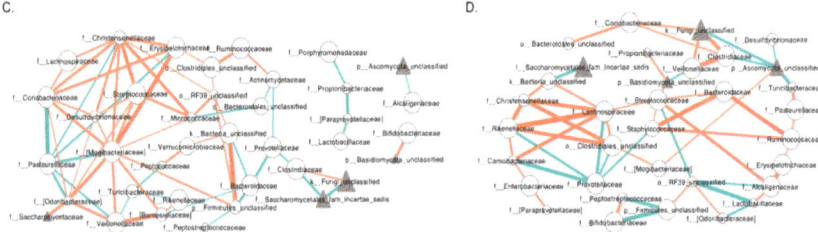

Figure 5. Microbial family (bacterial and fungal) co-occurrence networks for four subgroups. (**A**) Normal weight (NW) controls. (**B**) Overweight or obese (OWOB) controls. (**C**) NW PWS children. (**D**) OWOB PWS children. Taxon pairs with Spearman's Rho ≥ 0.3 or ≤ −0.3 with *p*-values < 0.05 were visualized. Circular nodes represent bacterial families, and triangular nodes represent fungal families. The size of the nodes indicates the occurrence frequency in each subgroup. Green lines indicate negative correlations, and orange lines indicate positive correlations. Connector line thickness represents the value of the Spearman correlation coefficient (ρ). Family names on the nodes represent the proposed taxonomy by the Greengenes database.

4. Discussion

The present study demonstrates that the fecal microbiota differs between children with and without PWS. In addition to differences in bacterial composition, for the first time, we show that the fecal mycobiota in PWS is also different from controls. The simultaneous analysis of both the bacterial and fungal microbiota enabled the elucidation of differences in the inter-kingdom interactions between patients with PWS and matched CON. By applying abundance analyses, we also identify taxa that are differentially abundant in PWS and CON subjects.

Loss of microbial diversity is a constant finding of intestinal dysbiosis, and seems to be associated with most chronic diseases, including obesity [19,20]. In our study, analysis of overall bacterial and fungal diversity found no difference between PWS and CON. In addition, no difference was found in the bacterial community structure between PWS and CON; however, patients with PWS showed a fungal community structure distinct from the matched controls. These differences might be merely the consequence of the disease, environmental factors, or covariates unrelated to PWS that are not examined here. Garcia-Ribera et al. also recently analyzed the fecal microbiota composition in children with PWS and observed higher phylogenetic diversity in normal weight subjects compared to those who were overweight or obese [21]. Our subgroup analyses, however, found no differences in microbial diversity between OWOB PWS and NW PWS. In contrast to the study by Olsson et al., which reported higher overall phylogenetic diversity in PWS adults with obesity compared to individuals with idiopathic obesity [7], the present study did not detect any difference between the OWOB PWS and OWOB CON groups. The discrepancies between these studies might be caused by differences in participant characteristics (age, diet, geography, socioeconomic status, and ethnicity), sample sizes, and analytic tools that were used. Olsson et al. additionally demonstrated that the phylogenetic diversity in subjects with PWS was similar to that of their non-obese, non-PWS parents, suggesting that the community is not likely shaped by PWS status or obesity in individuals with PWS, but instead by environmental factors. Microbiota diversity is potentially important in gut health and temporal stability; further studies are needed to investigate the compositional, and more importantly, functional diversity in the gut microbiota of individuals with PWS.

The LEfSe and random forest analyses demonstrated that gut bacterial and fungal microbiota were characterized by differences in their compositions in PWS, with certain taxa showing higher or lower abundance in children with PWS compared to controls. Both methods detected a higher abundance of *Prevotella* in PWS compared to CON, while subgroup analyses found its abundance was lower in OWOB PWS relative to NW PWS. There is human evidence linking gut bacteria and appetite, showing that microbiota activity is associated with changes in plasma levels of appetite-regulating hormones, such as glucagon-like peptide 1, peptide YY, and ghrelin [22]. Previously, the abundance of *Prevotella* species was found to be positively correlated with ghrelin, while negatively correlated with leptin in rat models [23]. *Prevotella* are well-known fiber degraders [24], and mechanistic studies suggest microbial metabolites produced during dietary fiber fermentation (i.e., short-chain fatty acids) as an important modulator of host metabolism [22]. Therefore, the increased abundance of *Prevotella* and its correlations with appetite and bodyweight in patients with PWS may deserve further study. However, *Oscillospira*, a genus that has been associated with lower BMI [25,26], was lower in abundance in PWS compared with CON. The RF model identified 10 additional genera, out of which four taxa (*Dorea*, *Akkermansia*, and genera classified in the *RF39* and *Christensenellaceae* families) had been previously reported by Olsson et al. Our study observed a lower abundance of *Dorea* in patients with PWS, which is in agreement with Olsson et al. showing significantly lower *Dorea* in subjects with PWS. Contrary to the enrichment of *Akkermansia* in PWS described in their report, we found a significantly lower abundance of this genus in children with PWS compared to controls. *Akkermansia*, in particular *Akkermansia muciniphila*, has been associated with intestinal integrity, and its abundance has been inversely correlated to obesity and metabolic dysfunction [27–32]. The change in the abundance of *Akkermansia* and its correlation with body weight and metabolic health in individuals with PWS might be worth exploring.

For differentially abundant fungi between PWS and CON, LEfSe analysis shows high concordance with results from RF: the same genera (*Mrakia*, *Candida*, *Saccharomyces*, and genera classified in the *Agaricomycetes* and *Basidiomycota* families) were obtained from both methods, with the exception of an unclassified *Ascomycota*. The major pathogenic *Candida* species in humans is *Candida albicans*, which, under normal conditions, behaves like commensal members of the gut microbiota, and its colonization is limited by other bacterial species [33]. Higher abundance of *Candida* might indicate disruptions in the microbial equilibrium, the intestinal mucosal barrier, or host's innate immune system in children with PWS [34]. Interestingly, a clear reduction in *Saccharomyces* was observed in the overall PWS group, but that could be due to lower consumption of fermented foods, such as bread. Overall, it should be considered that fungi are an overlooked kingdom of the microbiome, and we are only beginning to understand their structure, role, and functions; thus, the biological and clinical significance of observed changes in the gut mycobiome in children with PWS remains to be determined.

Dialister and *Bifidobacterium* were consistently enriched in OWOB subjects within the PWS and CON groups, shown in both the random forest models and LEfSe. Higher abundance of *Dialister* has been associated with failure to lose body weight in an intervention program [35]. *Bifidobacterium* is generally reported to be correlated with healthy status, but its effect on body weight is strain-specific, as reported previously in a mouse study [36]. Increased abundance of this genus in OWOB subjects may, therefore, reflect the enrichment of some strains that are able to induce increases in body weight.

Fungi and bacteria coexist in the gut; thus, their interaction networks may be altered in the disease state [37]. Alterations in bacteria–fungi interaction networks have been previously reported in colorectal cancer [38], inflammatory bowel disease [39,40], and ankylosing spondylitis [41]. In this study, we also noted a PWS-specific pattern for the inter-kingdom network. Children with PWS had more densely connected inter-kingdom co-occurrence networks compared to the CON, and those networks were largely positive, suggesting more collaboration between bacterial and fungal communities in PWS. Overall, these findings indicate that inter-kingdom interactions in the gut are an underappreciated, but potentially important component of human disease that deserves more research attention.

Analysis of macronutrient intakes revealed a significantly lower dietary carbohydrate intake in PWS, which might be linked to variation identified above. However, a logistic regression model showed that only unclassified *Christensenellaceae* was significantly associated with CHO. For most of the differentially abundant genera, these factors had no influence, suggesting that diet or PWS per se, or their interaction, was not a strong determinant of microbiota composition, which is in accordance with previous studies [42,43]. One study reported that in healthy Israeli individuals, non-genetic factors (age, sex, BMI, smoking status, and dietary patterns) and genetic factors explain only about

10% of the observed variation in the gut microbiome [42], and another study in northern Germany found that effects of specific environmental factors, such as diet, medication, and anthropometric measurements account for approximately 20% of the variation [43]. Overall, these results suggest that host and environment make only a small contribution to interindividual microbiota variation, implying some unknown sources of variance.

In this study, we report for the first time correlations between hyperphagic symptoms and microbiome features observed in patients with PWS. Specifically, mycobiota diversity was strongly and positively correlated with behavior scores. One possible explanation for this positive association is that these children might consume a greater variety and larger amounts of foods, as a result of bargaining, seeking, stealing, and foraging for food [4]. Further analysis of hyperphagia and fungal genus-level data revealed a negative correlation between the abundance of an unclassified *Ascomycota* and hyperphagia severity scores among the study dataset. The abundance of this fungal taxon was reduced in the PWS group and in OWOB subjects compared to NW subjects within the PWS and the CON groups. These results suggest a link between PWS-specific gut microbial features and hyperphagic symptoms. Further work studying changes in the gut microbiota throughout the lifespan and course of the disease are needed to determine whether diversity and abundance differences exacerbate hyperphagic symptoms, merely as a consequence of disease progression, or potentially driven by environmental factors.

One of the strengths of our study lies in the inclusion of normal weight and overweight/obese patients with PWS. Many children with PWS nowadays are able to maintain a normal body weight, since early diagnosis followed by rapid start of treatment, such as growth hormone replacement therapy and energy-restricted diet, may reduce the risk of early-onset obesity. An added advantage of our study is the analysis of the correlation between hyperphagia and dietary intake data and microbial abundances. Hyperphagia is the most striking clinical feature of PWS, but its symptoms vary greatly among patients. This study is the first to identify microbial taxa significantly associated with hyperphagia in PWS, which may represent a signature of varied appetite regulation. A limitation of this study was the small size of the PWS group, which is a common barrier in all rare disease studies; however, it was large enough for us to study the differences in the gut microbiota in children with and without PWS. We also note that the cross-sectional design limited interpretation of the results, particularly with respect to hyperphagia. Another limitation was that gut microbiota of family members of PWS were not analyzed in this study like in previous studies [7]. Including these data may facilitate understanding of the extent to which genetics contribute to the PWS-associated gut microbiota. In addition, the Hyperphagia Questionnaire, specifically designed for PWS, is not a valid instrument for use in healthy individuals, which might limit the conclusions reached. The species-level profiles generated by the amplicon sequencing methods used in this study were not reliable. Considering the zero-inflated nature of species/OTU-level abundance and the importance of precise taxonomic assignments, we used genus-level or above data in the analyses regarding comparisons of microbial abundances or the correlation between microbial abundances and phenotypes. Using additional methodologies, such as shotgun metagenomic sequencing and high-throughput culturomics, will facilitate strain-level dissection of the microbiome, and will allow us to identify specific functional bacterial and fungal strains and gain mechanistic insight into their role in the onset and progression of hyperphagia in PWS.

Although our study detected differences in the gut microbiota in children suffering from PWS as compared to healthy controls, our analysis does not provide any information as to whether such differences are causal or contributory to disease, rather than a consequence, or if they constitute compensatory beneficial responses. In this respect, it is important to point out that previous research on the role of the gut microbiota in PWS resulted in contradictory findings. Using experiments where human microbiota was transplanted into germ-free mice, Zhang et al. reported a causal contribution of gut dysbiosis to obesity in children with PWS [6], while Olsson et al. suggested that PWS-associated microbial features might play a role in the prevention of metabolic complications [7]. These discrepancies might stem from the inability of human microbiota-associated mice to make accurate predictions about causal claims [44,45]. With the limited evidence, it is too early to attribute any phenotypic effects to the microbiome without more robust investigation. More complex analysis, such as multi-omics and time-series measurements, and an interventionist framework are likely required if we want to approach an assertion about causality [44]. For example, the differences detected by us and the previous studies in microbiota composition could be targeted by nutritional or microbial-based approaches, in an attempt to improve outcomes in PWS patients. Should this be possible, microbiota features are likely to contribute or prevent pathology in PWS.

In conclusion, gut microbiota composition of patients with PWS differs from matched controls. In addition to differences in the relative abundance of certain bacterial taxa, our findings reveal differences in the gut fungal community and bacteria–fungi interkingdom interactions in PWS. Moreover, we identified several interesting links between gut microbes and hyperphagia in PWS. However, further work that includes a time-series of samples over the course of the disease and multi-omics data is required for the evaluation of the role of gut microbiome in the modulation of hyperphagic symptoms in PWS. While the implications of the present findings remain to be refined, they pave the way for the elucidation of characteristics of a PWS-specific gut microbiome, and lay the groundwork needed for future study of microbiota-based treatment strategies for individuals with PWS.

Supplementary Materials: The following are available online at http://www.mdpi.com/2073-4425/11/8/904/s1. Supplementary Table S1. Median values of α-diversity indices. Supplementary Table S2. Median abundance and occurrence frequency of differentially abundant bacterial and fungal taxa. Supplementary Table S3. Median values of nutrition intakes. Supplementary Table S4. Logistic regression for the association between CHO intake, group, and dichotomized abundance of differentially abundant bacterial and fungal taxa. Supplementary Table S5. Logistic regression for the association between hyperphagia scores, group, and dichotomized abundance of differentially abundant bacterial and fungal taxa. Supplementary Figure S1. Importance of predictors. Importance of the identified taxa in models for (A) differentially abundant bacterial genera: PWS vs. CON; (B) differentially abundant bacterial genera: OWOB CON vs. NW CON; (C) differentially abundant bacterial genera: OWOB PWS vs. NW PWS; (D) differentially abundant fungal genera: PWS vs. CON; (E) differentially abundant fungal genera: OWOB CON vs. NW CON; (F) differentially abundant fungal genera: OWOB PWS vs. NW PWS; (G) predicting PWS using selected bacterial and fungal genera markers; (H) predicting OWOB in CON subjects using selected bacterial and fungal genera markers; and (I) predicting OWOB in PWS subjects using bacterial and fungal genera markers. Predictors with grey labels in A–F were those with importance between the 80% and 90% quantile in each model, and were not included in the final models. Supplementary Figure S2. Performance of the model for differentiating PWS from CON subjects using bacterial genera markers. Supplementary Figure S3. Performance of the model for differentiating OWOB CON from NW CON subjects using bacterial genera markers. Supplementary Figure S4. Performance of the model for differentiating OWOB PWS from NW PWS subjects using bacterial genera markers. Supplementary Figure S5. Performance of the model for differentiating PWS from CON subjects using the identified fungal genera markers. Supplementary Figure S6. Performance of the model for differentiating OWOB CON from NW CON subjects using the identified fungal species markers. Supplementary Figure S7. Performance of the model for differentiating OWOB PWS from NW PWS subjects using the identified fungal genera. Supplementary Figure S8. Performance of the model for differentiating PWS from CON subjects using the identified bacterial and fungal genera. Supplementary Figure S9. Performance of the model for differentiating OWOB CON from NW CON subjects using the identified bacterial and fungal genera. Supplementary Figure S10. Performance of the model for differentiating OWOB PWS from NW PWS subjects using the identified bacterial and fungal genera. Supplementary Figure S11. Correlation between dietary intake and microbiota in the whole dataset. (A) Correlation of dietary intake with bacterial genus-level abundance. (B) Correlation of dietary intake with bacterial species-level diversity. (C) Correlation of dietary intake with fungal genus-level abundance. (D) Correlation of dietary intake with fungal species-level diversity. The *q*-values were generated using the Bonferroni method. + indicates *q*-values between 0.05 and 0.1; * indicates *q*-values less than 0.05.

Author Contributions: A.M.H.: conceptualization, resources, funding acquisition, writing—review and editing, and supervision. H.M.T.: conceptualization, methodology, writing—review and editing, and supervision. Y.P.: methodology, formal analysis, visualization, and writing—review and editing. Q.T.: formal analysis, writing—original draft, and writing—review and editing. S.A.: investigation, data curation, and formal analysis. E.C.D.: formal analysis and writing—review and editing. S.L.: formal analysis. M.G.: methodology and writing—review and editing. L.T.: data curation, formal analysis, and writing—review and editing. K.L.M.: writing—review and editing. J.W.: methodology and writing—review and editing. All authors have read and agreed to the published version of the manuscript.

Funding: This research was funded by the Weston Family Microbiome Initiative, the Prader–Willi Syndrome Association (United States) and Women and Children's Health Research Institute.

Conflicts of Interest: The authors declare no conflict of interest.

Appendix A

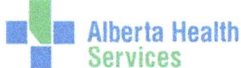 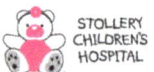 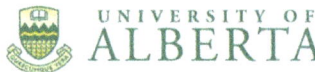

Hyperphagia Questionnaire

Study ID#

Study: "Profiling of the gut microbiome in children with PWS: a fiber intervention to target hyperphagia"
(AIM 1) Haqq, A (PI)

Instructions:
The following items refer to the person in your care and assessment of his/her food-related behavior during the past 2 weeks.

(1) How upset does your child generally become when denied a desired food?
___ Not particularly upset at all
___ A little upset
___ Somewhat upset
___ Very upset
___ Extremely upset

(2) How often does your child try to bargain or manipulate to get more food at meals?
___ A few times a year
___ A few times a month
___ A few times a week
___ Several times a week
___ Several times a day

(3) Once your child has food on their mind, how easy is it for you or others to re-direct your child away from food to other things?
___ Extremely easy, takes minimal effort to do so
___ Very easy, takes just a little effort to do so
___ Somewhat hard, takes some effort to do so
___ Very hard, takes a lot of work to do so
___ Extremely hard, takes sustained and hard work to do so

(4) How often does your child forage through the trash for food?
___ Never
___ A few times a year
___ 1–2 times a month
___ 1–3 times a week
___ 4 to 7 times a week

(5) How often does your child get up at night to food seek?
___ Never
___ A few nights a year
___ 1–2 nights a month

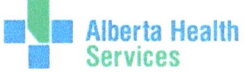 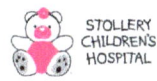 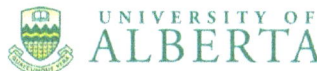

___ 1–3 nights a week
___ 4 to 7 nights a week

(6) How persistent is your child in asking or looking for food after being told "no" or "no more"?
___ Lets go of food ideas quickly and easily
___ Lets go of food ideas pretty quickly and easily
___ Somewhat persistent with food ideas
___ Very persistent with food ideas
___ Extremely persistent with food ideas

(7) Outside of normal meal times, how much time does your child spend talking about food or engaged in food-related behaviors?
___ Less than 15 minutes a day
___ 15 to 30 minutes a day
___ 30 minutes to an hour
___ 1 to 3 hours a day
___ more than 3 hours a day

(8) How often does your child try to steal food (that you are aware of?)
___ A few times a year
___ A few times a month
___ A few times a week
___ Several times a week
___ Several times a day

(9) When others try to stop your child from talking about food or engaging in food-related behaviors, it generally leads to:
___ No distress or upset
___ Mild distress or upset
___ Moderate distress or upset
___ Severe distress or upset
___ Extreme distress, behaviors can't usually be stopped

(10) How clever or fast is your child in obtaining food?
___ Not particularly clever or fast
___ A little clever or fast
___ Somewhat clever or fast
___ Very clever or fast
___ Extremely clever of fast

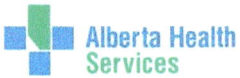 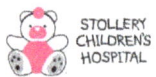 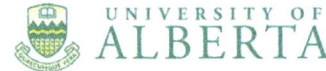

(11) To what extent to food-related thoughts, talk, or behavior interfere with your child's normal daily routines, self-care, school, or work?

____ No interference

____ Mild interference; occasional food-related interference in completing school, work, or hygiene tasks

____ Moderate interference; frequent food-related interference in completing school, work, or hygiene tasks

____ Severe interference; almost daily food-related interference in completing school, work, or hygiene tasks

____ Extreme interference, often unable to participate in hygiene tasks or to get to school or work due to food-related difficulties

References

1. Butler, M.G.; Miller, J.L.; Forster, J.L. Prader-Willi Syndrome-Clinical Genetics, Diagnosis and Treatment Approaches: An Update. *Curr. Pediatr. Rev.* **2019**, *15*, 207–244. [CrossRef] [PubMed]
2. Irizarry, K.A.; Miller, M.; Freemark, M.; Haqq, A.M. Prader Willi Syndrome: Genetics, Metabolomics, Hormonal Function, and New Approaches to Therapy. *Adv. Pediatr.* **2016**, *63*, 47. [CrossRef] [PubMed]
3. Kim, S.J.; Miller, J.L.; Kuipers, P.J.; German, J.R.; Beaudet, A.L.; Sahoo, T.; Driscoll, D.J. Unique and atypical deletions in Prader-Willi syndrome reveal distinct phenotypes. *Eur. J. Hum. Genet.* **2012**, *20*, 283–290. [CrossRef] [PubMed]
4. Miller, J.L.; Lynn, C.H.; Driscoll, D.C.; Goldstone, A.P.; Gold, J.A.; Kimonis, V.; Dykens, E.; Butler, M.G.; Shuster, J.J.; Driscoll, D.J. Nutritional phases in Prader-Willi syndrome. *Am. J. Med. Genet. Part A* **2011**, *155*, 1040–1049. [CrossRef]
5. Heymsfield, S.B.; Avena, N.M.; Baier, L.; Brantley, P.; Bray, G.A.; Burnett, L.C.; Butler, M.G.; Driscoll, D.J.; Egli, D.; Elmquist, J.; et al. Hyperphagia: Current concepts and future directions proceedings of the 2nd international conference on hyperphagia. *Obesity* **2014**, *22*, 1–35. [CrossRef]
6. Zhang, C.; Yin, A.; Li, H.; Wang, R.; Wu, G.; Shen, J.; Zhang, M.; Wang, L.; Hou, Y.; Ouyang, H.; et al. Dietary Modulation of Gut Microbiota Contributes to Alleviation of Both Genetic and Simple Obesity in Children. *EBioMedicine* **2015**, *2*, 968–984. [CrossRef]
7. Olsson, L.M.; Poitou, C.; Tremaroli, V.; Coupaye, M.; Aron-Wisnewsky, J.; Bäckhed, F.; Clément, K.; Caesar, R. Gut microbiota of obese subjects with Prader-Willi syndrome is linked to metabolic health. *Gut* **2019**, *69*, 1229–1238. [CrossRef]
8. Limon, J.J.; Skalski, J.H.; Underhill, D.M. Commensal Fungi in Health and Disease. *Cell Host Microbe* **2017**, *22*, 156–165. [CrossRef]
9. Dykens, E.M.; Maxwell, M.A.; Pantino, E.; Kossler, R.; Roof, E. Assessment of hyperphagia in prader-Willi syndrome. *Obesity* **2007**, *15*, 1816–1826. [CrossRef]
10. Willett, W.C.; Howe, G.R.; Kushi, L.H. Adjustment for total energy intake in epidemiologic studies. *Am. J. Clin. Nutr.* **1997**, *65*, 1220S–1228S. [CrossRef]
11. Centers for Disease Control and Prevention. Available online: https://www.cdc.gov/nchs/data/nhanes/nhanes_07_08/manual_an.pdf (accessed on 21 November 2016).
12. de Onis, M.; Onyango, A.W.; Borghi, E.; Siyam, A.; Nishida, C.; Siekmann, J. Development of a WHO growth reference for school-aged children and adolescents. *Bull World Health Organ.* **2007**, *85*, 660–667. [CrossRef] [PubMed]
13. Anderson, E.L.; Li, W.; Klitgord, N.; Highlander, S.K.; Dayrit, M.; Seguritan, V.; Yooseph, S.; Biggs, W.; Venter, J.C.; Nelson, K.E.; et al. A robust ambient temperature collection and stabilization strategy: Enabling worldwide functional studies of the human microbiome. *Sci. Rep.* **2016**, *6*, 1–10. [CrossRef] [PubMed]

14. Kozich, J.J.; Westcott, S.L.; Baxter, N.T.; Highlander, S.K.; Schloss, P.D. Development of a dual-index sequencing strategy and curation pipeline for analyzing amplicon sequence data on the miseq illumina sequencing platform. *Appl. Environ. Microbiol.* **2013**, *79*, 5112–5120. [CrossRef] [PubMed]

15. Schloss, P.D.; Westcott, S.L.; Ryabin, T.; Hall, J.R.; Hartmann, M.; Hollister, E.B.; Lesniewski, R.A.; Oakley, B.B.; Parks, D.H.; Robinson, C.J.; et al. Introducing mothur: Open-source, platform-independent, community-supported software for describing and comparing microbial communities. *Appl. Environ. Microbiol.* **2009**, *75*, 7537–7541. [CrossRef] [PubMed]

16. Afgan, E.; Baker, D.; Batut, B.; Van Den Beek, M.; Bouvier, D.; Ech, M.; Chilton, J.; Clements, D.; Coraor, N.; Grüning, B.A.; et al. The Galaxy platform for accessible, reproducible and collaborative biomedical analyses: 2018 update. *Nucleic Acids Res.* **2018**, *46*, W537–W544. [CrossRef]

17. Tun, H.M.; Bridgman, S.L.; Chari, R.; Field, C.J.; Guttman, D.S.; Becker, A.B.; Mandhane, P.J.; Turvey, S.E.; Subbarao, P.; Sears, M.R.; et al. Roles of birth mode and infant gut microbiota in intergenerational transmission of overweight and obesity from mother to offspring. *JAMA Pediatr.* **2018**, *172*, 368–377. [CrossRef] [PubMed]

18. Kim, B.R.; Shin, J.; Guevarra, R.B.; Lee, J.H.; Kim, D.W.; Seol, K.H.; Lee, J.H.; Kim, H.B.; Isaacson, R.E. Deciphering diversity indices for a better understanding of microbial communities. *J. Microbiol. Biotechnol.* **2017**, *27*, 2089–2093. [CrossRef]

19. Mosca, A.; Leclerc, M.; Hugot, J.P. Gut microbiota diversity and human diseases: Should we reintroduce key predators in our ecosystem? *Front. Microbiol.* **2016**, *7*, 455. [CrossRef]

20. McBurney, M.I.; Davis, C.; Fraser, C.M.; Schneeman, B.O.; Huttenhower, C.; Verbeke, K.; Walter, J.; Latulippe, M.E. Establishing What Constitutes a Healthy Human Gut Microbiome: State of the Science, Regulatory Considerations, and Future Directions. *J. Nutr.* **2019**, *149*, 1882–1895. [CrossRef]

21. Garcia-Ribera, S.; Amat-Bou, M.; Climent, E.; Llobet, M.; Chenoll, E.; Corripio, R.; Ibáñez, L.; Ramon-Krauel, M.; Lerin, C. Specific dietary components and gut microbiota composition are associated with obesity in children and adolescents with prader–willi syndrome. *Nutrients* **2020**, *12*, 1063. [CrossRef]

22. Cani, P.D.; Knauf, C. How gut microbes talk to organs: The role of endocrine and nervous routes. *Mol. Metab.* **2016**, *5*, 743–752. [CrossRef] [PubMed]

23. Queipo-Ortuño, M.I.; Seoane, L.M.; Murri, M.; Pardo, M.; Gomez-Zumaquero, J.M.; Cardona, F.; Casanueva, F.; Tinahones, F.J. Gut Microbiota Composition in Male Rat Models under Different Nutritional Status and Physical Activity and Its Association with Serum Leptin and Ghrelin Levels. *PLoS ONE* **2013**, *8*, e65465. [CrossRef] [PubMed]

24. Fehlner-Peach, H.; Magnabosco, C.; Raghavan, V.; Scher, J.U.; Tett, A.; Cox, L.M.; Gottsegen, C.; Watters, A.; Wiltshire-Gordon, J.D.; Segata, N.; et al. Distinct Polysaccharide Utilization Profiles of Human Intestinal Prevotella copri Isolates. *Cell Host Microbe* **2019**, *26*, 680–690. [CrossRef] [PubMed]

25. Goodrich, J.K.; Waters, J.L.; Poole, A.C.; Sutter, J.L.; Koren, O.; Blekhman, R.; Beaumont, M.; Van Treuren, W.; Knight, R.; Bell, J.T.; et al. Human genetics shape the gut microbiome. *Cell* **2014**, *159*, 789–799. [CrossRef] [PubMed]

26. Konikoff, T.; Gophna, U. Oscillospira: A Central, Enigmatic Component of the Human Gut Microbiota. *Trends Microbiol.* **2016**, *24*, 523–524. [CrossRef] [PubMed]

27. Depommier, C.; Everard, A.; Druart, C.; Plovier, H.; Van Hul, M.; Vieira-Silva, S.; Falony, G.; Raes, J.; Maiter, D.; Delzenne, N.M.; et al. Supplementation with Akkermansia muciniphila in overweight and obese human volunteers: a proof-of-concept exploratory study. *Nat. Med.* **2019**, *25*, 1096–1103. [CrossRef]

28. Plovier, H.; Everard, A.; Druart, C.; Depommier, C.; Van Hul, M.; Geurts, L.; Chilloux, J.; Ottman, N.; Duparc, T.; Lichtenstein, L.; et al. A purified membrane protein from Akkermansia muciniphila or the pasteurized bacterium improves metabolism in obese and diabetic mice. *Nat. Med.* **2017**, *23*, 107–113. [CrossRef]

29. Dao, M.C.; Everard, A.; Aron-Wisnewsky, J.; Sokolovska, N.; Prifti, E.; Verger, E.O.; Kayser, B.D.; Levenez, F.; Chilloux, J.; Hoyles, L.; et al. Akkermansia muciniphila and improved metabolic health during a dietary intervention in obesity: Relationship with gut microbiome richness and ecology. *Gut* **2016**, *64*, 531–537. [CrossRef]

30. Derrien, M.; Belzer, C.; de Vos, W.M. Akkermansia muciniphila and its role in regulating host functions. *Microb. Pathog.* **2017**, *106*, 171–181. [CrossRef]

31. Caesar, R.; Tremaroli, V.; Kovatcheva-Datchary, P.; Cani, P.D.; Bäckhed, F. Crosstalk between gut microbiota and dietary lipids aggravates WAT inflammation through TLR signaling. *Cell Metab.* **2015**, *22*, 658–668. [CrossRef]

32. Karlsson, C.L.J.; Önnerfält, J.; Xu, J.; Molin, G.; Ahrné, S.; Thorngren-Jerneck, K. The microbiota of the gut in preschool children with normal and excessive body weight. *Obesity* **2012**, *20*, 2257–2261. [CrossRef] [PubMed]

33. Bassetti, M.; Taramasso, L.; Nicco, E.; Molinari, M.P.; Mussap, M.; Viscoli, C. Epidemiology, species distribution, antifungal susceptibility and outcome of nosocomial candidemia in a tertiary care hospital in Italy. *PLoS ONE* **2011**, *6*, e24198. [CrossRef] [PubMed]

34. Yan, L.; Yang, C.; Tang, J. Disruption of the intestinal mucosal barrier in Candida albicans infections. *Microbiol. Res.* **2013**, *168*, 389–395. [CrossRef] [PubMed]

35. Muñiz Pedrogo, D.A.; Jensen, M.D.; Van Dyke, C.T.; Murray, J.A.; Woods, J.A.; Chen, J.; Kashyap, P.C.; Nehra, V. Gut Microbial Carbohydrate Metabolism Hinders Weight Loss in Overweight Adults Undergoing Lifestyle Intervention With a Volumetric Diet. *Mayo Clin. Proc.* **2018**, *93*, 1104–1110. [CrossRef] [PubMed]

36. Yin, Y.N.; Yu, Q.F.; Fu, N.; Liu, X.W.; Lu, F.G. Effects of four Bifidobacteria on obesity in high-fat diet induced rats. *World J. Gastroenterol.* **2010**, *16*, 3394. [CrossRef] [PubMed]

37. Van Dijck, P.; Jabra-Rizk, M.A. Fungal-bacterial interactions: In health and disease. In *Candida Albicans: Cellular and Molecular Biology*, 2nd ed.; Springer: New York, NY, USA, 2017; pp. 115–143. [CrossRef]

38. Coker, O.O.; Nakatsu, G.; Dai, R.Z.; Wu, W.K.K.; Wong, S.H.; Ng, S.C.; Chan, F.K.L.; Sung, J.J.Y.; Yu, J. Enteric fungal microbiota dysbiosis and ecological alterations in colorectal cancer. *Gut* **2019**, *68*, 654–662. [CrossRef]

39. Sokol, H.; Leducq, V.; Aschard, H.; Pham, H.P.; Jegou, S.; Landman, C.; Cohen, D.; Liguori, G.; Bourrier, A.; Nion-Larmurier, I.; et al. Fungal microbiota dysbiosis in IBD. *Gut* **2017**, *66*, 1039–1048. [CrossRef]

40. Hoarau, G.; Mukherjee, P.K.; Gower-Rousseau, C.; Hager, C.; Chandra, J.; Retuerto, M.A.; Neut, C.; Vermeire, S.; Clemente, J.; Colombel, J.F.; et al. Bacteriome and mycobiome interactions underscore microbial dysbiosis in familial Crohn's disease. *MBio* **2016**, *7*. [CrossRef]

41. Li, M.; Dai, B.; Tang, Y.; Lei, L.; Li, N.; Liu, C.; Ge, T.; Zhang, L.; Xu, Y.; Hu, Y.; et al. Altered Bacterial-Fungal Interkingdom Networks in the Guts of Ankylosing Spondylitis Patients. *mSystems* **2019**, *4*. [CrossRef]

42. Rothschild, D.; Weissbrod, O.; Barkan, E.; Kurilshikov, A.; Korem, T.; Zeevi, D.; Costea, P.I.; Godneva, A.; Kalka, I.N.; Bar, N.; et al. Environment dominates over host genetics in shaping human gut microbiota. *Nature* **2018**, *555*, 210–215. [CrossRef]

43. Wang, J.; Thingholm, L.B.; Skiecevičie, J.; Rausch, P.; Kummen, M.; Hov, J.R.; Degenhardt, F.; Heinsen, F.A.; Rühlemann, M.C.; Szymczak, S.; et al. Genome-wide association analysis identifies variation in Vitamin D receptor and other host factors influencing the gut microbiota. *Nat. Genet.* **2016**, *48*, 1396–1406. [CrossRef] [PubMed]

44. Walter, J.; Armet, A.M.; Finlay, B.B.; Shanahan, F. Establishing or Exaggerating Causality for the Gut Microbiome: Lessons from Human Microbiota-Associated Rodents. *Cell* **2020**, *180*, 221–232. [CrossRef] [PubMed]

45. Nguyen, T.L.A.; Vieira-Silva, S.; Liston, A.; Raes, J. How informative is the mouse for human gut microbiota research? *Dis. Model. Mech.* **2015**, *8*, 1–16. [CrossRef] [PubMed]

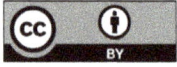 © 2020 by the authors. Licensee MDPI, Basel, Switzerland. This article is an open access article distributed under the terms and conditions of the Creative Commons Attribution (CC BY) license (http://creativecommons.org/licenses/by/4.0/).

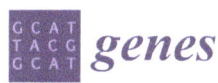

Article

A 24-Week Physical Activity Intervention Increases Bone Mineral Content without Changes in Bone Markers in Youth with PWS

Daniela A. Rubin [1,*], Kathleen S. Wilson [1], Camila E. Orsso [2], Erik R. Gertz [3], Andrea M. Haqq [2,4], Diobel M. Castner [1] and Marilyn Dumont-Driscoll [5]

[1] Department of Kinesiology, California State University Fullerton, 800 N. State College Blvd., Fullerton, CA 92831, USA; kswilson@fullerton.edu (K.S.W.); dmendozacastner@gmail.com (D.M.C.)
[2] Department of Agricultural, Food, and Nutritional Science, University of Alberta, 8602 112 Street, Edmonton, AB T6G 2E1, Canada; camilaorsso@gmail.com (C.E.O.); Andrea.Haqq@albertahealthservices.ca (A.M.H.)
[3] Obesity and Metabolism Unit, Western Human Nutrition Research Center, U.S. Department of Agriculture, 430 W Health Sciences Drive, Davis, CA 95616, USA; erik.gertz@usda.gov
[4] Division of Pediatric Endocrinology, University of Alberta, 8440-112 Street, Edmonton, AB T6G 2B7, Canada
[5] Academic General Pediatrics, University of Florida, Gainesville, 1699 SW 16th Avenue, Gainesville, FL 32608, USA; dumonmd@peds.ufl.edu
* Correspondence: drubin@fullerton.edu; Tel.: +1-657-278-4704

Received: 21 July 2020; Accepted: 19 August 2020; Published: 24 August 2020

Abstract: Bone mineral density (BMD) is of concern in Prader-Willi syndrome (PWS). This study compared responses to a physical activity intervention in bone parameters and remodeling markers in youth with PWS ($n = 45$) and youth with non-syndromic obesity (NSO; $n = 66$). Measurements occurred at baseline (PRE) and after 24 weeks (POST) of a home-based active games intervention with strengthening and jumping exercises (intervention group = I) or after a no-intervention period (control group = C). Dual x-ray absorptiometry scans of the hip and lumbar spine (L1-L4) determined BMD and bone mineral content (BMC). Bone markers included fasting bone-specific alkaline phosphatase (BAP) and C-terminal telopeptide of type I collagen (CTx). Both I and C groups increased their hip BMD and BMC ($p < 0.001$). Youth with PWS-I increased their spine BMC from PRE to POST ($p < 0.001$) but not youth with PWS-C ($p = 1.000$). Youth with NSO (I and C) increased their spine BMC between PRE and POST (all $p < 0.001$). Youth with PWS showed lower BAP (108.28 ± 9.19 vs. 139.07 ± 6.41 U/L; $p = 0.006$) and similar CTx (2.07 ± 0.11 vs.1.84 ± 0.14 ng/dL; $p = 0.193$) than those with NSO regardless of time. Likely, the novelty of the intervention exercises for those with PWS contributed to gains in spine BMC beyond growth. Bone remodeling markers were unaltered by the intervention.

Keywords: games; parents; home; exercise; bone health

---

1. Introduction

Prader-Willi syndrome (PWS) is a complex neurodevelopmental disorder characterized by hypotonia, developmental delay, poor motor competence, and commonly low levels of spontaneous physical activity (PA) [1]. PWS is the best characterized form of syndromic pediatric obesity, and previous studies have shown that adolescents and adults with PWS exhibit lower bone mineral density (BMD) for the whole body and the lumbar spine by dual x-ray absorptiometry (DXA) when compared to sex and body mass index matched controls [2,3]. In adults with PWS, the high incidence of osteopenia and osteoporosis is likely multifactorial and a consequence of the low peak bone mass attained during adolescence and early adulthood [1]. Specifically, hypothalamic hypogonadism, central hypothyroidism, and growth hormone deficiency, common features of the syndrome, may contribute to short stature and poor bone mineralization [1]. This poor bone density was shown in previous studies in which most adults with PWS had not been on growth hormone replacement therapy (GHRT) [2,3].

The reduced levels of PA frequently described in individuals with PWS may also contribute to the low BMD phenotype. In a recent study in youth with PWS who had been on GHRT for at least two years, we showed that youth with PWS showed lower BMD at the hips than height-matched controls with obesity [4]. This finding is potentially due to insufficient ambulatory activity and stimulus for bone formation [5]. Weight-bearing exercise applies mechanical forces on the bones through the ground reaction forces and the contractile activity of the muscles [6]. These physical forces induce strain in the bone and depending on the magnitude of such strain may serve to prevent bone loss or induce bone mass accumulation. This mechanical deformation of the bone is sensed by osteocytes which, in turn, release different molecules such as Wnt, sclerotin, and nitric oxide to regulate the activity of osteoclasts (bone resorption) and osteoblasts (bone formation) [6,7]. The general consensus is that PA is associated with bone accrual and bone strength during childhood but the exact duration and intensity required are yet to be determined [8].

Another approach to monitor bone development other than using body composition techniques is to evaluate changes in blood bone markers related to bone formation and bone resorption. Compared to obese controls, adults with PWS who have not been on GHRT exhibited higher concentrations of bone turnover markers, such as bone-specific alkaline phosphatase (BAP; released by osteoblasts) [2,3] and cross-linked C-terminal telopeptide of type I collagen (CTX-1; bone resorption marker) [3]. Specifically, the increase in the levels of both markers suggests an augmented activity of both formation and resorption. While bone markers change with pharmaceutical interventions [9,10], it is unknown whether blood bone markers are sensitive to PA interventions in PWS.

From what is known, it appears that lean mass and not fat mass is the most important factor for bone health in youth with obesity [11]. This factor can be problematic in PWS as the syndrome is characterized by lower lean mass than expected even in those exposed to GHRT [4]. A recent systematic review and meta-analysis demonstrated that youth with obesity have higher bone mineral content (BMC) and BMD than their normal weight peers [12]. However, from what has been shown, youth with PWS have either lower or similar BMD compared to their obese peers [2–4]. This previously mentioned meta-analysis with focus on PA interventions also showed that 50% of the included articles presented with a positive effect on bone health as measured by DXA while bone markers were unaltered [12]. To date, there are no studies that evaluated the effect of a PA intervention on bone parameters in youth with PWS. Thus, this study aim was two-fold: (1) To examine and contrast changes in BMC and BMD in response to a home-based 24-week PA intervention in youth with and without PWS; and (2) to examine changes in blood bone markers (BAP and CTx) in a sub-sample of youth who completed the intervention. It was hypothesized that both groups of youth would demonstrate improvements in BMD and BMC (particularly in the spine, hips, and femoral neck) in response to the intervention. No changes were expected for CTx and possible increases in BAP.

2. Materials and Methods

2.1. Study Design

2.1.1. Bone Parameters Study Design

Participants were pseudo-randomized to either an intervention group that completed a 24-week PA intervention or a waitlist control group [13]. The control group eventually received the intervention after serving as a control for 24 weeks. The group allocation took place based on the participants' availability to attend the planned study visits [13]. Measurements took place at baseline and after 24 weeks (post).

2.1.2. Bone Markers Study Design

This sub-study included measurements completed at pre-intervention (PRE) and post-intervention (POST) for a sub-sample of participants who completed the intervention (regardless of their initial assigned group).

2.1.3. Intervention Description

At the beginning of the intervention, parents and their children were trained in using a PA curriculum that contained four pre-planned sessions of PA 25–45+ minutes long per week for 24 weeks. Sessions for two days included bone and muscle strengthening exercises and playground-based games. Sessions for the other two days included interactive console-based games using the Nintendo Wii gaming system (one day playing Wii Fit Plus and the other playing Just Dance 2 or 3). The bone and muscle strengthening exercises included resistance exercises using the body weight and jumping. The playground-based games included running and jumping, as well as activities requiring coordination and balance. Participants were provided with all materials and equipment for implementing the curriculum at home. Parents also received communications via phone or email from study staff to check with the progress of the intervention and address any barriers. Every six weeks parents filled in and submitted checklists for the sessions their child completed, which were used to evaluate their child's adherence with the intervention [14]. The results of the intervention for the PA outcomes and compliance with the PA sessions have been reported elsewhere [15]. In brief, participants' compliance with the intervention sessions was 68.2% and the intervention did not increase levels of moderate-to-vigorous intensity or total PA [15]. The main intervention goals were to increase levels of PA and improve motor skills. Hence, while it included some high impact and strengthening exercises, it was not designed for bone health.

2.1.4. Participants

Forty-five children with PWS and sixty-six children with non-syndromic obesity (NSO) participated. The sex distribution of participants included 54% males (PWS, $n = 25/45$, and obese, $n = 35/66$). Youth with NSO presented with a body fat percentage greater than the 95th percentile based on age and sex [16]. PWS diagnosis was confirmed by documentation of appropriate molecular and cytogenetic testing (i.e., chromosomes, FISH 15, DNA methylation, and/or DNA polymorphism studies). The genetic diagnosis for PWS included: deletion ($n = 20$), uniparental disomy ($n = 8$), DNA methylation ($n = 13$), and unknown type ($n = 4$). As GHRT is the standard of care in PWS, 33 youth were currently and had been using GHRT for more than 2 years, nine used GHRT in the past, and three never used GHRT. PWS participants also presented with hip dysplasia ($n = 2$), scoliosis ($n = 14$), and hypothyroidism ($n = 8$). Youth with NSO were excluded if they were currently using lipid-lowering, diabetes, or blood pressure medications or were pregnant.

2.2. Ethical Statement

The study protocol was approved by the institutional review boards at California State University, Fullerton HSR-16-0135, University of Florida Gainesville original submission 201702437, and the Human Subjects Research Protection Office from the U.S. Army Research and Materiel Command HRPO A-16501a. All youth signed the approved assent and their parents signed the consent forms. This trial was registered at ClinicalTrials.gov under registration number NCT02058342.

2.3. Outcome Variables

2.3.1. Medical History and Anthropometrics

Parents filled out a medical history form that included current or past signs and symptoms of disease and drug and/or supplement use. Pubertal development was estimated from parents' responses to a modified version of the Pubertal Developmental Scale [17]. Body mass to the nearest 0.01 kg was obtained using a digital scale (ES200L; Ohaus, Pinewood, NJ, USA) with the subject wearing a t-shirt, shorts, and no shoes. Height was measured to the nearest 0.1 cm using a wall-mounted stadiometer (Seca, Ontario, CA, USA) at the end of inhalation. Body mass index (BMI) z-scores were derived from the Centers for Disease Control and Prevention website [18].

2.3.2. Body Composition

All measurements were assessed by DXA with participants positioned following manufacturer's indication (Lunar Prodigy Advance, GE Healthcare, Madison, WI, USA). Total body fat and lean tissue were expressed as mass in kilograms and as percentage of soft tissue mass. Bone measurements included BMC (grams), and areal BMD (g/cm^2) for the lumbar spine (L1–L4), left and right hips (hip), bilateral femoral necks and total body minus the head (TBLH). Two technicians completed all scans (lumbar spine, hips, whole body) in the same Lunar Prodigy scanner. The same technician completed all DXA scans for the same participant over time and also completed the subsequent in-software analyses using the Paediatric Encore software version 12.30.008 (GE Healthcare Inc., Madison, WI, USA). The facility least significance change (LSC) in absolute and percent units was calculated using the procedures outlined by the International Society for Clinical Densitometry [19]. The calculated facility LSC for BMD at the L1–L4 were 0.030 g/cm^2 and 1.713% and for the hip were 0.020 g/cm^2 and 1.073%.

2.3.3. Nutritional Intake

Parents of youth participants were trained by a registered dietitian with experience in PWS for food record completion. Parents were instructed to log their child's meals including beverages (e.g., food description and preparation, amount consumed, and consumption location) in real time during one weekend day and two weekdays. Food records were screened to check for compliance in the recording resulting in 63 of 111 food records to be included in the analyses. Food records data and nutritional supplements used were then entered into The Food Processor software, version 10.12.0.0 (ESHA Research, Salem, OR, USA) to determine average daily intake of total kilocalories, vitamin D, and calcium.

2.3.4. Blood Bone Markers

An enzyme-linked immunoassay (ELISA) kit from Quidel Corporation (San Diego, CA, USA) was used to determine BAP concentrations, with an overall coefficient of variation (CV) of 1.63%. An ELISA kit from Immunodiagnostics Systems Inc. (Gaithersburg, MD, USA) was used to determine CTx concentrations with a CV of 2.41%. The LSC was calculated using inter-assay and intra-assay CV with values of 4.52% and 6.67% for BAP and CTx, respectively.

2.4. Statistical Analyses

Mean and standard error of the mean values were computed for all participant characteristics, bone and nutrition measurements. Baseline values were compared between treatment groups (intervention vs. control) and youth with PWS and those with NSO using two by two analyses of variance. Generalized estimated equations (GEE) were used to compare changes over time between the control and the intervention groups as well as between those with PWS and those with NSO for all bone parameters (hip, femoral neck, spine, and TBLH BMC, and BMD). Height was included as a covariate for all BMC analyses and baseline values were included as a covariate for all variables [20]. These covariates were selected based on recommendations by the literature and based on differences at baseline between youth or intervention groups in our sample. GEE models were also evaluated to determine changes PRE to POST in the subsample for BAP and CTx. Statistical significance was set at $p < 0.050$. Analyses were conducted using Statistical Package for the Social Sciences version 26.0 for Windows (SPSS, Chicago, IL, USA).

3. Results

3.1. Participant Baseline Differences

Baseline participant characteristics are presented in Table 1. Youth with PWS were older than those with NSO ($p = 0.001$). Youth in the intervention group were taller than those in the control group ($p = 0.030$). Youth with PWS had lower BMI percentile scores ($p < 0.001$) and z-scores ($p = 0.002$) than youth with NSO at baseline. Youth with PWS were in the prepubertal ($n = 6$), early pubertal ($n = 12$), mid-pubertal ($n = 17$), and late pubertal ($n = 7$) stages. Youth with NSO were in the prepubertal ($n = 17$), early pubertal ($n = 13$), mid-pubertal ($n = 28$), and late pubertal ($n = 7$) stages. There were no differences for body fat % or lean mass between those with and without PWS ($p > 0.050$). Baseline data were analyzed in 111 participants for hip parameters and 107 participants for spine parameters as four participants had metal from spine surgery which precluded spine films. Data were available in 28 youth with PWS and 52 with NSO for TBLH parameters. At baseline, youth with PWS presented lower hip and femoral neck BMC ($p = 0.030$) and BMD ($p < 0.001$) than youth with NSO. Several variables also differed between intervention and control groups including height ($p = 0.030$), hip BMC ($p = 0.031$), femoral neck BMC ($p = 0.026$), femoral neck BMD ($p = 0.026$), spine BMD ($p = 0.050$), and TBLH BMC ($p = 0.004$).

Table 1. Baseline characteristics of participants with Prader-Willi syndrome (PWS) and with non-syndromic obesity (NSO).

	Intervention		Control		*p*-Value		
	PWS (*n* = 34)	NSO (*n* = 43)	PWS (*n* = 11)	NSO (*n* = 23)	G	I	G × I
Age (years)	10.9 (2.5)	10.0 (1.0)	10.8 (2.3)	9.2 (1.0)	0.001	0.242	0.354
Weight (kg)	58.46 (21.48)	62.98 (19.04)	62.44 (33.18)	59.90 (15.93)	0.828	0.921	0.438
Height (cm)	145.85 (11.84)	148.17 (8.63)	140.99 (13.58)	143.20 (9.11)	0.313	0.030	0.982
BMI z-score	1.719 (0.864)	2.087 (0.468)	1.759 (1.091)	2.322 (0.306)	0.002	0.344	0.502
Body Fat (%)	46.3 (9.9)	44.1 (6.2)	47.0 (9.1)	45.5 (4.8)	0.274	0.528	0.831
Lean Mass (kg)	28.68 (8.51)	32.91 (7.91)	29.82 (12.82)	31.12 (7.29)	0.138	0.861	0.429
Hip							
BMC (g)	19.82 (7.12)	24.07 (6.67)	17.61 (7.296)	20.03 (5.18)	0.022	0.031	0.525
BMD (g/cm²)	0.837 (0.151)	0.927 (0.132)	0.778 (0.146)	0.870 (0.116)	0.003	0.053	0.959
Femoral neck							
BMC (g)	3.34 (1.05)	3.89 (0.93)	2.97 (1.20)	3.33 (0.69)	0.030	0.026	0.662
BMD (g/cm²)	0.817 (0.149)	0.914 (0.132)	0.742 (0.138)	0.858 (0.108)	0.001	0.026	0.740
Spine							
BMC (g)	36.38 (14.79)	34.89 (9.19)	32.76 (8.31)	29.40 (6.41)	0.309	0.057	0.695
BMD (g/cm²)	0.929(0.170)	0.904 (0.138)	0.901 (0.082)	0.812 (0.091)	0.061	0.050	0.297
TBLH							
BMC (g)	1311.7 (580.3)	1438.0 (394.9)	864.2 (214.5)	1185.2 (241.9)	0.064	0.004	0.416
BMD (g/cm²)	0.866 (0.129)	0.893 (0.088)	0.788 (0.133)	0.865 (0.068)	0.071	0.066	0.385

Data are presented as mean (standard error of the mean). Abbreviations: BMC = bone mineral content, BMD = bone mineral density, TBLH = total body less head, G = group (PWS vs. NSO), I = intervention treatment allocation (intervention vs. waitlist control), G × I = group by intervention interaction.

3.2. Hip and Femoral Neck Changes

Based on the youth (PWS vs. NSO) or intervention group differences at baseline, all analyses included the baseline values as a covariate. Additionally, height was included as a covariate for BMC outcomes. Because baseline values were included as a covariate, there were no differences between treatments or groups at baseline for any parameter. Table 2 presents outcomes for the hip, femoral neck, spine, and TBLH parameters. There were no group by intervention by time interactions for any of the following parameters: hip BMC ($p = 0.414$), hip BMD ($p = 0.473$), femoral neck BMC ($p = 0.760$) or femoral neck BMD ($p = 0.258$). Youth with PWS showed overall lower hip BMC than those with NSO (21.62 ± 0.13 vs. 22.09 ± 0.08 g, $p = 0.002$). The hip BMC intervention-by-time interaction showed a trend toward statistical significance ($p = 0.071$). Pairwise comparisons showed both the intervention ($p < 0.001$) and control groups ($p = 0.001$) significantly increased from baseline to post in hip BMC ($p < 0.001$); and there were no differences at post ($p = 0.709$). Inspection of means showed a slightly greater increase in the intervention group (7.05% change) than control group (4.75% change). Hip BMD increased from baseline to post regardless of group or intervention (0.873 ± 0.001 vs. 0.894 ± 0.005 g/cm^2; $p < 0.001$).

Table 2. Changes in bilateral hip ($n = 111$), spine ($n = 107$) and total body less head ($n = 80$) bone parameters by intervention groups in youth with Prader-Willi syndrome (PWS) and youth with non-syndromic obesity (NSO).

	Hip		Femoral neck		Spine		TBLH	
	BMC [1,2,3]	BMD [2]	BMC [1,2,4]	BMD [2]	BMC [1,2,3,4,5]	BMD	BMC [2,4]	BMD [1,2,4]
Intervention								
PWS Pre	21.22 (0.02)	0.874 (0.001)	3.50 (0.00)	0.855 (0.001)	33.69 (0.13)	0.886 (0.001)	1314.7 (2.9)	0.871 (0.000)
PWS Post	22.33 (0.13)	0.906 (0.018)	3.64 (0.03)	0.872 (0.004)	36.38 (0.47)	0.917 (0.006)	1390.9 (18.9)	0.886 (0.004)
NSO Pre	21.20 (0.03)	0.871 (0.001)	3.50 (0.00)	0.852 (0.001)	33.54 (0.06)	0.887 (0.000)	1311.3 (2.1)	0.871 (0.000)
NSO Post	23.08 (0.18)	0.899 (0.005)	3.73 (0.03)	0.880 (0.006)	36.79 (0.65)	0.917 (0.009)	1443.5 (16.1)	0.897 (0.003)
Overall Pre	21.21 (0.02)	0.873 (0.000)	3.50 (0.00)	0.854 (0.000)	33.61 (0.07)	0.887 (0.001)	1313.0 (1.5)	0.871 (0.000)
Overall Post	22.70 (0.11)	0.902 (0.009)	3.68 (0.02)	0.876 (0.004)	36.59 (0.39)	0.917 (0.005)	1417.2 (12.6)	0.892 (0.002)
Control								
PWS Pre	21.27 (0.05)	0.876 (0.002)	3.51 (0.01)	0.857 (0.002)	33.96 (0.24)	0.887 (0.000)	1329.7 (7.6)	0.873 (0.001)
PWS Post	21.64 (0.47)	0.883 (0.008)	3.59 (0.08)	0.871 (0.009)	32.71 (1.32)	0.867 (0.043)	1420.9 (25.8)	0.884 (0.006)
NSO Pre	21.25 (0.03)	0.873 (0.001)	3.51 (0.005)	0.854 (0.001)	33.77 (0.09)	0.887 (0.001)	1318.0 (3.0)	0.871 (0.000)
NSO Post	22.85 (0.27)	0.891 (0.001)	3.71 (0.04)	0.863 (0.007)	36.28 (0.33)	0.919 (0.0007)	1445.5 (22.3)	0.894 (0.005)
Overall Pre	21.26 (0.03)	0.874 (0.001)	3.51 (0.01)	0.855 (0.001)	33.86 (0.13)	0.887 (0.001)	1322.4 (5.1)	0.872 (0.001)
Overall Post	22.25 (0.27)	0.887 (0.005)	3.65 (0.04)	0.867 (0.006)	34.49 (0.69)	0.893 (0.022)	1433.2 (17.4)	0.889 (0.004)

1 = group effect. 2 = time effect. 3 = intervention × time effect. 4 = group × time effect. 5 = group×intervention×time effect. Abbreviations: BMC = bone mineral content (g), BMD = bone mineral density (g/cm^2), TBLH = total body less head, Pre = baseline. Estimated means (standard error of the mean) are presented. BMC is adjusted for baseline values and height; BMD is adjusted for baseline values.

Femoral neck BMC increased from baseline to post regardless of group or intervention (3.50 ± 0.000 vs. 3.67 ± 0.022 g, $p < 0.001$). Follow-up pairwise comparisons for the group by time interaction ($p = 0.021$) showed a trend toward statistical significance for an increase in youth with PWS ($p = 0.064$) and a significant increase in the youth with NSO ($p < 0.001$). The means were similar for the groups at post ($p = 0.151$). Femoral neck BMD increased from baseline to post regardless of group or intervention (0.855 ± 0.001 vs. 0.871 ± 0.003 g/cm^2; $p < 0.001$).

3.3. Spine and Total Body Changes

For spine BMC there was a significant group by intervention by time interaction ($p = 0.050$). In youth with PWS, the intervention group showed an increase in BMC from baseline to post ($p < 0.001$) but the control group showed no significant change ($p = 1.000$). For those with PWS, intervention and control groups showed similar spine BMC at post ($p = 0.266$). Youth with NSO showed increased spine BMC between baseline and post regardless of intervention or control ($p < 0.001$ for both). There were no differences between the intervention and control groups at post ($p = 1.000$ for both). There were no significant effects of the intervention, time or group in spine BMD ($p > 0.109$).

For total body BMC, there also was a significant group by time interaction ($p = 0.032$). The pairwise comparisons showed that youth with PWS and those with NSO increased TBLH BMC from baseline to post (PWS: 1320.7 ± 4.7 vs. 1405.9 ± 15.8 g [6.45% change] and NSO: 1314.6 ± 1.5 vs. 1444.5 ± 13.7 g [8.88% change], $p < 0.001$ for both). There were no group differences at post ($p = 0.358$). There was no group by time by intervention interaction ($p = 0.992$) for TBLH BMD. There was a significant group by time interaction for TBLH BMD ($p = 0.008$). Pairwise comparisons showed that youth with PWS increased TBLH BMD from baseline to post (0.872 ± 0.001 vs. 0.885 ± 0.003 g/cm^2 (1.49% change), $p < 0.001$) and so did the youth with NSO (0.871 ± 0.001 vs. 0.896 ± 0.003 g/cm^2 (2.87% change), $p < 0.001$). There were no differences at post between youth groups ($p = 0.097$). Table 3 presents all percent changes by group and treatment and the percent improvement of the intervention over the control groups for comparison purposes.

Table 3. Bone parameters percent change (%) as well as percent improvement (%) of the intervention over the control group presented by youth groups.

	Youth with PWS			Youth with NSO		
	% Change		% Improvement	% Change		% Improvement
	Intervention	Control		Intervention	Control	
Hip						
BMC	5.25	1.72	3.53	8.85	7.53	1.32
BMD	3.66	0.80	2.86 *	3.21	2.06	1.15 *
Femoral neck						
BMC	3.88	2.22	1.66	6.58	5.70	0.88
BMD	1.99	1.63	0.36	3.29	1.05	2.24
Spine						
BMC	7.99	−3.69	11.68	9.70	7.44	2.26
BMD	3.50	3.61	−0.11	3.38	0.68	2.7 *
TBLH						
BMC	5.80	6.86	−1.06	10.08	9.67	0.41
BMD	1.72	1.26	0.46	2.99	2.64	0.35

* Percent improvement of the intervention over the control condition is above the facility least significance change (LSC) calculated for hip and spine BMD. Abbreviations: BMC = bone mineral content, BMD = bone mineral density, TBLH = total body less head, PWS = Prader-Willi syndrome, NSO = non-syndromic obesity.

3.4. Blood Bone Markers

There were no group-by-time interactions for any bone marker ($p > 0.425$), or time effects ($p > 0.209$). Youth with NSO had overall higher BAP (139.07 ± 6.41 vs. 108.28 ± 9.19 U/L; $p = 0.006$) and similar CTx (2.07 ± 0.11 vs.1.84 ± 0.14 ng/dL; $p = 0.193$) than those with PWS. Values for BAP for youth with PWS were: pre = 107.40 ± 8.73 and post = 109.15 ± 13.43 U/L, and for youth with NSO were: pre = 144.42 ± 7.56 and post = 133.72 ± 7.71 U/L. Values for CTx for youth with PWS were: pre = 1.77 ± 0.13 and post = 1.91 ± 0.19 U/L, and for youth with NSO were: pre = 2.02 ± 0.13 and post = 2.12 ± 0.11 U/L.

3.5. Nutritional Intake

Twenty three and 40 food records were analyzed in youth with PWS and with NSO. Youth with PWS consumed lower daily calories (1289 ± 67 vs. 1581 ± 64, $p = 0.002$) and higher calcium (1083.1 ± 133.3 vs. 769.0 ± 30.2 mg, $p = 0.022$) and vitamin D (588.6 ± 143.5 vs. 265.4 ± 33.8 IUD, $p = 0.028$) intakes than those with NSO. Calcium intake increased over time (887.4 ± 70.5 to 964.6 ± 70.0 mg, $p = 0.017$) in both youth groups. Regarding nutritional manipulation, 16/23 and 13/23 youth with PWS reported caloric restriction and using nutritional supplementation (multivitamin and calcium), respectively compared to 3/40 and 7/40 of youth with NSO, respectively.

4. Discussion

We hypothesized that completion of a 24-week PA intervention could lead to increases in BMC and BMD in youth with PWS and those with NSO. Our results show that completion of the intervention led to significant increases in BMC in the spine for those with PWS and a small non-significant increase in hip BMC. The intervention had no significant effect in bone parameters in youth with NSO. Percent improvements are discussed below.

In youth with PWS, sustained GHRT not only helps with normalization of height, but also improving BMD [21]. Potentially the role of GH is multifaceted as it may influence bone by normalizing height, increasing lean mass, but also increasing osteocalcin in osteoblasts (bone forming cells) through an IGF-1-mediated pathway. However, as children with PWS fail to go through full puberty, BMD begins to decline despite GHRT, demonstrating the important role for sex hormones inhibiting osteoclast activity [21]. To contribute to the problem is the prescribed hypocaloric diet, which is necessary for weight regulation in PWS [22]. This hypocaloric diet also likely contributes to poor bone mineralization as calcium and vitamin intake are positively related to caloric intake [23,24]. Hence, if individuals with PWS do not supplement their diet with calcium, they likely will not attain the necessary calcium for healthy bone accrual during growth. Thus, all these factors may combine during childhood and adolescence and result in low bone mass and BMD explaining why in this study the group with PWS showed lower BMD and BMC at almost every site compared to youth with obesity.

In youth, recommendations for PA include muscle and bone strengthening exercises at least three days a week in addition to 60 min a day of moderate-to-vigorous PA (MVPA). Reviews evaluating the efficacy of exercise interventions in bone parameters have postulated that effective osteogenic doses can be achieved with interventions that generate a ground reaction force in one leg equal to 3.5 times the body mass delivered three days a week over at least seven months [25]. A recent study by Gabel and collaborators added that the frequency of the stimulus (when of certain intensity such as vigorous intensity [VPA]) and not the total volume is in fact associated with higher bone accrual over time [26]. In prepubertal youth, a meta-analysis including twenty-two studies that used bone loading exercise (resistance training, jumping, and/or high impact activities) showed that the percent improvement for the intervention over the control condition were of 0.8% for total body BMC, 1.5% for femoral neck BMC and 1.7% for spine BMC [27]. However, much larger doses may be needed in youth going through puberty as suggested by the results of this meta-analyses demonstrating no effect of the intervention over the control in the children who were early or post-pubertal [27]. A window of opportunity has been proposed for youth in pre-puberty or early puberty as they experience larger changes compared to when they enter puberty [25]. The hormonal changes that occur during puberty may override the potential effect of exercise on the bone explaining why small changes are observed in interventions in youth during or post puberty [25]. Lastly, the results of a 9-month intervention delivered through the school five days a week showed that children with obesity exhibited less improvement in BMD when compared to those of normal weight [28]. Hence, in the present study, several factors may have contributed to a lack of an effect of the intervention in youth with NSO including an insufficient dose, insufficient intervention length, potentially their pubertal stage as 62% of them were in early or mid-puberty, obesity, and low statistical power (i.e., our study was not a-priori powered to detect changes in bone parameters but powered for other outcomes reported elsewhere [13]). Additionally, compliance with completion of all sessions and activities might have influenced the outcomes [14]. However, the percent improvements, although small, were above the facility computed LSC for BMDs in the hip and spine (1.15% and 2.7%, respectively), indicating that changes in these variables were real and due to the intervention and not measurement errors. Furthermore, these percent changes were above those shown in the previously mentioned meta-analyses [27].

There are not many studies that have evaluated changes in bone parameters in people with PWS. An early study showed no changes in BMD in adults with PWS in response to a four-week exercise intervention delivered at four different times during the year [29]. Likely, the discontinuous nature of the intervention and the lack of routine strengthening or bone building exercises in the routine explain why this early study showed no change in BMD. Thus, our results show promise as we demonstrated increased BMC at the spine by ~8% in the group with PWS in response to this home-based intervention. Our results do not show the same degree of increase in BMC at the hip, but a small non-significant improvement in BMD (~3%) which may be important considering the lower BMD in those with PWS. The risk for low BMD during childhood is problematic because it is such a critical stage for bone acquisition. As BMD during childhood and adolescence tracks over time [30], a poor BMD during growth may increase the risk of future osteoporotic fractures. The small (3.5%) improvement in the hip BMC suggests that the protocol was perhaps insufficient; we only included bone strengthening exercises twice a week. However, the exercises used did not have the dose of jumping interventions (such as jumping from a platform 61 cm high with two feet 100 times) previously tested in youth without PWS [31]. Despite this lack of exercise dose, likely the novelty of the exercises done in addition to a minimum frequency and quantity was sufficient to induce a small effect. Additionally, as we have shown before, youth with PWS were only achieving 30 min of MVPA a day [15] which is less than the recommended 40 min [32].

As more exercise studies are developed for people with PWS, specific exercises must be incorporated to target bone remodeling in those with PWS. The challenge resides in the characteristics needed for the exercise load to have an osteogenic impact [25]. In youth with PWS some limitations exist related to poor muscular strength, running speed, and agility and balance [33]. These factors may limit the ability of individuals with PWS to complete, for example, jumping tasks at a frequency needed. It is possible that to observe larger changes in BMD in the hip, longer interventions with a minimum of three days a week of bone building exercises are needed. In addition, a preparatory period may be allocated to building the minimum motor proficiency to engage in bone-building tasks. We have demonstrated that our intervention strategy improved muscular strength and running speed and agility but did not improve balance in six months [13]. In the action of drop landing or jumping, all three aspects are needed: muscular strength, agility, and dynamic balance. Thus, for youth with PWS to engage in higher impact activities such as running, jumping, or drop landing from elevated platforms [25] basic aspects of their motor skills and proficiency may need to be built first. Of consideration, a plausible approach may be to use a combination of strategies including exercise and whole-body vibration therapy. This combination has been successfully used in youth with severe burns [34].

Our results showed higher BAP in youth without PWS than in those with PWS and no differences in CTx. This lower BAP in those with PWS could be related lower osteoblast activity in those with PWS [35]. The comparable levels of CTx-1 between those with and without PWS is similar to the findings of another study in children and adults with PWS [36]. Our results showed no changes in either BAP or CTx over the 24 weeks. Mostly, changes in bone blood markers have been shown in response to pharmacotherapy [9,10] so the lack of increase in BAP and decrease in CTx is not surprising. The concomitant low concentration of BAP and bone parameters in PWS compared to NSO suggests that perhaps the combination of pharmacotherapy and exercise could be considered to increase bone formation in this population.

By design our group with PWS had an older range of participants compared to those with obesity—this is one reason why we included height as a covariate to assess changes in BMC. Our intervention strategy, while it included bone-building activities twice a week, did not have the recommended optimal dose of three days a week and was not at least seven months long. Our bone blood markers analysis had major limitations as we did not include a control group and the analysis only assesses a snapshot in time. While we tracked changes in diet over time, this was not the main purpose of the study. Therefore, we had no control over dietary changes which resulted in a small increase in calcium intake regardless of youth or treatment allocations. This intervention strategy had a main aim to improve motor proficiency and levels of MVPA and was effective at improving motor proficiency [13] but did not increase ambulation of moderate-to-vigorous intensity [15]. Hence, while some activities might have been novel, likely the osteogenic stimulus might not have been sufficient. Lastly, our study was not powered to detect statistical differences between treatment or youth groups for bone parameters, and we had uneven and relatively small sample sizes for those with PWS. This last aspect, coupled with hip measurements not being the most reliable site for measurement in growing children [37], might have influenced our hip results.

5. Conclusions

This study confirmed results from earlier studies showing lower BMC and BMD in youth with PWS compared to those with obesity. It extended previous characterization studies by showing that youth with PWS (most of them on GHRT) showed lower levels of a marker for bone absorption. Importantly, the results of this study showed increased BMC in youth with PWS after completing a novel 24-week home-based intervention that had a twice-a-week muscle and bone building exercise routine. Future studies aiming to improve bone health in PWS should consider longer intervention strategies that first built upon muscular strength, agility, and dynamic balance that will allow for completion of targeted exercises of higher impact for the bone.

Author Contributions: Conceptualization, D.A.R., K.S.W., C.E.O. and A.M.H.; methodology, D.A.R., K.S.W. and C.E.O.; formal analysis, K.S.W.; data curation, D.M.C. and E.R.G.; investigation, D.A.R., D.M.C., M.D.-D. and E.R.G.; writing—original draft preparation, D.A.R.; writing—review and editing, K.S.W., C.E.O., E.R.G., A.M.H., D.M.C. and M.D.-D.; visualization, D.A.R.; project administration, D.M.C.; funding acquisition, D.A.R., K.S.W. and M.D.-D. All authors have read and agreed to the published version of the manuscript.

Funding: This research was funded by the US army medical research and materiel command, grants numbers W81XWH11-1-076 and W81XWH-09-1-0682.

Acknowledgments: The authors would like to thank the study staff at the California State University Fullerton and University of Florida Gainesville, and the youth participants and their parents for completing the study.

Conflicts of Interest: The authors declare no conflict of interest. The funders had no role in the design of the study; in the collection, analyses, or interpretation of data; in the writing of the manuscript, or in the decision to publish the results.

References

1. Cassidy, S.B.; Schwartz, S.; Miller, J.L.; Driscoll, D.J. Prader-Willi syndrome. *Genet. Med.* **2012**, *14*, 10–26. [CrossRef] [PubMed]
2. Butler, M.G.; Haber, L.; Mernaugh, R.; Carlson, M.G.; Price, R.; Feurer, I.D. Decreased bone mineral density in Prader-Willi syndrome: Comparison with obese subjects. *Am. J. Med. Genet.* **2001**, *103*, 216–222. [CrossRef] [PubMed]
3. Vestergaard, P.; Kristensen, K.; Bruun, J.M.; Ostergaard, J.R.; Heickendorff, L.; Mosekilde, L.; Richelsen, B. Reduced bone mineral density and increased bone turnover in Prader-Willi syndrome compared with controls matched for sex and body mass index—A cross-sectional study. *J. Pediatr.* **2004**, *144*, 614–619. [CrossRef] [PubMed]
4. Rubin, D.A.; Cano-Sokoloff, N.; Castner, D.L.; Judelson, D.A.; Wright, P.; Duran, A.; Haqq, A.M. Update on body composition and bone density in children with Prader-Willi syndrome. *Horm. Res. Paediatr.* **2013**, *79*, 271–276. [CrossRef]
5. Duran, A.T.; Wilson, K.S.; Castner, D.M.; Tucker, J.M.; Rubin, D.A. Association between physical activity and bone in children with Prader-Willi syndrome. *J. Pediatr. Endocrinol. Metab.* **2016**, *29*, 819–826. [CrossRef]
6. Klein-Nulend, J.; Bacabac, R.G.; Bakker, A.D. Mechanical loading and how it affects bone cells: The role of the osteocyte cytoskeleton in maintaining our skeleton. *Eur. Cell Mater.* **2012**, *24*, 278–291. [CrossRef]
7. Galea, G.L.; Lanyon, L.E.; Price, J.S. Sclerostin's role in bone's adaptive response to mechanical loading. *Bone* **2017**, *96*, 38–44. [CrossRef]
8. Janz, K.F.; Baptista, F. Bone Strength and Exercise During Youth-The Year That Was 2017. *Pediatr. Exerc. Sci.* **2018**, *30*, 28–31. [CrossRef]
9. Bauer, D.C.; Black, D.M.; Bouxsein, M.L.; Lui, L.Y.; Cauley, J.A.; de Papp, A.E.; Grauer, A.; Khosla, S.; McCulloch, C.E.; Eastell, R.; et al. Treatment-Related Changes in Bone Turnover and Fracture Risk Reduction in Clinical Trials of Anti-Resorptive Drugs: A Meta-Regression. *J. Bone Miner. Res.* **2018**, *33*, 634–642. [CrossRef]
10. Bianchi, M.L.; Colombo, C.; Assael, B.M.; Dubini, A.; Lombardo, M.; Quattrucci, S.; Bella, S.; Collura, M.; Messore, B.; Raia, V.; et al. Treatment of low bone density in young people with cystic fibrosis: A multicentre, prospective, open-label observational study of calcium and calcifediol followed by a randomised placebo-controlled trial of alendronate. *Lancet Respir. Med.* **2013**, *1*, 377–385. [CrossRef]
11. Sioen, I.; Lust, E.; De Henauw, S.; Moreno, L.A.; Jimenez-Pavon, D. Associations Between Body Composition and Bone Health in Children and Adolescents: A Systematic Review. *Calcif. Tissue Int.* **2016**, *99*, 557–577. [CrossRef] [PubMed]
12. Chaplais, E.; Naughton, G.; Greene, D.; Dutheil, F.; Pereira, B.; Thivel, D.; Courteix, D. Effects of interventions with a physical activity component on bone health in obese children and adolescents: A systematic review and meta-analysis. *J. Bone Miner. Metab.* **2018**, *36*, 12–30. [CrossRef] [PubMed]
13. Rubin, D.A.; Wilson, K.S.; Dumont-Driscoll, M.; Rose, D.J. Effectiveness of a Parent-led Physical Activity Intervention in Youth with Obesity. *Med. Sci. Sports Exerc.* **2019**, *51*, 805–813. [CrossRef]
14. Rubin, D.A.; Wilson, K.S.; Honea, K.E.; Castner, D.M.; McGarrah, J.G.; Rose, D.J.; Dumont-Driscoll, M. An evaluation of the implementation of a parent-led, games-based physical activity intervention: The Active Play at Home quasi-randomized trial. *Health Educ. Res.* **2019**, *34*, 98–112. [CrossRef] [PubMed]

15. Rubin, D.A.; Wilson, K.S.; Castner, D.M.; Dumont-Driscoll, M.C. Changes in Health-Related Outcomes in Youth With Obesity in Response to a Home-Based Parent-Led Physical Activity Program. *J. Adolesc. Health* **2019**. [CrossRef]

16. McCarthy, H.D.; Cole, T.J.; Fry, T.; Jebb, S.A.; Prentice, A.M. Body fat reference curves for children. *Int. J. Obes. (Lond.)* **2006**, *30*, 598–602. [CrossRef]

17. Petersen, A.C.; Crockett, L.; Richards, M.; Boxer, A. A self-report measure of pubertal status: Reliability, validity, and initial norms. *J. Youth Adolesc.* **1988**, *17*, 117–133. [CrossRef]

18. Centers for Disease Control and Prevention. Z-scores data files. Available online: https://www.cdc.gov/growthcharts/zscore.htm (accessed on 19 March 2011).

19. Crabtree, N.J.; Arabi, A.; Bachrach, L.K.; Fewtrell, M.; El-Hajj Fuleihan, G.; Kecskemethy, H.H.; Jaworski, M.; Gordon, C.M.; International Society for Clinical Densitometry. Dual-energy X-ray absorptiometry interpretation and reporting in children and adolescents: The revised 2013 ISCD Pediatric Official Positions. *J. Clin. Densitom.* **2014**, *17*, 225–242. [CrossRef]

20. Wasserman, H.; O'Donnell, J.M.; Gordon, C.M. Use of dual energy X-ray absorptiometry in pediatric patients. *Bone* **2017**, *104*, 84–90. [CrossRef]

21. Bakker, N.E.; Kuppens, R.J.; Siemensma, E.P.; Tummers-de Lind van Wijngaarden, R.F.; Festen, D.A.; Bindels-de Heus, G.C.; Bocca, G.; Haring, D.A.; Hoorweg-Nijman, J.J.; Houdijk, E.C.; et al. Bone mineral density in children and adolescents with Prader-Willi syndrome: A longitudinal study during puberty and 9 years of growth hormone treatment. *J. Clin. Endocrinol. Metab.* **2015**, *100*, 1609–1618. [CrossRef]

22. Eiholzer, U.; Whitman, B.Y. A comprehensive team approach to the management of patients with Prader-Willi syndrome. *J. Pediatr. Endocrinol. Metab.* **2004**, *17*, 1153–1175. [CrossRef] [PubMed]

23. Rubin, D.A.; Nowak, J.; McLaren, E.; Patino, M.; Castner, D.M.; Dumont-Driscoll, M.C. Nutritional intakes in children with Prader-Willi syndrome and non-congenital obesity. *Food Nutr. Res.* **2015**, *59*, 29427. [CrossRef] [PubMed]

24. Jeukendrup, A.; Gleeson, M. *Sport Nutrition*, 3rd ed.; Human Kinetics: Champaign, IL, USA, 2019.

25. Gunter, K.B.; Almstedt, H.C.; Janz, K.F. Physical activity in childhood may be the key to optimizing lifespan skeletal health. *Exerc. Sport Sci. Rev.* **2012**, *40*, 13–21. [CrossRef]

26. Gabel, L.; Macdonald, H.M.; Nettlefold, L.; McKay, H.A. Bouts of Vigorous Physical Activity and Bone Strength Accrual During Adolescence. *Pediatr. Exerc. Sci.* **2017**, *29*, 465–475. [CrossRef]

27. Specker, B.; Thiex, N.W.; Sudhagoni, R.G. Does Exercise Influence Pediatric Bone? A Systematic Review. *Clin. Orthop. Relat. Res.* **2015**, *473*, 3658–3672. [CrossRef]

28. Kondiboyina, V.; Raine, L.B.; Kramer, A.F.; Khan, N.A.; Hillman, C.H.; Shefelbine, S.J. Skeletal Effects of Nine Months of Physical Activity in Obese and Healthy Weight Children. *Med. Sci. Sports Exerc.* **2020**, *52*, 434–440. [CrossRef] [PubMed]

29. Grolla, E.; Andrighetto, G.; Parmigiani, P.; Hladnik, U.; Ferrari, G.; Bernardelle, R.; Lago, M.D.; Albarello, A.; Baschirotto, G.; Filippi, G.; et al. Specific treatment of Prader-Willi syndrome through cyclical rehabilitation programmes. *Disabil. Rehabil.* **2011**, *33*, 1837–1847. [CrossRef] [PubMed]

30. Kalkwarf, H.J.; Gilsanz, V.; Lappe, J.M.; Oberfield, S.; Shepherd, J.A.; Hangartner, T.N.; Huang, X.; Frederick, M.M.; Winer, K.K.; Zemel, B.S. Tracking of bone mass and density during childhood and adolescence. *J. Clin. Endocrinol. Metab.* **2010**, *95*, 1690–1698. [CrossRef]

31. Fuchs, R.K.; Bauer, J.J.; Snow, C.M. Jumping improves hip and lumbar spine bones in prepubescent children: A randomized controlled trial. *J. Bone Miner. Res.* **2001**, *16*, 148–156. [CrossRef]

32. Janz, K.F.; Burns, T.L.; Levy, S.M.; Torner, J.C.; Willing, M.C.; Beck, T.J.; Gilmore, J.M.; Marshall, T.A. Everyday activity predicts bone geometry in children: The iowa bone development study. *Med. Sci. Sports Exerc.* **2004**, *36*, 1124–1131. [CrossRef]

33. Lam, M.Y.; Rubin, D.A.; Duran, A.T.; Chavoya, F.A.; White, E.; Rose, D.J. A characterization of movement skills in obese children with and without Prader-Willi Syndrome. *Res. Q. Exerc. Sport* **2016**, *87*, 245–253. [CrossRef] [PubMed]

34. Edionwe, J.; Hess, C.; Fernandez-Rio, J.; Herndon, D.N.; Andersen, C.R.; Klein, G.L.; Suman, O.E.; Amonette, W.E. Effects of whole-body vibration exercise on bone mineral content and density in thermally injured children. *Burns* **2016**, *42*, 605–613. [CrossRef] [PubMed]

35. Cox, G.; Einhorn, T.A.; Tzioupis, C.; Giannoudis, P.V. Bone-turnover markers in fracture healing. *J. Bone Jt. Surg. Br.* **2010**, *92*, 329–334. [CrossRef] [PubMed]

36. Brunetti, G.; Grugni, G.; Piacente, L.; Delvecchio, M.; Ventura, A.; Giordano, P.; Grano, M.; D'Amato, G.; Laforgia, D.; Crino, A.; et al. Analysis of Circulating Mediators of Bone Remodeling in Prader-Willi Syndrome. *Calcif. Tissue Int.* **2018**, *102*, 635–643. [CrossRef] [PubMed]

37. Baim, S.; Leonard, M.B.; Bianchi, M.L.; Hans, D.B.; Kalkwarf, H.J.; Langman, C.B.; Rauch, F. Official Positions of the International Society for Clinical Densitometry and executive summary of the 2007 ISCD Pediatric Position Development Conference. *J. Clin. Densitom.* **2008**, *11*, 6–21. [CrossRef] [PubMed]

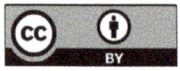 © 2020 by the authors. Licensee MDPI, Basel, Switzerland. This article is an open access article distributed under the terms and conditions of the Creative Commons Attribution (CC BY) license (http://creativecommons.org/licenses/by/4.0/).

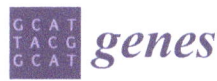

Article

Genetic Subtype-Phenotype Analysis of Growth Hormone Treatment on Psychiatric Behavior in Prader-Willi Syndrome

Andrea S. Montes [1], Kathryn E. Osann [2], June Anne Gold [1], Roy N. Tamura [3], Daniel J. Driscoll [4], Merlin G. Butler [5] and Virginia E. Kimonis [1,*]

[1] Division of Genetics and Genomics Medicine, Department of Pediatrics, University of California, Irvine, CA 92868, USA; andrea.sm021@gmail.com (A.S.M.); goldj@uci.edu (J.A.G.)
[2] Department of Medicine, University of California, Irvine, CA 92868, USA; kosann@hs.uci.edu
[3] Health Informatics Institute, University of South Florida, Tampa, FL 33620, USA; Roy.Tamura@epi.usf.edu
[4] Department of Pediatrics, University of Florida, Gainesville, FL 32610, USA; driscdj@peds.ufl.edu
[5] Departments of Psychiatry, Behavioral Sciences, and Pediatrics, University of Kansas Medical Center, Kansas City, KS 66160, USA; mbutler4@kumc.edu
* Correspondence: vkimonis@uci.edu; Tel.: +714-456-5791; Fax: +714-456-5330

Received: 25 August 2020; Accepted: 20 October 2020; Published: 23 October 2020

Abstract: Prader-Willi syndrome (PWS) is a complex multisystemic condition caused by a lack of paternal expression of imprinted genes from the 15q11.2–q13 region. Limited literature exists on the association between molecular classes, growth hormone use, and the prevalence of psychiatric phenotypes in PWS. In this study, we analyzed nine psychiatric phenotypes (depressed mood, anxiety, skin picking, nail picking, compulsive counting, compulsive ordering, plays with strings, visual hallucinations, and delusions) recognized in PWS and investigated associations with growth hormone treatment (GHT), deletions (DEL) and uniparental disomy (UPD) in a cohort of 172 individuals with PWS who met the criteria for analysis. Associations were explored using Pearson chi-square tests and univariable and multivariable logistic regression analyses to control for confounding exposures. This observational study of the largest dataset of patients with PWS to date suggested the following genetic subtype and phenotype correlations in psychiatric behaviors: (1) skin picking was more frequent in those with DEL vs. UPD; (2) anxiety was more common in those with UPD vs. DEL; and (3) an increased frequency of anxiety was noted in the UPD group treated with GHT compared to the DEL group. No other significant associations were found between the genetic subtype or GHT including for depressed mood, nail picking, compulsive counting, compulsive ordering, playing with strings, and visual hallucinations. Further studies will be required before any conclusions can be reached.

Keywords: Prader-Willi syndrome (PWS); PWS molecular classes; PWS genetic subtype–phenotype correlations; natural history; psychiatric behavioral phenotype; growth hormone treatment

---

1. Introduction

Prader-Willi syndrome (PWS) is a multisystemic neurogenetic disorder that affects approximately 1/15,000 live births. PWS is found across all races and affects both genders equally [1,2]. Clinical manifestations change dramatically with age. Infants present with severe hypotonia, feeding problems, poor weight gain, and overall failure to thrive. As the individual enters early childhood, they develop hyperphagia with aggressive and obsessive food-seeking behaviors including hoarding and stealing food and eating non-food items or food from the floor or garbage. These behaviors typically lead to morbid obesity and the associated complications of diabetes, obstructive sleep apnea,

Genes **2020**, *11*, 1250; doi:10.3390/genes11111250   www.mdpi.com/journal/genes

and right-sided heart failure if the caloric intake is not externally controlled. Individuals with PWS develop hypothalamic dysfunction, which often leads to endocrinopathies including growth hormone deficiency, hypogonadism, and hypothyroidism [3,4]. PWS also has a unique cognitive and behavioral profile which typically presents with delayed motor and language skills, learning disabilities, and an average intelligence quotient (IQ) of 65 [4]. Severe behavioral problems are common and often present as stubbornness, defiance, easy frustrations, and quickness to anger. They often have mood disorders, a striking inability to control their emotions, obsessive tendencies, autistic traits, and are at high risk of developing psychoses in late adolescence or early adulthood, particularly those with uniparental disomy (UPD) [4–6].

Prader-Willi syndrome is a genetically heterogeneous disorder caused by three main molecular mechanisms by which the loss of the paternally expressed genes in the 15q11.2–q13 region occurs, generally by paternal interstitial deletions followed by maternal uniparental disomy 15 and imprinting center defects (ICD) [7–10]. Depending on the molecular mechanism causing the disorder, significant differences in the clinical presentation, primarily related to the behavioral and psychiatric phenotype, may occur [4,10–14]. Those with deletions (DEL) are more likely to have severe behavioral problems, such as self-injury, food-stealing, and compulsive behaviors as well as speech articulation deficits, yet they often have a particular strength with visual-perceptual skills and jigsaw puzzles [4]. Individuals with UPD tend to have significantly higher verbal IQ scores and a higher likelihood to develop psychotic disorders than those with DEL [4,15].

All individuals with Prader-Willi syndrome are at increased risk for psychiatric comorbidities. Lifetime risk for psychotic illness is reported to be up to 60% in those with UPD and 20% in those with deletions, while the general population risk is less than 3.5% [3]. Common psychiatric disorders seen in those with PWS include affective disorders, compulsions, autistic disorders, and psychoses [4]. The mechanisms for psychiatric disturbances in PWS are not well understood; however, growth hormone and insulin-like growth factor (IGF-I) which are important hormones or peptides involving brain and axonal growth with myelination, are deficient in 40–100% of individuals with PWS [16]. Treating these deficiencies with growth hormone therapy is thought to strengthen neuronal signaling, long-term potentiation, and plasticity in hippocampal and other brain regions, thus improving brain growth and resulting in improved cognition [3].

There is no cure for the Prader-Willi syndrome, so treatment is based on the individual's symptoms. Recombinant growth hormone therapy (GHT) for PWS was approved in the United States in 2000 and has since been widely recognized as a beneficial treatment for the multiple co-morbidities associated with the syndrome [17–20]. GHT improves linear growth, body composition and lean muscle mass, metabolism and energy expenditure, bone mineral density, and cardiovascular health across all ages of PWS patients [4,16,18]. In addition to the physical improvements, GHT may improve behavior and cognition. Significant improvements in motor development as well as other markers of development, such as language and cognitive ability, have been observed in infants and toddlers treated with growth hormone compared to those who were untreated [17–21].

This study explored the association between PWS genetic subtypes, growth hormone use, and the prevalence of nine psychiatric behaviors using data from a large multi-site cohort.

2. Materials and Methods

An 8-year longitudinal observational study was conducted through the Rare Disease Clinical Research Network's (RDCRN) Natural History PWS and Morbid Obesity Clinical Protocol. This study was reviewed and approved by the Institutional Review Board of the participating sites prior to enrollment (i.e., University of California Office of Research, Irvine (HS# 2007-5605)). Individuals with PWS (*n* = 355) were recruited by experts in this disorder at four research sites: University of Florida (lead site), University of Kansas Medical Center, University of California at Irvine, and Vanderbilt University. Informed consent was obtained from all individuals or their parents or legal representatives. Funding for this study was provided through the Rare Disease Clinical Research Network (RDCRN) by the National Institutes of Health (NIH)/National Institute of Child Health and Human Development (NICHD) [22].

Data on clinical, cognitive, behavioral, PWS genetic subtypes, physical, and body composition measures were collected over multiple visits. The same questionnaires were used at each of the four clinical sites to collect information on screening eligibility, demographics and diagnosis, medication history and concomitant medications, as well as behavior. Data were collected on each participant's current and past psychiatric behaviors using yes/no responses which represented parent/guardian assessments and were not necessarily diagnosed by mental health professionals.

Participants were enrolled in this study from 7 September 2006 to 31 July 2014. They were invited to return every year until the age of 3 years and biennially if they were over the age of 3 years. Fifty percent of participants came for one visit. Data were entered and stored at the Data Management Coordinating Center (DMCC) at the University of South Florida in Tampa, Florida. The DMCC provided electronic forms for data entry and performed data retrieval and statistical analyses [22].

This study used the largest dataset on patients with PWS to date to explore the association between growth hormone use and the prevalence of nine psychiatric behaviors (depressed mood, anxiety, skin picking, nail picking, compulsive counting, compulsive ordering, plays with strings, visual hallucinations, and delusions) seen in PWS (Table 1). A comparison between growth hormone users and non-growth hormone users was performed and potential dosage effects were assessed by analyzing ages of growth hormone treatment (GHT) initiation and the duration of GHT. The effects of GHT use on PWS genetic subtypes were also investigated. Exclusion criteria included participants under the age of 8 years as the onset of psychiatric disorders is typically in late childhood or adolescence, as well as those who began GHT after their first visit [23]. In this cohort, 172 participants met the criteria for this study.

Table 1. Psychiatric behaviors grouped into three categories.

Depressive Disorders	Compulsions	Psychoses
Depressed mood	Skin picking	Visual hallucinations
Anxiety	Nail picking	Delusions
	Compulsive counting	
	Compulsive ordering	
	Plays with strings	

Study participants were divided into two cohorts, DEL vs. UPD, as well as those who used GHT at any point in their lives and those who had not, and were analyzed with respect to demographics, medications, and the presence of psychiatric phenotypes at their initial visit using descriptive statistics. Although information was also collected on whether the participant had ever experienced psychiatric behaviors, the data were often incomplete so they were not included in the analysis. Changes in psychiatric phenotype at subsequent visits were also not analyzed as half of the participants came to only one visit. Categorical variables (use of growth hormone, psychiatric medication or sex hormone and PWS genetic subtypes) were described with frequencies and percentages, and continuous variables (age at first visit, age at GHT initiation, and GHT duration) were described using the mean and standard deviation. Associations between the use of GHT and psychiatric phenotypes were explored using Pearson chi-square tests. To further explore associations between GHT use, other exposures, and the risk of psychiatric outcome, univariable and multivariable logistic regression analyses were employed. Multivariable logistic regression was used to control for other independent risk factors and possible confounding exposures when a univariable analysis suggested associations between GHT and psychiatric outcomes with a significance level of $p \leq 0.05$. The following covariates were tested: (1) age at visit 1, (2) age at GHT initiation, (3) psychiatric medication use, (4) PWS genetic subtype, (5) sex of participant, (6) sex hormone use, and (7) GHT duration. Age at GHT initiation was strongly correlated with age at visit 1 ($r = 0.837$) making it uninformative as an independent contributor to outcome risk; therefore, it was dropped from the multivariable analyses. Sex hormone use and the sex of the participant were also not shown to be associated with any of the outcomes by univariable analyses, so these variables were dropped from multivariable analyses. To determine whether the growth hormone had a different effect on outcome risks for different PWS genetic subtypes, an interaction variable was added to the multivariable model between the GHT and PWS genetic subtypes (DEL vs. UPD). The following interaction variables were created: GH*Del (DEL = 1 and UPD = 0) for phenotypes which showed a positive association with the deletion subtype and GH*UPD (UPD = 1 and DEL = 0) for phenotypes which showed a positive association with the UPD subtype. Statistical analyses were performed using SPSS Statistics Software (IBM SPSS Statistics for Windows, Version 21.0 (IBM Corp., Armonk, NY, USA). The data supporting the findings in this paper are available upon request from the corresponding author, Dr. Virginia Kimonis.

3. Results

Variables

Among our cohort of 172 participants with PWS that met our inclusion criteria, 107 (62%) had DEL, 57 (33%) had UPD, and 8 (5%) had ICD. Of those with DEL or UPD (n = 164), 116 (71%) were on GHT (73% vs. 67%, respectively; p = 0.40). Psychiatric phenotype frequencies for those with DEL vs. UPD were as follows: depressed mood (30% vs. 30%; p = 0.98), anxiety (57% vs. 74%; p = 0.04), skin picking (82% vs. 63%; p = 0.008), nail picking (49% vs. 39%; p = 0.30), compulsive counting (19% vs. 16%; p = 0.69), compulsive ordering (43% vs. 40%; p = 0.74), playing with strings (20% vs. 18%; p = 0.66), visual hallucinations (2% vs. 6%; p = 0.21), and delusions (5% vs. 7%; p = 0.52) (Table 2). There were no significant differences in age between the DEL and UPD subgroups (p = 0.09) (Table 3).

Table 2. Presence of psychiatric phenotypes by deletion (DEL) and uniparental disomy (UPD) subtypes.

Phenotype	Presence of Phenotype at Visit 1	DEL		UPD		Totals		Pearson Chi-Square p-Value
		n *	%	n *	%	n *	%	
Depressed Mood n = 155 *	Yes	31/102	30	16/53	30	47	30	0.98
Anxiety n = 157 *	Yes	59/103	57	40/54	74	99	63	0.04
Skin Picking n = 162 *	Yes	86/105	82	36/57	63	122	75	0.008
Nail Picking n = 127 *	Yes	42/86	49	16/41	39	58	46	0.30
Compulsive Counting n = 158 *	Yes	19/102	19	9/56	16	28	18	0.69
Compulsive Ordering n = 158 *	Yes	44/103	43	22/55	40	66	42	0.74
Plays with Strings n = 160 *	Yes	21/103	20	10/57	18	31	19	0.66
Visual Hallucinations n = 156 *	Yes	2/103	2	3/53	6	5	3	0.21
Delusions n = 156 *	Yes	5/102	5	4/54	7	9	6	0.52

* Total number of participants varies for each phenotype depending on whether the data were provided or left incomplete on the questionnaire.

Table 3. Age groups at visit 1 by deletions (DEL) and uniparental disomy (UPD) genotypes.

Age Groups at Visit 1 (Years)	DEL		UPD		Totals		Pearson Chi-Square p-Value
	n = 107	%	n = 57	%	n = 164	%	
8–13	29	27	25	44	54	33	
14–18	26	24	7	12	33	20	
19–26	27	25	11	19	38	23	0.09
27–62	25	23	14	25	39	24	

After adjusting for the effects of confounding variables, GHT was significantly associated with increased presence of anxiety (OR = 2.7, 95% CI: 1.006–7.426, p = 0.05) and delusions (OR = 14.0, 95% CI: 1.262–155.638, p = 0.03) (see Table 4). As the number of participants with delusions was low (n = 9), the model was run without the additional covariable of psychiatric medication use, and GHT use remained a significant association (p = 0.04). PWS individuals with UPD had a higher presence of anxiety than those with DEL (OR = 7.4, 95% 1.760–31.309, p = 0.006) and there was a significant interaction between the GHT use and genotype (p = 0.04). GHT use was associated with a 3.25-fold increased presence of anxiety in those with UPD vs. a 2.73-fold increased presence in those with DEL.

Table 4. Covariables included in the multivariable model for anxiety and delusions.

Anxiety (n = 99)	Delusions (n = 9)
GHT use (OR = 2.7, CI: 1.0–7.4; p = 0.05)	GHT use (OR = 14.0, CI: 1.3–155.6, p = 0.03)
Age at visit 1 (OR = 1.0, 95% CI: 0.9–1.0; p = 0.03)	Age at visit 1 (OR = 1.1, 95% CI: 1.0–1.1; p = 0.08)
Psychiatric medication use (OR = 3.9, CI: 1.6–9.2; p = 0.002)	Psychiatric medication use (OR = 3.4, 95% CI: 0.91–12.8; p = 0.07)
UPD genotype (OR = 7.6, CI:1.8–32.1; p = 0.006)	
Interaction between GHT use and genotype (OR = 0.2, CI: 0.03–0.9; p = 0.04)	

OR = odds ratio; CI = confidence interval.

Age at GHT initiation was intended to be a measure of dosage; however, it was too strongly correlated with age (r = 0.837, p < 0.001) to clearly interpret. Individuals who used GHT were significantly younger at visit 1 than those who did not use GHT: 5 (9%) no GHT vs. 50 (91%) GHT were <13 y., 5 (14%) no GHT vs. 30 (86%) GHT were 14–18 y., 15 (35%) no GHT vs. 28 (65%) GHT were 19–26 y., and 27 (69%) no GHT vs. 12 (31%) GHT were >27 y. (p < 0.001) (Table 5). Thus, as age at first visit increased, so did the age of GHT initiation. Among participants with ages 8–13 years at visit 1, 57% started GHT by the age of 2 years and 78% started GHT by the age of 6 years. For those aged 19 years or older, none started GHT by the age of 2 years and only 4% started GHT by the age of 6 years.

Table 5. Descriptive data by growth hormone treatment use.

Descriptive Data		Growth Hormone Treatment Use						Pearson Chi-Square p-Value
		No		Yes		Total		
		n = 52	%	n = 120	%	n = 172	%	
Sex	Male	19	37	59	49	78	45	0.13
	Female	33	63	61	51	94	55	
Genetic Subtype	DEL	29	56	78	65	107	62	0.33
	UPD	19	36	38	32	57	33	
	ICD	4	8	4	3	8	5	
Age Group at Visit 1 (Years)	8–13	5	10	50	42	55	32	<0.001
	14–18	5	10	30	25	35	20	
	19–26	15	28	28	23	43	25	
	27–62	27	52	12	10	39	23	

DEL = deletion; UPD = uniparental disomy; ICD = imprinting center defect.

GHT duration was also investigated in order to measure dosage. Of the 113 individuals in the GHT cohort who provided data on their duration of treatment, 32 (25%) were on GHT for 0.1–3 years, 31 (24%) for 4–9 years, 35 (27%) for 10–12 years, and 15 (24%) for 13–19 years. As anxiety and delusions had statistically significant associations with GHT use, GHT duration was expected to provide additional supporting evidence. No significant associations, however, were found to support this hypothesis (anxiety: p = 0.06; delusions: p = 0.54) (see Figures 1–4).

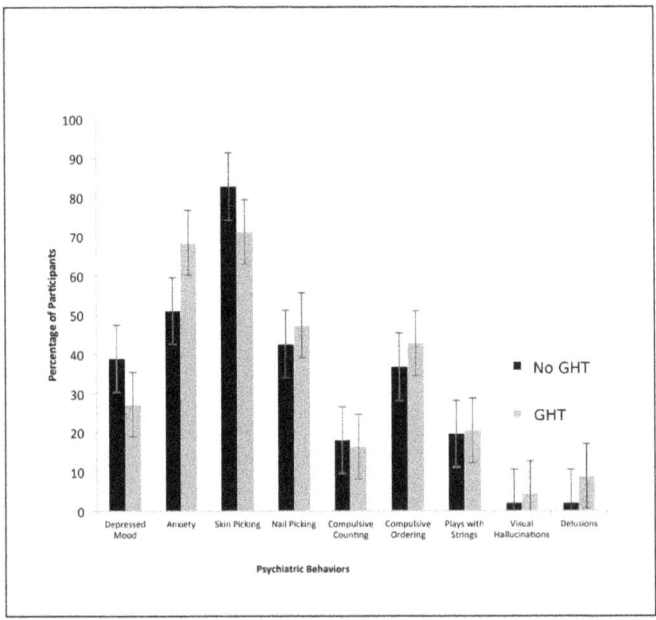

Figure 1. Association between psychiatric behavior and growth hormone treatment use. Percentage of GHT users and non-GHT users who reported the presence of each psychiatric behavior (unadjusted for confounders) at their first visit. There was a significantly higher prevalence of anxiety in GHT users over non-GHT users ($p = 0.03$).

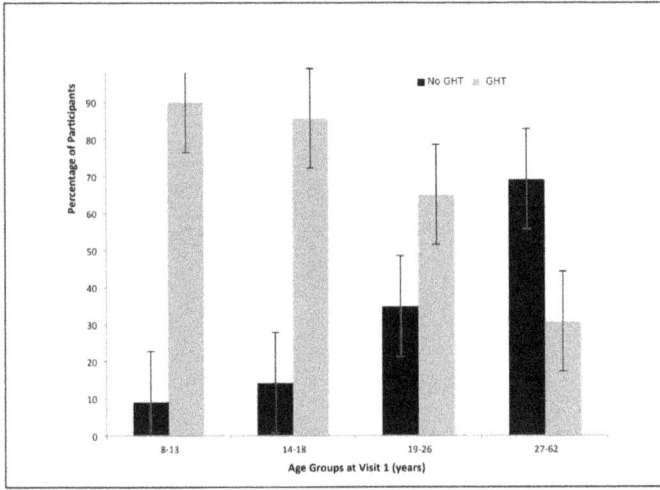

Figure 2. Growth hormone treatment (GHT) use by age group at visit 1. Individuals who used GHT were significantly younger at visit 1 than those who did not use GHT.

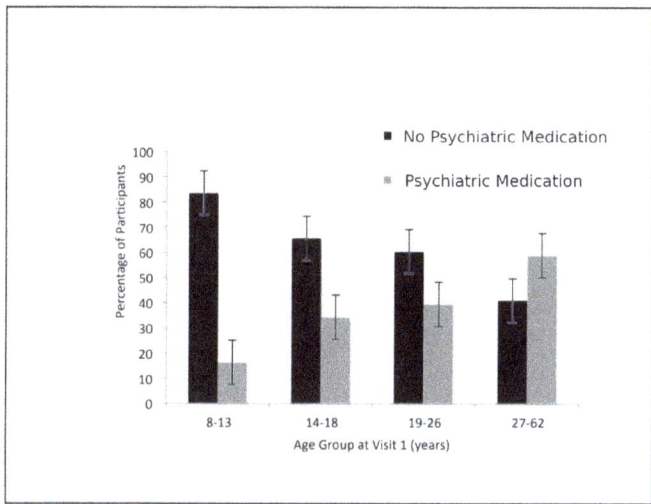

Figure 3. Psychiatric medication use by age group at visit 1. Individuals who used psychiatric medications were significantly older at visit 1 than those who did not use psychiatric medications.

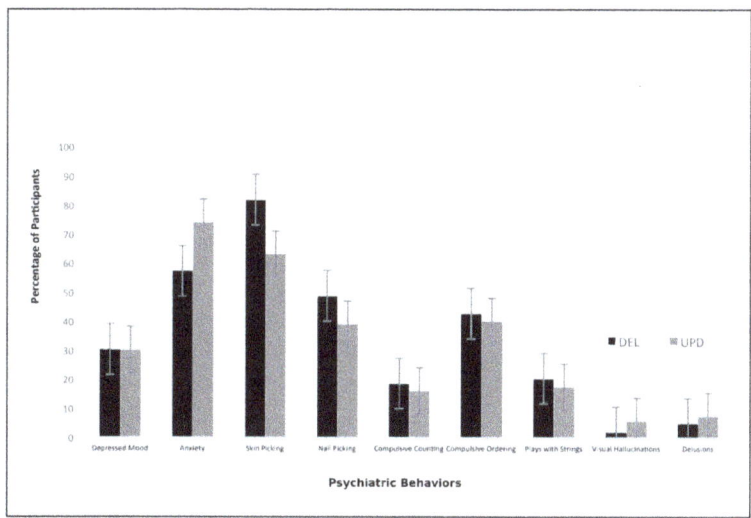

Figure 4. Prader-Willi syndrome (PWS) genetic subtype–phenotype associations (DEL = deletion; UPD = uniparental disomy). Comparison between individuals with DEL and UPD for nine psychiatric phenotypes.

4. Discussion

This study adds to the existing literature regarding PWS genetic subtype–phenotype associations in Prader-Willi syndrome. According to this dataset, UPD is significantly associated with a higher risk for anxiety and deletions are significantly associated with a higher risk of skin picking. These findings are supported by the literature, which reports that those with UPD have greater vulnerability for developing psychoses [24], and those with deletions have higher rates of developing compulsions and self-injury [10,11,14,25].

Based on reports that growth hormone treatment may improve cognition and behavior in individuals with PWS, we speculated that growth hormone treatment would also contribute to a decreased risk of psychiatric behaviors. This hypothesis, however, was not supported by the data in our study. After adjusting for confounding variables, anxiety and delusions were outcomes that had a significant association with growth hormone treatment use, and the data suggested that GHT use was associated with a 2.7 times increased association with anxiety (CI: 1.0–7.4; $p = 0.05$) and a 14.0 times increased association with delusions (CI: 1.3–155.6; $p = 0.03$). These findings were unexpected as there are no documented associations between psychiatric behaviors and GHT. While these findings may be true, they may also be due to chance or other confounding variables that were not captured by the study. One possible explanation is that those receiving growth hormone treatment may also be receiving superior medical care in which psychiatric symptoms are more likely to be detected. It is also plausible that younger individuals experience more anxiety-inducing situations as they transition through school and different living arrangements, whereas older individuals may have more consistency in their routine. Perhaps the most important limitation is that psychiatric behaviors were not necessarily diagnosed by a mental health professional; instead, the data were provided entirely by a parent/guardian report. Notably, out of 164 participants in the study with DEL or UPD, only nine reported delusions, which explains the wide confidence interval, and along with the modest p values for both anxiety and delusions, increases the possibility that these may be chance findings.

It was also hypothesized that growth hormone would have a different effect on the deletion vs. UPD subtypes based on reports of psychiatric differences due to genotype. This hypothesis was supported by the data, which suggests that GHT use has a greater effect on increased risk for anxiety for those with UPD than for those with DEL. These findings have not been previously reported in the literature. While this finding may be true, it may also be due to chance or other confounding variables that were not captured by the study.

In order to support the association between exposure and outcome, we investigated age at GHT initiation and GHT duration for the possible evidence of a consistent dosage effect. Age at GHT initiation was uninformative, however, because it was too strongly correlated to age. This is largely because the GHT was FDA approved for PWS patients in 2000 and there was a lag in GHT being adopted as the standard of treatment. Consequently, individuals had a greater chance of initiating GHT at an earlier age if born after 2000, while individuals born prior did not receive GHT at a younger age as the treatment was not available or approved. Therefore, age at growth hormone initiation was found to be a poor measure of dosage and it was dropped from the analysis. As anxiety and delusions had statistically significant associations with GHT use, GHT duration was expected to provide additional supporting evidence. No significant associations, however, were found to support this hypothesis. Although GHT could be associated with anxiety and delusions without treatment duration effects, the finding of a dosage effect typically supports the association between exposure and outcome. It is possible that dosage truly does have an effect on the outcome, but that duration of treatment is not a good stand-alone measure of dosage. Notably, the type of growth hormone treatment and the dosage of each treatment was not included in the analysis. Another possibility is that GHT duration truly is associated with the outcome, but the sample was not large enough to produce a statistically significant association. The lack of an association with GHT duration, however, suggests that the association of GHT use and an increased risk of anxiety and delusions may be a chance finding.

Psychiatric behaviors are complex and often due to a combination of several genetic and environmental factors [26]. Measuring the effects of one exposure on psychiatric outcome is therefore complicated, as one must attempt to eliminate the effects of all other confounding variables. The strengths of this study include the large longitudinal sample size and the amount of information gathered on each patient using standardized protocols which allowed for the evaluation of several possible confounding variables; however, many additional potential confounders were not included in the data collection and therefore not controlled in the analyses. Potential confounders include race, culture, socioeconomic status (SES), family history, and comorbidities. It is estimated that children and adolescents from families with low SES are up to three times more likely to develop mental health problems than their peers from families with high SES [27]. Access to GHT is also associated with SES due to the expense and not all families have equal access due to variable health care coverage throughout the nation [28]. Additionally, controlling for the co-occurrence of sleep disturbances is also important, as it is common in individuals with Prader-Willi syndrome. Sleep is an important psychophysiological process to promote healthy brain function and mental health, possibly making it a confounding variable [29].

In this study, information on psychiatric diagnosis was gathered by guardian report and data were obtained through medical records rather than through a formal psychiatric evaluation. Psychiatric disorders are highly stigmatized which may lead to the underreporting of symptoms [30]. Stigma regarding mental health disorders has been reported to vary among individuals and families from different races and cultures [31]. Differences in reporting by race and/or culture were not assessed in the analyses in this study, as 85% of the study participants were white; therefore, an important confounding factor for psychiatric behavior reporting may have been missed. A better evaluation of psychiatric disorders in the family history is also recommended, as psychiatric disorders are highly heritable.

5. Conclusions

This observational study of the largest dataset of PWS patients to date suggested differences in psychiatric phenotype exist between genetic subtypes, namely those with DEL were more likely to exhibit skin picking while those with UPD were more likely to experience anxiety. The data also suggested the association of GHT and psychiatric phenotype may differ by genetic subtype as an increased frequency of anxiety was found in the UPD group treated with GHT compared to the DEL group. However, in order to better understand the effects of GHT on psychiatric behavior in PWS, the limitations of this study must be addressed. Future analyses should include detailed information on the age of onset of psychiatric symptoms as well as the duration and the frequency of episodes. It would also be important to determine when, and if, symptoms started in relation to growth hormone use. Increasing the sample size to include more adolescent and adult individuals would also be beneficial in order to give the study greater statistical power over a wider age range of individuals with PWS. The authors encourage more controlled studies and prospective investigations in a large PWS cohort similarly treated and assessed to further characterize or validate our preliminary observations of GHT effects on psychiatric behavioral phenotypes in PWS.

Author Contributions: All authors have participated in revising it critically and give their final approval of the version to be submitted. Conceptualization: A.S.M., V.E.K., D.J.D.; methodology: D.J.D.; acquisition of data: J.A.G., V.E.K., M.G.B., D.J.D.; validation: K.E.O., R.N.T.; analysis and interpretation of data: A.S.M., K.E.O., R.N.T., V.E.K.; formal analysis: A.S.M., K.E.O., R.N.T.; investigation, resources: D.J.D.; writing—original draft preparation: A.S.M.; data curation, critical revision: A.S.M., K.E.O., M.G.B., D.J.D., V.E.K.; writing—review and editing: A.S.M., K.E.O., M.G.B., D.J.D., R.N.T.; visualization: A.S.M., V.E.K.; supervision: V.E.K., M.G.B., D.J.D.; project administration: V.E.K., M.G.B., D.J.D.; funding acquisition: D.J.D. All authors have read and agreed to the published version of the manuscript.

Funding: This research was funded by a grant from the Prader-Willi Syndrome Association (USA); NIH/NCATS Clinical and Translational Science Award of Florida (UL1 TR000064); and National Institutes of Health (NIH) Rare Disease Clinical Research Network (RDCRN) (U54 HD06122).

Acknowledgments: We thank the patients and families for their contribution to this study. We acknowledge support from the Prader-Willi Syndrome Association (USA) and the Angelman, Rett and Prader-Willi Syndromes Consortium (U54 HD06122) which was part of the National Institutes of Health (NIH) Rare Disease Clinical Research Network (RDCRN) supported through collaboration between the NIH Office of Advancing Translational Science (NCATS) and the National Institute of Child Health and Human Development (NICHD). We thank Emily Curtin and Mabel Tang for administrative assistance.

Conflicts of Interest: The authors have no conflict of interest.

References

1. Butler, M.G. Prader-Willi Syndrome: Current Understanding of Cause and Diagnosis. *Am. J. Med Genet.* **1990**, *35*, 319–332. [CrossRef] [PubMed]

2. Cassidy, S.B. Prader-Willi syndrome. *J. Med Genet.* **1997**, *34*, 917–923. [CrossRef] [PubMed]

3. Lukoshe, A.; White, T.; Schmidt, M.N.; van der Lugt, A.; Hokken-Koelega, A.C. Divergent structural brain abnormalities between different genetic subtypes of children with Prader-Willi syndrome. *J. Neurodev. Disord.* **2013**, *5*, 31. [CrossRef] [PubMed]

4. Butler, M.G.; Hanchett, J.M.; Thompson, T. Clinical findings and natural history of Prader-Willi syndrome. In *Management of Prader-Willi Syndrome*; Springer: New York, NY, USA, 2006; pp. 3–48.

5. Dykens, E.; Shah, B. Psychiatric disorders in Prader-Willi syndrome: Epidemiology and management. *CNS Drugs* **2003**, *17*, 167–178. [CrossRef]

6. Zhang, Y.; Zhao, H.; Qiu, S.; Tian, J.; Wen, X.; Miller, J.; Liu, Y. Altered functional brain networks in Prader-Willi syndrome. *NMR Biomed.* **2013**, *26*, 622–629. [CrossRef] [PubMed]

7. Bittel, D.C.; Butler, M.G. Prader-Willi syndrome: Clinical genetics, cytogenetics and molecular biology. *Expert Rev. Mol. Med.* **2005**, *7*, 1–20. [CrossRef] [PubMed]

8. Butler, M.G.; Sturich, J.; Myers, S.E.; Gold, J.A.; Kimonis, V.; Driscoll, D. Is gestation in Prader-Willi syndrome affected by the genetic subtype? *J. Assist. Reprod. Genet.* **2009**, *26*, 461. [CrossRef]

9. Cheon, C.K. Genetics of Prader-Willi syndrome and Prader-Will-Like syndrome. *Ann. Pediatr. Endocrinol. Metab.* **2016**, *12*, 126–135. [CrossRef]

10. Butler, M.G.; Bittel, D.C.; Kibiryeva, N.; Talebizadeh, Z.; Thompson, T. Behavioral differences among subjects with Prader-Willi syndrome and type I or type II deletion and-maternal-disomy. *Pediatrics* **2004**, *113 Pt 1*, 565–573. [CrossRef]

11. Zarcone, J.; Napolitano, D.; Peterson, C.; Breidbord, J.; Ferraioli, S.; Caruso-Anderson, M.; Holsen, L.; Butler, M.G.; Thompson, T. The relationship between compulsive behavior and academic achievement across the three genetic subtypes of Prader-Willi syndrome. *J. Intellect. Disabil. Res.* **2007**, *51*, 478–487. [CrossRef]

12. Dykens, E.M.; Roof, E. Behavior in Prader-Willi syndrome: Relationship to genetic subtypes and age. *J. Child Psychol. Psychiatry* **2008**, *49*, 1001–1008. [CrossRef]

13. Yang, L.; Zhan, G.; Ding, J.; Wang, H.; Huang, G.; Zhou, W. Psychiatric Illness and Intellectual Disability in the Prader-Willi Syndrome with Different Molecular Defects—A Meta Analysis. *PLoS ONE* **2013**, *8*, e72640. [CrossRef] [PubMed]

14. Manzardo, A.M.; Weisensel, N.; Ayala, S.; Hossain, W.; Butler, M.G. Prader-Willi syndrome genetic subtypes and clinical neuropsychiatric diagnoses in residential care adults. *Clin. Genet.* **2018**, *93*, 622–631. [CrossRef] [PubMed]

15. Grugni, G.; Sartorio, A.; Crino, A. Growth hormone therapy for Prader-Willi syndrome: Challenges and solutions. *Ther. Clin. Risk Manag.* **2016**, *12*, 873–888. [CrossRef] [PubMed]

16. Burman, P.; Ritzen, E.M.; Lindgren, A.C. Endocrine Dysfunction in Prader-Willi Syndrome: A Review with Special Reference to GH. *Endocr. Rev.* **2001**, *22*, 787–799. [CrossRef]

17. Höybye, C.; Thorén, M.; Böhm, B. Cognitive, emotional, physical and social effects of growth hormone treatment in adults with Prader-Willi syndrome. *J. Intellect. Disabil. Resour.* **2005**, *49*, 245–252. [CrossRef]

18. Myers, S.E.; Whitman, B.Y.; Carrel, A.L.; Moerchen, V.; Bekx, M.T.; Allen, D.B. Two years of growth hormone therapy in young children with Prader-Willi syndrome: Physical and neurodevelopmental benefits. *Am. J. Med Genet.* **2007**, *143A*, 443–448. [CrossRef] [PubMed]

19. Siemensma, E.; Tummers-de Lind van Wijngaarden, R.; Festen, D.; Troeman, Z.; van Alfen-vander Velden, A.A.E.M.; Otten, B.; Rotteveel, J.; Hokken-Koelega, A. Beneficial Effects of Growth Hormone Treatment on Cognition in Children with Prader-Willi Syndrome: A Randomized Controlled Trial and Longitudinal Study. *J. Clin. Endocrinol. Metab.* **2012**, *97*, 2307–2314. [CrossRef]

20. Butler, M.G.; Matthews, N.A.; Patel, N.; Surampalli, A.; Gold, J.; Khare, M.; Thompson, T.; Cassidy, S.B.; Kimonis, V.E. Impact of genetic subtypes of Prader-Willi syndrome with growth hormone therapy on intelligence and body mass index. *Am. J. Med. Genet.* **2019**, *179*, 1826–1835. [CrossRef]

21. Festen, D.; Wevers, M.; Lindgren, A.C.; Bohn, B.; Otten, B.; Wit, J.; Duivenvoorden, H.; Hokken-Koelega, A. Mental and motor development before and during growth hormone treatment in infants and toddlers with Prader-Willi syndrome. *Clin. Endocrinol.* **2008**, *68*, 919–925. [CrossRef]

22. Montes, A. A Genotype-Phenotype Analysis of the Effects of Growth Hormone Treatment on Psychiatric Behavior in Prader-Willi Syndrome. Ph.D. Thesis, UC Irvine, Irvine, CA, USA, 2019. Available online: https://escholarship.org/uc/item/0w14g4dm (accessed on 8 January 2020).
23. Kessler, R.C.; Amminger, G.P.; Aguilar-Gaxiola, S.; Alonso, J.; Lee, S.; Üstün, T.B. Age of onset of mental disorders: A review of recent literature. *Curr. Opin. Psychiatry* **2007**, *20*, 359–364. [CrossRef] [PubMed]
24. Roof, E.; Stone, W.; MacLean, W.; Feurer, I.D.; Thompson, T.; Butler, M.G. Intellectual characteristics of Prader-Willi syndrome: Comparison of genetic subtypes. *J. Intellect. Disabil. Res.* **2001**, *44*, 25–30. [CrossRef] [PubMed]
25. Krefft, M.; Frydecka, D.; Adamowski, T.; Misiak, B. From Prader-Willi syndrome to psychosis: Translating parent-of-origin effects into schizophrenia research. *Epigenomics* **2014**, *6*, 677–688. [PubMed]
26. Tsuang, M.T.; Bar, J.L.; Stone, W.S.; Faraone, S.V. Gene-environment interactions in mental disorders. *World Psychiatry* **2004**, *3*, 73–83.
27. Reiss, F.; Meyrose, A.K.; Otto, C.; Lampert, T.; Klasen, F.; Ravens-Sieberer, U. Socioeconomic status, stressful life situations and mental health problems in children and adolescents: Results of the German BELLA cohort-study. *PLoS ONE* **2019**, *14*, e0213700. [CrossRef] [PubMed]
28. Dykens, E.M.; Roof, E.; Hunt-Hawkins, H. Cognitive and adaptive advantages of growth hormone treatment in children with Prader-Willi syndrome. *J. Child Psychol. Psychiatry* **2017**, *58*, 64–74. [PubMed]
29. Baglioni, C.; Nanovska, S.; Regen, W.; Spiegelhalder, K.; Feige, B.; Nissen, C.; Reynolds, C., III; Riemann, D. Sleep and Mental Disorders: A Meta-Analysis of Research. *Psychol. Bull.* **2017**, *142*, 969–990. [CrossRef]
30. Takayanagi, Y.; Spira, A.P.; Roth, K.B.; Gallo, J.J.; Eaton, W.W.; Mojtabai, R. Accuracy of reports of lifetime mental and physical disorders: Results from the Baltimore Epidemiological Catchment Area study. *JAMA Psychiatry* **2014**, *71*, 273–280. [CrossRef]
31. Anglin, D.M.; Link, B.G.; Phelan, J.C. Racial differences in stigmatizing attitudes toward people with mental illness. *Psychiatr. Serv.* **2006**, *57*, 857–862. [CrossRef]

Publisher's Note: MDPI stays neutral with regard to jurisdictional claims in published maps and institutional affiliations.

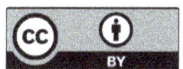 © 2020 by the authors. Licensee MDPI, Basel, Switzerland. This article is an open access article distributed under the terms and conditions of the Creative Commons Attribution (CC BY) license (http://creativecommons.org/licenses/by/4.0/).

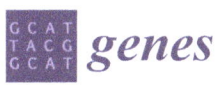

Case Report

Pharmacogenetic Testing of Cytochrome P450 Drug Metabolizing Enzymes in a Case Series of Patients with Prader-Willi Syndrome

Janice Forster [1,*], Jessica Duis [2] and Merlin G. Butler [3]

[1] Pittsburgh Partnership, PWS, Pittsburgh, PA 15218, USA
[2] Section of Genetic and Inherited Metabolic Disease, Department of Pediatrics, Children's Hospital Colorado, Aurora, CO 80045, USA; jessica.duis@childrenscolorado.org
[3] Division of Research and Genetics, Departments of Psychiatry & Behavioral Sciences and Pediatrics, University of Kansas Medical Center, Kansas City, KS 66160, USA; mbutler4@kumc.edu
* Correspondence: janiceforstermd@aol.com

Abstract: Prader-Willi syndrome (PWS) is associated with co-morbid psychiatric symptoms (disruptive behavior, anxiety, mood disorders, and psychosis) often requiring psychotropic medications. In this clinical case series of 35 patients with PWS, pharmacogenetic testing was obtained to determine allele frequencies predicting variations in activity of cytochrome (CYP) P450 drug metabolizing enzymes 2D6, 2B6, 2C19, 2C9, 3A4, and 1A2. Results were deidentified, collated, and analyzed by PWS genetic subtype: 14 deletion (DEL), 16 maternal uniparental disomy (UPD) and 5 DNA-methylation positive unspecified molecular subtype (PWS Unspec). Literature review informed comparative population frequencies of CYP polymorphisms, phenotypes, and substrate specificity. Among the total PWS cohort, extensive metabolizer (EM) activity prevailed across all cytochromes except CYP1A2, which showed greater ultra-rapid metabolizer (UM) status ($p < 0.05$), especially among UPD. Among PWS genetic subtypes, there were statistically significant differences in metabolizing status for cytochromes 2D6, 2C19, 2C9, 3A4 and 1A2 acting on substrates such as fluoxetine, risperidone, sertraline, modafinil, aripiprazole, citalopram, and escitalopram. Gonadal steroid therapy may further impact metabolism of 2C19, 2C9, 3A4 and 1A2 substrates. The status of growth hormone treatment may affect CYP3A4 activity with gender specificity. Pharmacogenetic testing together with PWS genetic subtyping may inform psychotropic medication dosing parameters and risk for adverse events.

Keywords: pharmacogenetic testing; cytochrome P450 enzymes; Prader-Willi syndrome; drug interactions; medication management

Citation: Forster, J.; Duis, J.; Butler, M.G. Pharmacogenetic Testing of Cytochrome P450 Drug Metabolizing Enzymes in a Case Series of Patients with Prader-Willi Syndrome. *Genes* **2021**, *12*, 152. https://doi.org/10.3390/genes12020152

Academic Editor: Domingo González-Lamuño

Received: 14 November 2020
Accepted: 21 January 2021
Published: 24 January 2021

Publisher's Note: MDPI stays neutral with regard to jurisdictional claims in published maps and institutional affiliations.

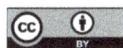

Copyright: © 2021 by the authors. Licensee MDPI, Basel, Switzerland. This article is an open access article distributed under the terms and conditions of the Creative Commons Attribution (CC BY) license (https://creativecommons.org/licenses/by/4.0/).

1. Introduction

1.1. Prader-Willi Syndrome (PWS)

PWS is a rare, complex genetic disorder recognized as the most common form of syndromic obesity. PWS is reported to affect between 350,000 and 400,000 individuals worldwide with an estimated prevalence of one in 10,000 to 38,000 individuals [1]. PWS results from errors in genomic imprinting with loss of expression of paternal genes in the chromosome 15q11–q13 region generally from a paternal deletion (DEL, 60% of cases) followed by maternal uniparental disomy 15 (UPD, 35% of cases) in which both chromosome 15 s are inherited from the mother. Imprinting center defects (IC) and chromosome 15 translocations or inversions are seen in the remaining patients [2]. This multi-system disorder is characterized by severe infantile hypotonia with a poor suck, weak cry, failure to thrive and feeding difficulties. Hypogonadism/hypogenitalism is noted at birth. Hypothalamic dysfunction causes growth and other hormone deficiencies, as well as dysregulation of body temperature, sleep and wakefulness, hunger, thirst, and stress response. Currently, growth hormone, usually started in the first year of life, is the only medication indicated for PWS to manage short stature, small hands and feet, global developmental delay and abnormalities of body composition consisting of excessive fat mass to lean body weight [3]. In early childhood there is an increased interest in food, and calories must be managed to avoid excess weight gain. Six nutritional phases have been described [4]. Excessive food intake leads to obesity, unless dietary management, environmental controls and mandatory exercise are implemented. Psychological food security helps to manage behavior difficulties presenting around food [5]. Temper tantrums emerge in early childhood and persist into adulthood. They are followed by the appearance of other behavior problems in middle childhood. These include manifestations of cognitive rigidity (e.g., repetitive asking, insistence on sameness, selective attention, difficulty with transitions), and anxiety (e.g., excessive and repetitive actions, emotional lability, and stress sensitivity) [6]. These characteristics define the behavioral phenotype of PWS and are often a focus of treatment from mental health professionals. Behavior management, psychological therapies and psychotropic medications are often prescribed. Symptoms of co-morbid psychiatric conditions (e.g., mood disorder and psychosis) often emerge in adolescence and require medication management [6]. There are some phenotypic differences that correlate with PWS genetic subtypes. Individuals with the deletion subtype are generally more affected with compulsions and self-injury and perform more poorly on cognitive and behavior instruments [7,8]. Those with UPD have higher verbal IQs than those with deletion, but they may be more prone to symptoms of autism spectrum disorder in early childhood and affective psychosis with onset in adolescence and young adult years [9,10]. There is an increased incidence of psychosis among both subtypes [10,11].

The NIH Rare Disease PWS Consortium Registry tracked 355 patients during clinic visits over ten years and recorded age of onset of use of psychotropic medication and pattern of sustained utilization [12]. A total of 265 patients were receiving 483 psychotropic medications. From these data, it appears that multiple medications were used for management of the complex symptoms and co-morbid conditions associated with PWS [13]. Selective serotonin reuptake inhibitors (SSRIs) were used in nearly 50% of the 5–12 year age group and in 70% of the 12–21 year age cohort. Atypical neuroleptics were the second most frequent class of medications used (34%), often in combination with SSRIs [13]. Polypharmacy, the use of more than one medication of a single class or multiple medications from different classes, increases the risk for drug-drug interactions and adverse effects, and this tendency is exacerbated at younger ages. Careful medication selection and informed medication management is required [14].

1.2. Pharmacogenetics of the Cytochrome P450 System

Pharmacogenetics examines the influence of DNA structural variations on genes coding for enzymes responsible for drug metabolism determining efficacy and tolerability. These protein-coding genes are diverse across the genome. The cytochrome P450 enzyme system (CYP) is a heme-based superfamily of proteins responsible for the oxidative phosphorylation of toxins and medications and the synthesis of lipids, steroids (hormones) and some vitamins [14]. This enzyme system is present in most body tissues including the liver and brain [15,16]. It is primarily positioned within the inner mitochondrial membrane or endoplasmic reticulum of the cell. Up to 80% of all drugs are metabolized in the liver by these six different cytochrome P450 enzymes: CYP1A2, CYP2B6, CYPC19, CYP2D6, CYP3A4 and CYP3A5 [17]. CYPD26 by itself may account for the breakdown of up to 25% of all medications [14]. Gene variants have clinically relevant impact on drug metabolism, drug efficacy, side effects, and drug-drug interaction in the clinical setting; they are also associated with susceptibility to cancer and disease [18]. Drugs undergoing metabolism often involve more than one cytochrome enzyme. This is graphically represented for most drugs [https://www.pharmgkb.org/pathways]. In addition, drugs may require first pass metabolism to generate the therapeutic agent for treatment effect. Also, cytochrome P450 genes and their encoded enzymes may be altered by the environment through inhibitors and inducers [14]. The chromosome location for genes encoding cytochrome P450 enzymes that are discussed in this article, their common polymorphisms, and phenotypic activity can be found in Table A1. The Variation (PharmVar) Consortium: Incorporation of the Human Cytochrome P450 (CYP) Allele Nomenclature Database [https://www.pharmgkb.org] is a helpful reference to understand and decode gene notation, population frequency and phenotypic expression.

Compared to all medications, psychotropic drugs are more selectively metabolized by cytochromes 2D6, 2B6, 3A4, 1A2, 2C19 and 2C9 [19]. These genes have many polymorphisms that produce enzymes of variable activity. Some alleles have enhanced activity while others are reduced or inactive. The cytochrome P450 phenotype is defined by the number and combination of alleles inherited from the parents. Gene function is described by four phenotypic categories: ultra-rapid metabolizer (UM); extensive metabolizer (EM); intermediate metabolizer (IM); and poor metabolizer (PM) for each cytochrome P450 gene. The typical or normal rate of activity is the extensive metabolizing phenotype.

Also, gene polymorphisms vary according to race, ethnicity, and geographical ancestry. A comprehensive list of gene polymorphisms and their phenotypic activity are reported at [https://www.pharmgkb.org]. Similar data, together with allelic frequencies and their racial and ethno-geographic frequency, can be found in the review article by Zhou et al. [20].

More than ten years ago at Vanderbilt University, a survey was completed by the parents or caregivers of 86 persons with PWS to ascertain the respondent's satisfaction with the use of SSRIs and/or atypical neuroleptics to manage behavioral symptoms related to PWS [21]. SSRIs were used in 33%, atypical neuroleptics were used in 11%, and a combination of SSRIs plus atypical antipsychotics was used in 17% of the study population. PWS genetic subtype was not specified. In this pilot study, research-based probes were used to identify phenotypes of CYP2D6 and CYP2C19; allelic frequencies were not reported. Although the EM phenotype predominated for cytochromes 2D6 and 2C19, 37% were IMs of CYP2D6, 2.5% were PMs of CYP2D6, and 3.2% were PMs of CYP2C19. The results of the Vanderbilt study indicated that in more than one-third of persons with PWS, the IM or PM status was noted for CYP2D6. It can be inferred that serum levels of antidepressant or antipsychotic medication metabolized by CYP2D6 would be higher than expected at typical doses, leading to clinical response at lower doses or adverse effects at typical doses. This finding is corroborated by clinical experience with SSRI medications in PWS, as described in the mood and behavioral activation case series reported by Durette et al. [22].

The aim of this clinical report was to examine and summarize pharmacogenetic results from a cohort of patients with PWS referred for evaluation and treatment of psychiatric and behavioral problems. Our approach was to identify differences in CYP genotypes and phenotypes in the referred cohort as a whole, correlate these findings with phenotypic frequencies among the PWS genetic subtypes, and compare these results to data from a normative population. These findings may inform our understanding of why many of our patients have a therapeutic response at low doses of SSRIs and adverse events at typical doses of psychotropic medications as reported by Gourash et al. [23]. This knowledge will be used in our daily clinical practice to guide selection and dose of psychotropic medication, to anticipate potential drug interactions, and to foresee vulnerability to adverse effects while treating the psychiatric and behavioral problems occurring in our patients with this rare genetic syndrome.

2. Methods

Thirty-five patients with PWS (14 DEL; 16 UPD; 5 Unspec-methylation positive, molecular subtype unspecified) were seen for evaluation and treatment at one of three regional centers by the physician authors who have extensive experience using psychotropic medications to manage psychiatric or behavior problems in patients with PWS. The clinical use of pharmacogenetic testing was discussed with and approved by the patient and/or guardian, and testing was ordered to determine cytochrome P450 function to guide the selection of medication and the dosage required for treatment. The authors collected buccal cells in the clinical setting and sent them to one of three CLIA approved and accredited, commercial laboratories: Genesight (GS) in Mason, Ohio (n = 29); Genelex (GL) in Seattle, Washington (n = 5); and Genomind (GM) in King of Prussia, Pennsylvania (n = 1). These laboratories undertake quality control testing required for accreditation to assure and maintain accuracy of laboratory testing results. DNA was extracted at the laboratories and analyzed for polymorphisms of *CYP2D6*, *CYP2B6*, *CYP2C19*, *CYP2C9*, *CYP3A4* and *CYP1A2* as well as other genes not included in this case report. Results were received by the authors and protected health information was removed (name, age, gender, race, ethnicity) prior to data pooling and sorting by genetic subtype of PWS. Psychiatric diagnosis, psychotropic medication history, and family psychiatric and treatment history were not available, although all the patients met medical necessity criteria indicating a failure of previous medications, either due to inefficacy or adverse effects, and/or the presence of psychiatric co-morbidities that would require treatment with multiple psychotropic medications.

When comparing the testing results from the three commercial laboratories, there were subtle differences noted. In some cases, different nomenclature was used for the same results, i.e., *CYP1A2 *1* and *1A* are both names for the wildtype gene, and *CYP1A2*1F* is the hyper-inducible-163 A/A polymorphism. Also, we found that the interpretation of phenotype from genotype may differ across the commercial laboratories, as each of them uses a combinatorial phenotype that is determined by a proprietary algorithm. For example, GL identifies any carrier of *CYP1A2*1F* as HI (hyper-inducible), while GS identifies *1F* heterozygotes as UM (ultrarapid metabolizers) and GM identifies them as EM (extensive metabolizers). Although we used the phenotypic nomenclature reported by the commercial companies designating metabolizing status as poor, intermediate, extensive and ultrarapid, we also analyzed the frequencies of alleles and diplotypes and compared them to published norms.

For *CYP2C19*, the pharmacogenomic companies reported *CYP2C19* phenotype as ultrarapid, extensive, intermediate, and poor metabolizing. However, the authors were aware that the current phenotypic nomenclature for *CYP2C19* has been changed to ultrarapid, rapid, normal, intermediate and poor metabolizing, as described at https://www.pharmgkb.org/page/cyp2c19RefMaterials, to more accurately describe the function of the *CYP2C19*17* rapid metabolizing allele. To calculate the phenotypic frequencies for *CYP2C19* from the normative data, we combined the frequencies for rapid and normal metabolizing phenotype and used this value for the normative extensive metabolizers, as discussed and implemented in Martis et al. [24]. Pharmacokinetic testing has indicated that there is minimal variance between the normal and rapid metabolizing phenotypes [25].

In this clinical case report, the frequency of phenotypes assigned by the commercial providers for each cytochrome P450 gene is displayed as a histogram for each PWS genetic subtype (DEL, UPD and PWS Unspec) and compared to frequencies found in the normative Caucasian population. Then, for each genetic subtype of PWS, the frequency of phenotypes for each CYP gene was calculated, compared to published normative data, and analyzed for significance using the chi-square test. p values of <0.05 were statistically significant. Next, for each cytochrome P450 polymorphism, the frequency of occurrence of the alleles and diplotypes was calculated for each genetic subtype of PWS and displayed graphically for comparison with normative population data.

For this case series normative data from the Caucasian population was referenced because the NIH PWS Registry found minimal racial/ethnic diversity (93% Caucasian) among 355 enrollees from regional clinics across the USA. The phenotypic frequency in the Caucasian population was obtained from https://www.pharmgkb.org for cytochromes *2D6*, *2B6*, *2C19*, and *2C9*, and Zhou et al. was used for *3A4* [20]. The values reported in the literature for the frequencies of CYP phenotypes for each cytochrome show some variability across studies even within designated ethnic categories. Normative data for the phenotypic frequency of *1A2* among Caucasians was not available, although the increased prevalence of the poor metabolizer phenotype among the Asian population is well documented in the literature. We elected to use the results of studies measuring urinary caffeine metabolites to report the normative metabolic phenotype of CYP1A2, a method that has been used for over 20 years and more recently correlated with genotype [26–28].

The patients in this clinical case series sought care at one of three specialty programs across the USA. They were evaluated by physician experts with over 80 years of collective clinical experience in treating patients with this rare disorder. These patients received pharmacogenetic testing as part of their medical evaluation because it was deemed as medically necessary. The clinical care described in this article was not part of a research project, so this report did not require ethical review or approval. Prior to the collation and analysis of data, all pertinent private or protected health information about each patient was eliminated or deidentified, except for the genetic subtype of PWS and the pharmacogenetic genotypes and phenotypes. The results of the analysis of this group data will not affect the patient's clinical care, nor does it have the potential to cause the patient any harm. It is the authors hope that this report will inform, improve, and advance the quality of medical and psychiatric care of patients with PWS.

3. Results

This case series represents the largest number of patients with known genetic subtype of PWS to receive pharmacogenetic testing with analysis of results that are summarized in Table 1. The frequencies of CYP phenotypes in the PWS cohort are itemized for each genetic subtype and compared to a normative (typical) Caucasian population. The list of substrates affected by these CYP phenotypic differences was derived from the frequency of medication use among 265 patients with PWS enrolled in the NIH PWS Registry [12,13]. The raw data obtained from the pharmacogenetic testing of this cohort of referred patients is displayed in the Appendix A. For each genetic subtype of PWS, the testing laboratory, cytochrome P450 genotype, and cytochrome P450 phenotype are specified in a series of tables: Deletion (Table A2), UPD (Table A3) and PWS Unspecified (Table A4). Table A5 shows the proportion of phenotypes for each cytochrome P450 gene according to the PWS genetic subtype.

Table 1. Frequencies of CYP phenotypes in PWS cohort compared to a typical population, and substrates most likely to be affected based on drug utilization data from the NIH PWS Registry.

CYP Gene/ Metabolizer Phenotype	CYP Phenotype Frequency						Substrate Frequency
	PWS Referred Cohort				Typical Population		PWS Clinic Patients
	DEL	UPD	Unspec	All PWS	Frequency/Reference	Reference	NIH PWS Registry [12,13]
CYP2D6	(n = 14)	(n = 16)	(n = 5)	(n = 35)	(n = 56,945)		(n = 265)
EM	28.5% †	56.3%	4	48.6%	63.6%	http://www.pharmgkb.org/page/cyp2d6RefMaterials	Fluoxetine (21.9%), Risperidone (14%), Sertraline (14%), Aripiprazole (9.8%), Citalopram (8.7%), Escitalopram (5.7%), Paroxetine (4.5%), Bupropion (4.5%), Amphetamine (4.2%), Clonidine (3%), Ziprasidone (3%)
IM	57.1% *	25.0%	0	34.0%	23.6%		
PM	14.3% †	18.8% *	1	17.1% *	2.2%		
CYP2B6	(n = 14)	(n = 15)	(n = 5)	(n = 34)	(n = 56,945)		
EM	50%	40%	5	53%	43%	http://www.pharmgkb.org/page/cyp2b6RefMaterials	Sertraline (14%), Bupropion (4.5%)
IM	50%	60%	0	47%	39%		
CYP2C19	(n = 14)	(n = 16)	(n = 5)	(n = 35)	(n = 56,945)		
EM	78.6%	100% †	3	85.7%	76.4%	http://www.pharmgkb.org/page/cyp2C19RefMaterials	Fluoxetine (21.9%), Sertraline (14%), Citalopram (8.7%), Escitalopram (5.7%)
IM	7.1%	0% †	2	8.6%	21.4%		
UM	14.3% †	0%	0	5.7%	0.74%		
CYP2C9	(n = 14)	(n = 16)	(n = 5)	(n = 35)	(n = 56,945)		
EM	76.9%	56.2% *	2	61.8% *	83.2%	http://www.pharmgkb.org/page/cyp2C9RefMaterials	Fluoxetine (21.9%), Sertraline (14%), Valproate (6.4%)
IM	23.0%	37.5% *	3	35.3% *	16.4%		
PM	0%	6.3% †	0	2.9%	0%		
CYP3A4	(n = 14)	(n = 15)	(n = 5)	(n = 34)	(n = 5789)		
EM	85.7% †	80.0% †	5	85.3% *	97.3%	Zhou et al., 2017 [20]	Risperidone (14%), Sertraline (14%), Modafinil (12.8%), Aripiprazole (9.8%), Citalopram (8.7%), Clonazepam (6.8%), Escitalopram (5.7%), Bupropion (4.5%), Ziprasidone (3%)
IM	14.3% †	20.0% †	0	14.7% *	2.7%		
CYP1A2	(n = 14)	(n = 16)	(n = 5)	(n = 35)	(n = 183)		
UM	42.9% *	62.5% *	2	51.4% *	0%	Muscat et al., 2008 [27]	Fluvoxamine (1.1%), Haloperidol (1.1%), Thioridazine (1.1%), Olanzapine (0.4%), Chlorpromazine (0.4%), Imipramine (0.4%)
EM/HI	57.1%	31.2%	3	45.7%	37.0%		
IM	0% †	6.25% †	0	2.85%	54.0%		
PM	0%	0%	0	0% †	10.0%		

KEY: Phenotype% = within group comparison; (*) = statistical significance by chi-square comparison, $p < 0.05$; (†) = statistical significance by chi-square, $p < 0.05$, but results may not be reliable due to small cell size. The frequency of psychotropic medications in this table is derived from the NIH PWS Registry [12,13]. Only the most frequently prescribed medications are listed for each cytochrome. This data reflects regional prescribing practices; it does not reflect treatment efficacy, nor does it constitute recommended treatment.

3.1. Cytochrome P450 Genotypes, Phenotypes and Genetic Subtype of PWS

The cytochrome P450 phenotypes for the combined group of patients with PWS in our referred cohort is shown in Figure 1. The distribution of frequencies of cytochrome P450 phenotypes is displayed as a percentage of the total cohort ($n = 35$) for ease of comparison with normative data.

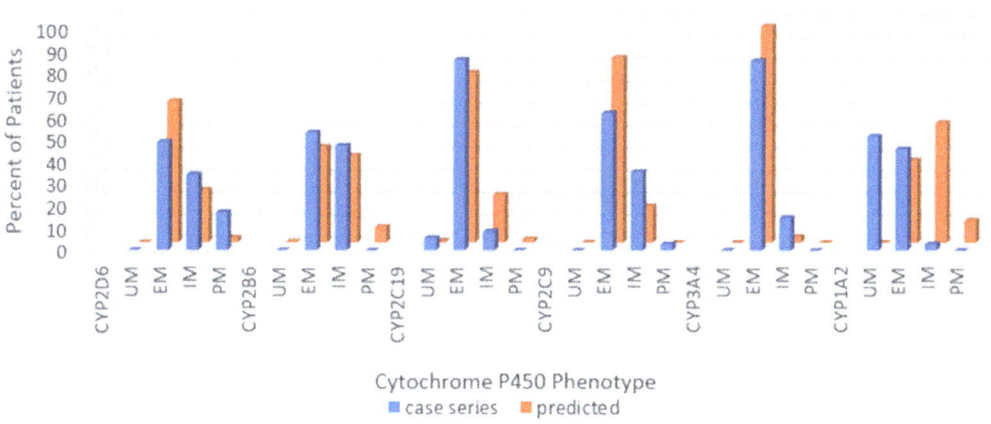

Figure 1. Distribution of Cytochrome P450 phenotypes among the combined PWS cohort ($n = 35$) compared to predicted, normative populations [https://www.pharmgkb.org/page/cyp2d6RefMaterials]; [https://www.pharmgkb.org/page/cyp2b6RefMaterials]; [https://www.pharmgkb.org/page/cyp2c19RefMaterials]; [https://www.pharmgkb.org/page/cyp2c9RefMaterials]; [20,27]. Key: UM—ultra-rapid metabolizer; EM—extensive metabolizer; IM—intermediate metabolizer; PM—poor metabolizer.

The normative data delineating the phenotypic frequencies for CYP1A2 activity (slow, intermediate and rapid) were derived from studies measuring caffeine and its metabolites in urine [27]. Al-Ahmad et al. have described the correlation between metabolic phenotypes and genotypes, e.g., rapid metabolizer phenotype corresponds to *1A/*1A (extensive metabolizer) genotype [28].

Across the combined cohort, the extensive metabolizing status prevailed in all but one cytochrome; for CYP1A2, the ultra-rapid phenotype was more common than the extensive metabolizing. Extensive metabolizing phenotype for the predicted normative data exceeded the PWS cohort for CYP2D6 and CYP2C9 but not for CYP2B6 or CYP2C19. Poor metabolizing status for CYP2D6 and intermediate metabolizing status for CYP2C9 were greater in the PWS cohort than predicted in normative populations. The following series of histograms display the cytochrome P450 enzyme phenotypes for each PWS genetic subtype (Figure 2—DEL, Figure 3—UPD, and Figure 4—PWS Unspecified) and compare these to the predicted normative data for CYP2D6, CYP2B6, CYP2C19 and CYP2C9.

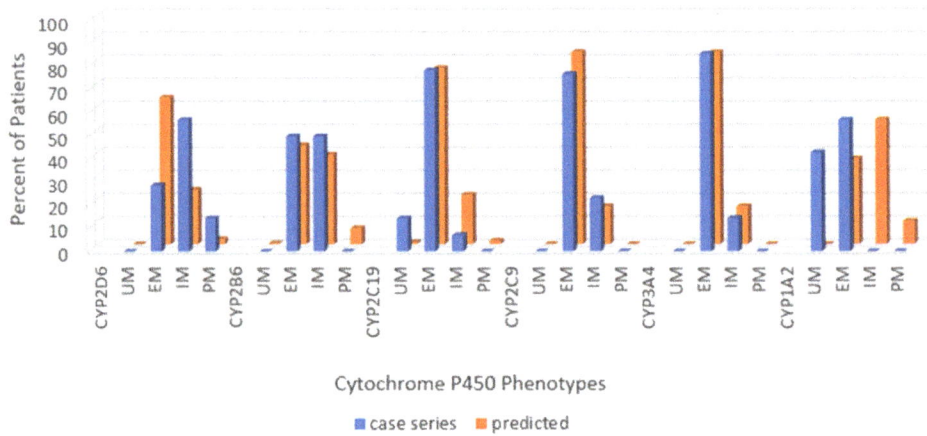

Figure 2. Distribution of Cytochrome P450 phenotypes among PWS DEL (*n* = 14) compared to normative populations [https://www.pharmgkb.org/page/cyp2d6RefMaterials]; [https://www.pharmgkb.org/page/cyp2b6RefMaterials]; [https://www.pharmgkb.org/page/cyp2c19RefMaterials]; [https://www.pharmgkb.org/page/cyp2c9RefMaterials]; [20,27]. Key: UM—ultra-rapid metabolizer; EM—extensive metabolizer; IM—intermediate metabolizer; PM—poor metabolizer.

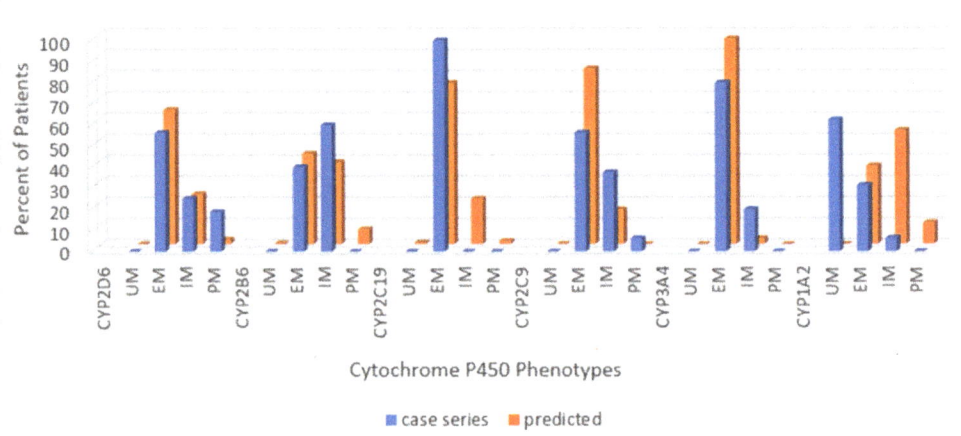

Figure 3. Distribution of Cytochrome P450 phenotypes among the PWS UPD cohort (*n* = 16) compared to normative populations [https://www.pharmgkb.org/page/cyp2d6RefMaterials]; [https://www.pharmgkb.org/page/cyp2b6RefMaterials]; [https://www.pharmgkb.org/page/cyp2c19RefMaterials]; [https://www.pharmgkb.org/page/cyp2c9RefMaterials]; [20,27]. Note: There were 15 results for cytochromes 2B6 and 3A4. Key: UM—ultra-rapid metabolizer; EM—extensive metabolizer; IM—intermediate metabolizer; PM—poor metabolizer.

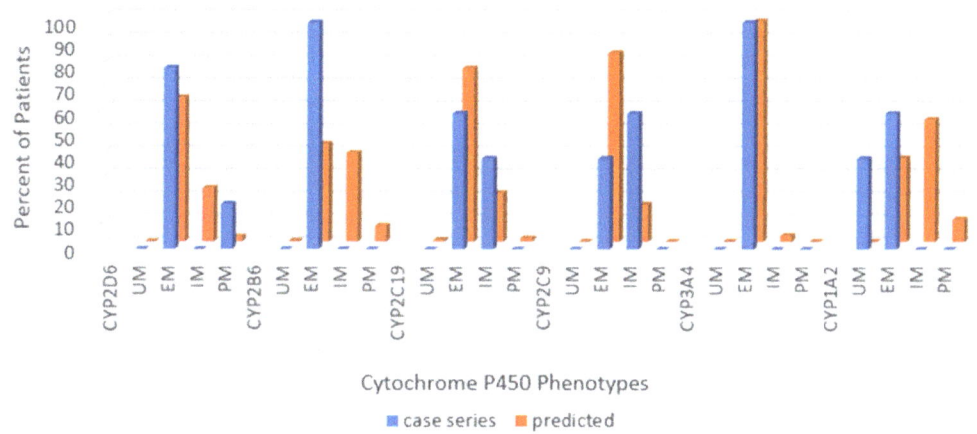

Figure 4. Distribution of Cytochrome P450 phenotypes among PWS Unspecified genetic subtype, (*n* = 5) compared to normative populations [https://www.pharmgkb.org/page/cyp2d6RefMaterials]; [https://www.pharmgkb.org/page/cyp2b6RefMaterials]; [https://www.pharmgkb.org/page/cyp2c19RefMaterials]; [https://www.pharmgkb.org/page/cyp2c9RefMaterials]; [20,27]. Key: UM—ultra-rapid metabolizer; EM—extensive metabolizer; IM—intermediate metabolizer; PM—poor metabolizer.

When the data sets for PWS genetic subtypes in our referred population were compared to each other, differences were found in the distribution of phenotypes for all cytochromes. In the following sections, the allelic frequencies of the cytochrome P450 gene polymorphisms are displayed for the PWS genetic subtypes. Also, when possible, the distribution of diplotypes is itemized and compared with normative data. The phenotypic action of the most common alleles for each cytochrome P450 gene is itemized in Table A1 (Appendix A).

3.2. CYP2D6

For CYP2D6 the data from our case report and the Vanderbilt study is compared to the normative American population referenced at [www.pharmgkb.org/page/cyp2b6 RefMaterials]. In our combined cohort of referred patients, 48.6% of had the extensive metabolizing phenotype compared to 63.6% among the normative American population; this was not significantly different by chi-square test ($p > 0.05$). The percentage of CYP2D6 intermediate metabolizers was 34%, and this is similar to the percentage reported in the Vanderbilt survey (37%); both values exceed the 23.6% found in the normative American population, but the chi-square value was not significant ($p > 0.05$). There were 17.1% poor metabolizers in the current cohort compared to 2.5% in the Vanderbilt survey and 2.2% in the normative American population, and the chi-square value was significant ($p < 0.05$). When comparing the current data to the Vanderbilt survey, it should be noted that the current cohort was derived from a clinically referred sample, where medical necessity dictated testing. There may have been more treatment failures or adverse events in the current cohort. Data from our referred cohort indicates that over half of the patients with PWS had the intermediate or poor metabolizing phenotype of *CYP2D6*, which could impact efficacy and tolerability of many of the psychotropic drugs used in treating patients with PWS.

When considering the PWS genetic subtypes, there were fewer extensive metabolizers, more intermediate metabolizers, and more poor metabolizers among those with DEL compared to the normative American population, and all values were statistically significant ($p < 0.05$). Among those with UPD, the ratio of EM:IM was roughly the same as in the normative American population, although the number of poor metabolizers was actually greater than among DEL, and both PM values were statistically significant ($p < 0.05$). Figure 5 displays the allelic distribution and frequencies of *CYP2D6* polymorphisms among PWS genetic subtypes in our referred cohort.

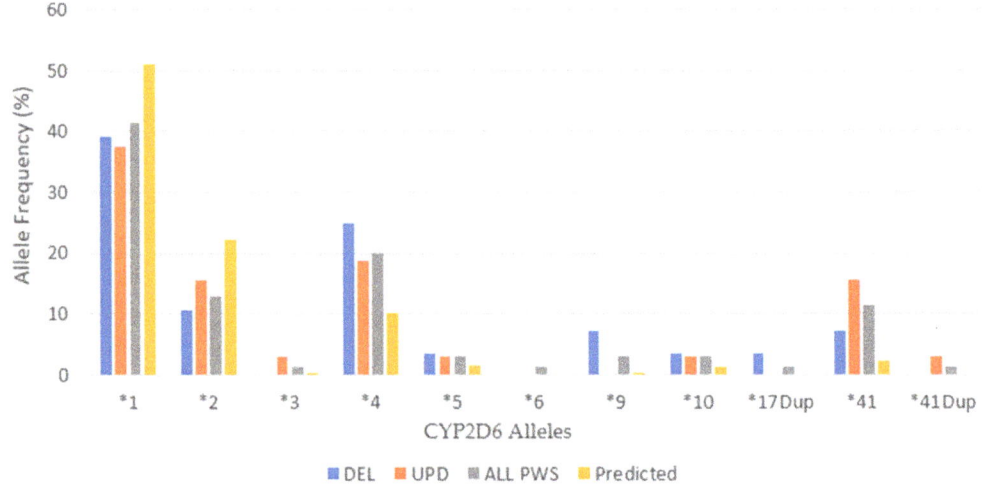

Figure 5. Cytochrome 2D6 allele frequencies among a referred cohort of patients with PWS DEL ($n = 14$), UPD ($n = 16$) and combined cohort (ALL PWS, $n = 35$) compared to predicted, American normative data [http://www.pharmgkb.org/page/cyp2d6RefMaterials].

In our cohort of patients, there is a lesser frequency than predicted for the most common CYP2D6 alleles *1 and *2 (both convey normal activity) and an increased frequency of alleles *4 (inactive) and *41 (reduced function). Further, the distribution of alleles includes others with a lower frequency of occurrence that are inactive or have reduced function. Subtle differences were noted in the number of alleles between the PWS genetic subtypes, but the DEL group had a higher frequency of *4 alleles, and the UPD group had a greater number of *41 alleles. See Figure 6 for *CYP2D6* diplotypes.

Among the total cohort of PWS, the wild type diplotype *1*1 occurs at a reduced rate, roughly two-thirds of the American normative population, but nearly equal to the frequency of the *1*4 diplotype, which codes for decreased activity, and exceeds the normative frequency by more than one-third. The most frequent CYP2D6 diplotypes among the DEL subtype are *1*4 and *1*9, both of which have decreased activity predicting intermediate metabolizer phenotype. The frequency of *1*1, which is the extensive metabolizing wild type, is equal in frequency to *1*9, which has decreased activity. These frequencies explain the predominance of intermediate metabolizer status among DEL. Among the UPD subtype, the highest frequencies are *1*2A (extensive metabolizing) and *1*4 (intermediate metabolizing), and the next most frequent are *1*41 (extensive metabolizing) and *4*41 (poor metabolizing), explaining the 9EM:4IM:3PM ratio of metabolizer phenotypes.

Because CYP2D6 metabolizes many antidepressants and antipsychotics often prescribed in PWS, it is not a surprise that our cohort of patients referred for treatment has alleles with reduced function contributing to decreased efficacy or adverse effects; conversely, they may respond to a lower dose [29,30]. Medications (in alphabetical order) most commonly used in PWS that are substrates of CYP2D6 include amphetamines, aripiprazole, bupropion, citalopram, clonidine, diphenhydramine, escitalopram, fluoxetine, fluvoxamine, haloperidol, olanzapine, quetiapine, risperidone, sertraline, trazadone and ziprasidone [31]. The CYP2D6 enzyme activity in our cohort showed a greater number of patients than predicted with poor metabolizer status among both PWS genetic subtypes, which could impact approximately 25% of all medications and 60–70% of behavioral/psychiatric prescribed drugs as discussed by Butler [18].

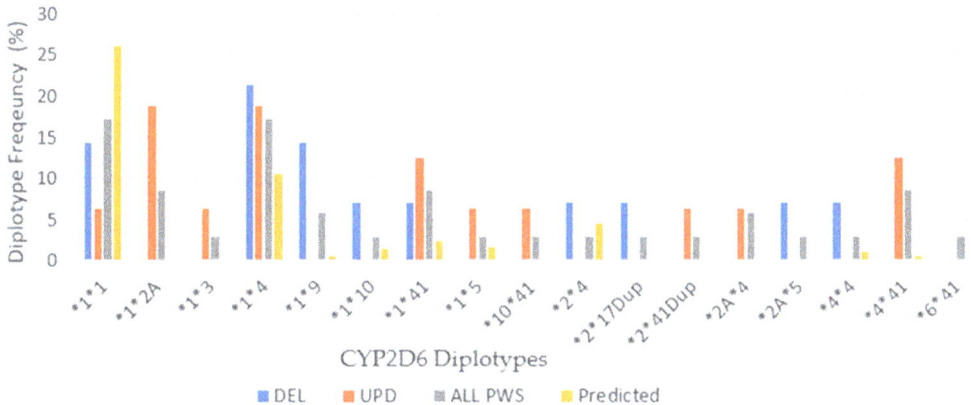

Figure 6. Cytochrome 2D6 diplotype frequencies among PWS DEL (*n* = 14), UPD (*n* = 16) and combined cohort (ALL PWS, *n* = 35) compared to predicted, American normative data [http://www.pharmgkb.org/page/cyp2d6RefMaterials].

3.3. CYP2B6

Among our total PWS cohort, 53% had the extensive metabolizer phenotype compared to 43% in a normative European population [www.pharmgkb.org/page/cyp2b6 RefMaterials]. The chi-square test was not significant (*p* > 0.05). Intermediate metabolizers were found in 47% of the patients with PWS compared with 39% in the European population, but again, the chi-square value was not significant (*p* > 0.05). There were no poor metabolizers among our patients with PWS. The intermediate metabolizing phenotype predominated among the UPD cohort, whereas the intermediate and extensive metabolizing phenotypes were equal among DEL. These results were not statistically significant by chi-square test (*p* > 0.05). The distribution of alleles for *CYP2B6* is shown in Figure 7.

There were 4 alleles identified in our cohort with a greater expression of the wild type allele (*CYP2B6*1*) that confers normal activity in the combined cohort (69%) compared to the normative European population (47%). In the combined cohort the expression of *6, an allele associated with decreased function, is nearly equal to the normative population. Comparing DEL and UPD genetic subtypes, there is a greater expression of *6 allele among the UPD cohort.

Differences in the distribution of diplotypes are noted among the PWS genetic subtypes. Among both DEL and UPD, the frequency of the *CYP2B6*1*6* diplotype, which is associated with the intermediate phenotype, is expressed more frequently than the *1*1 diplotype, which has the extensive metabolizer phenotype. In the UPD cohort, *1*6 is expressed almost twice as frequently as *1*1, and this explains the greater number of intermediate metabolizers among the UPD group. The diplotype *CYP2B6*1*5*, which is associated with normal function, occurs more frequently among DEL than the normative population, but is not found at all among UPD.

Among the total cohort of PWS, both the *1*1 and *1*6 diplotypes are expressed at nearly twice the frequency of the European normative population. This explains the distribution of phenotypic activity among our cohort where the extensive and intermediate metabolizer status are nearly equal. These results would suggest caution when prescribing medications metabolized by CYP2B6, such as bupropion and sertraline among the UPD group.

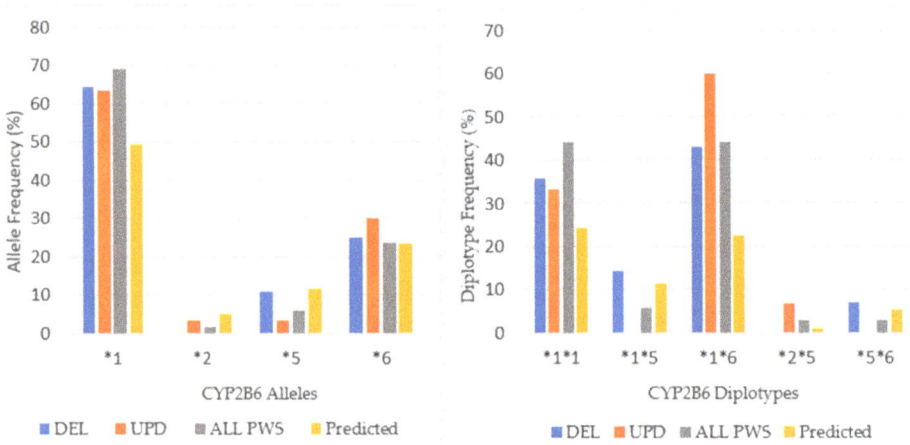

Figure 7. Cytochrome *2B6* allele frequency and diplotype distribution in a referred cohort with PWS DEL (*n* = 14), UPD (*n* = 15) and combined cohort (ALL PWS, *n* = 34) compared to the predicted, European normative data [http://www.pharmgkb.org/page/cyp2b6RefMaterials].

3.4. CYP2C19

Eighty-six percent of the PWS combined cohort had the extensive metabolizer phenotype of CYP2C19, and this is higher than expected from American normative data (76.4%) but not significantly different by chi-square test ($p > 0.05$). Less than 10% in the current study were intermediate metabolizers compared to 21.4% for the American population, which again was not significant by chi-square ($p > 0.05$). Ultra-rapid metabolizers were seen in 5.7% of the patients with PWS compared to 0.7% for the American data, which was not significant by chi-square ($p > 0.05$). There were no poor metabolizers among the current cohort compared to 3.2% in the Vanderbilt survey. For CYPC19, there were PWS subtype group differences. Among those with deletion, there were more ultra-rapid metabolizers compared to the normative population ($p < 0.05$). The UPD cohort displayed 100% extensive metabolizer phenotype and no intermediate metabolizers, and both results were statistically significant ($p < 0.05$) compared to the normative population of 76.4% and 21.4%, respectively. The frequency of alleles and diplotypes are compared with normative American data in Figure 8.

Among our cohort of referred patients with PWS, there is a lesser frequency of the most common *CYP2C19* alleles *1 and *2 that have normal function and an increased frequency of *17 allele, which is associated with increased function; there was one person in the PWS Unspecified diagnostic group with *8 allele (inactive). Differences were noted between the PWS genetic subtypes with the *17 allele being highest among DEL. The allelic frequency of *17 in our combined cohort was more than twice that predicted in the American population (8.6%), and three times higher among the DEL. This is the reason for the increased frequency of ultra-rapid metabolizers among DEL and among the total cohort as well.

The frequency of the normal functioning diplotype *1*1 is less than predicted by normative data except among the UPD group. Among the UPD cohort, only extensive metabolizers were found. The number with increased function *1*17 is more frequent due to the presence of *17 allele, especially among DEL. Also, the ultra-rapid functioning diplotype *17*17 is noted among DEL but not UPD. Overall, the extensive metabolizer phenotype of CYP2C19 prevails in our PWS cohort largely due to the increased expression of the *1 and *17 alleles.

Many psychotropic medications used in patients with PWS are substrates for CYP2C19, including (but not limited to) citalopram, clomipramine, doxepin, escitalopram, fluoxetine, imipramine, and sertraline [32]. It is inferred that these medications would have been well tolerated by most of our referred cohort. However, gonadal steroids (estradiol and testosterone), which are replaced commonly in PWS due to delayed or absent puberty, are substrates for CYP2C19, indicating a potential for drug interactions. This is discussed more fully in Sections 4.1 and 4.2.

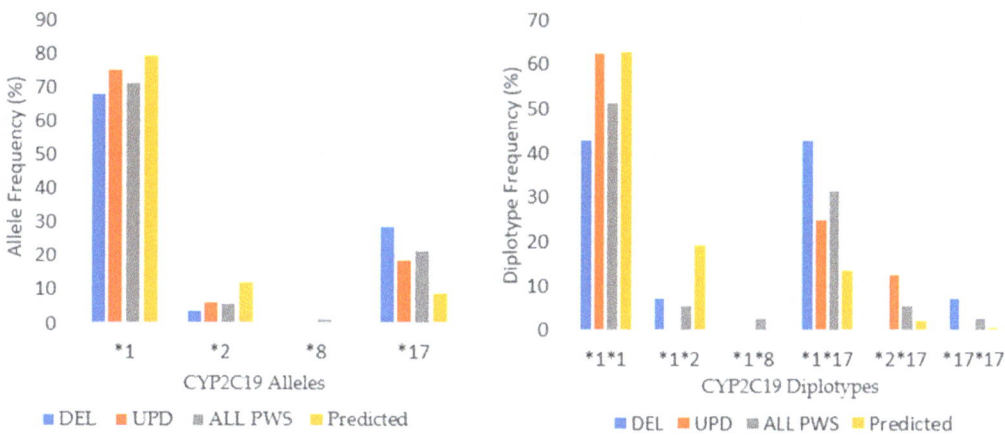

Figure 8. *CYP2C19* allele frequency and distribution of diplotypes in PWS DEL (*n* = 14), UPD (*n* = 16) and combined cohort (ALL PWS, *n* = 35) compared to the predicted normative American data [http://www.pharmgkb.org/page/cyp2c19RefMaterials].

3.5. CYP2C9

The prevailing phenotype of CYP2C9 in our cohort was extensive metabolizing (61.8%), which was decreased in comparison to American normative data (83.2%) and was significantly different by chi-square test, $p < 0.05$. The intermediate metabolizing phenotype was found in 35% of the combined cohort, and this is twice the number predicted in the American population (16.4%) and significantly different also by chi-square test ($p < 0.05$). For CYP2C9 the DEL cohort was 76.9% extensive metabolizer and 23.1% for intermediate, remarkably similar to American normative data at 83.2% and 16.4%, respectively. But for the UPD cohort, extensive metabolizer was 56.3%, intermediate 37.5%, and poor 6.3%; all of these values were statistically significant by chi-square ($p < 0.05$).

Among our cohort of patients with PWS, the distribution of alleles in Figure 9 shows a predominance of *CYP2C9*1*, which confers normal activity at a lesser frequency than in the normative American population. There is a greater occurrence of the *CYP2C9*2* allele (16.2% of ALL PWS) compared to the frequency in the American population (3.3%) with greatest prevalence among UPD (18.8%). Alleles *2 and *3 have decreased activity, and there were no *CYP2C9*3* alleles among DEL. Among the UPD cohort, the frequency of

CYP2C9*1 allele was less than DEL, and the CYP2C9*2 allele frequency was nearly twice that found among DEL.

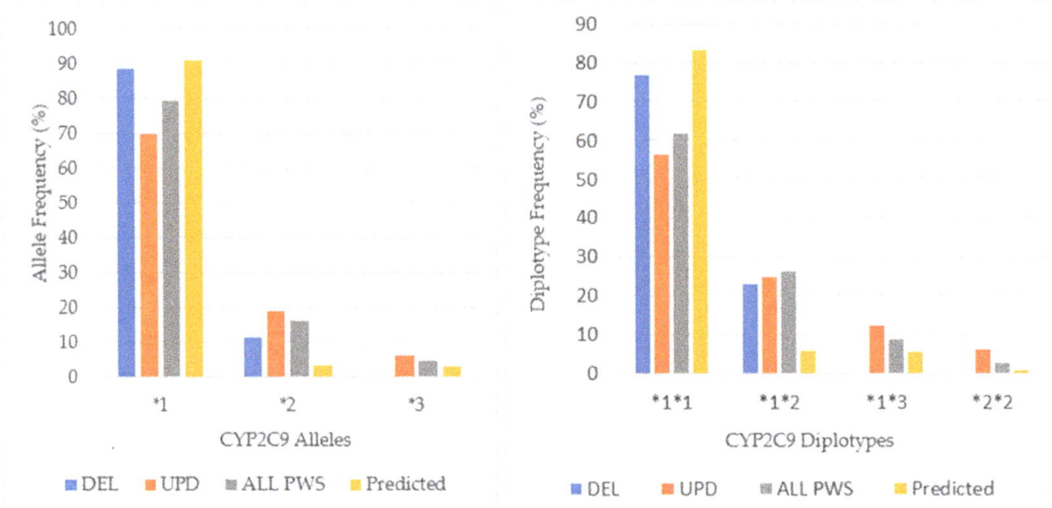

Figure 9. CYP2C9 allele and diplotype frequencies in PWS DEL ($n = 13$), UPD ($n = 16$) and combined cohort (ALL PWS, $n = 34$) compared to American normative, predicted data [http://www.pharmgkb.org/page/cyp2c9RefMaterials].

The CYP2C9*1*1 diplotype that confers the normal phenotype has the greatest frequency across all PWS genetic subtypes, although it occurs more frequently among DEL than UPD. All other pairs are intermediate metabolizing, and there is a greater proportion of these pairs in UPD compared to DEL. This likely contributes to the greater number of intermediate metabolizers among UPD, twice as many as DEL. More than half of patients with UPD in this cohort may have required dosage adjustment for drugs such as amitriptyline, fluoxetine, and sertraline especially when used with concurrent oral contraceptives, methylphenidate, modafinil and omeprazole [31].

3.6. CYP3A4

In the admixed American population, 97.3% had the extensive metabolizing phenotype of CYP3A4 [20]. Across all PWS genetic subtypes the predominate phenotype of CYP3A4 was extensive metabolizing; there were only 5 patients who had intermediate metabolizing status. CYP3A4 has over 30 polymorphisms, most of which occur at low allelic frequencies. The distribution of alleles and diplotypes is found in Figure 10.

There were only three alleles present in the analysis of CYP3A4: *1A, *22, and *1B across PWS genetic subtypes in our cohort of referred patients. The wildtype gene, CYP3A4*1A, was the major allele expressed with a frequency of 92.6% that compared favorably with Caucasian population norms of 92.1% [33]. CYP3A4*22 is a reduced function allele. The allelic frequency for CYP3A4*22 in this study was 5.9%, and this was consistent with population norms of 5–7% [35]. CYP3A4*1B was expressed only among the PWS UPD subtype at a frequency of 3.3%, which is less than allele frequencies of 7.9% reported among Caucasians [33]. This value was not statistically significant by chi-square, $p > 0.05$. CYP3A4*1B has been associated with patients who have cancer, and recently Swiechowski et al. found that compared to controls, patients suffering from recurrent major depressive disorder were more likely to have the heterozygous (AG) CYP3A4*1B genotype [36]. In this study comparing 102 patients with 90 controls, the G allele frequency was higher among patients than controls, and those with the homogeneous (GG) genotype, although fewer in number, reported an earlier age of onset of depression. Even though CYP3A4 is involved in the metabolism of many antidepressant medications, such as tricyclics, SSRIs, SNRIs, and mirtazapine, the phenotypic results did not support any differences in metabolism [36].

The distribution of diplotypes finds that the frequency of the wildtype alleles *1A*1A predominates across all PWS genetic subtypes at nearly typical frequency. The occurrence of the reduced function *1*22 diplotype is greater than predicted among all PWS genetic subtypes [34].

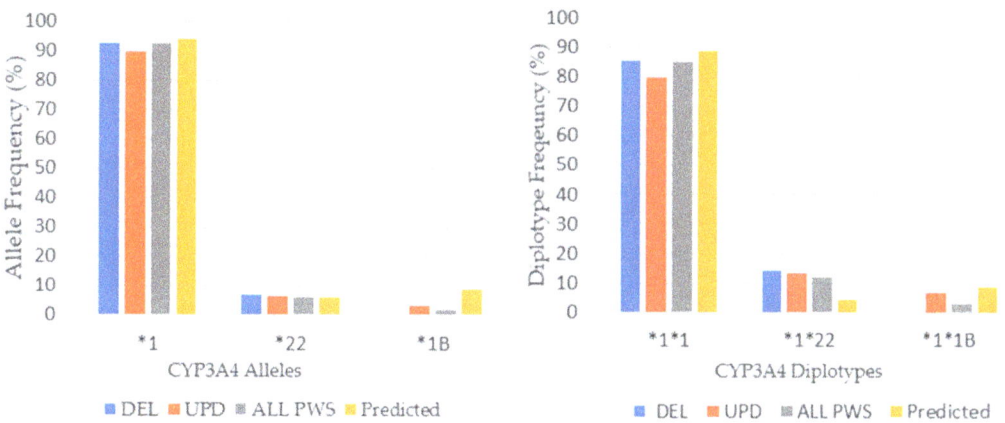

Figure 10. *CYP3A4* allele and diplotype frequencies among PWS DEL (*n* = 14), UPD (*n* = 15), and combined cohort (ALL PWS, *n* = 34) compared to Caucasian normative, predicted data [33,34].

3.7. CYP1A2

For *CYP1A2*, the frequency of ultra-rapid metabolizing phenotype exceeded the extensive metabolizing among the total cohort, and this most likely reflects the influence of the 2:1 frequency of ultra-rapid metabolizers to extensive metabolizers among patients with UPD. Further there is a low frequency of intermediate metabolizers, and there are no poor metabolizers. Compared to other cytochromes, *CYP1A2* appears to be unique in the number of polymorphisms, the variety of inherited allelic combinations, and the capacity for induction from medicinal, dietary, gender, hormonal, and lifestyle factors [14].

Across all PWS subtypes, there was an increase in the number of ultrarapid metabolizers, especially among UPD ($p < 0.05$), and there were no poor metabolizers across the total PWS cohort compared to the normative population ($p < 0.05$). A significant difference was noted by chi-square test ($p < 0.05$) when comparing the frequency of CYP1A2 IM metabolic phenotype to the normative population (54%) in our patients with DEL (0%) and UPD (6.25%) [27].

There were six alleles present in the analysis of *CYP1A2* in our cohort (*1A, *1B, *1C, *1D, *1E*, and *1F*) and their frequencies among each genetic subtype are presented in Figure 11 and compared to predicted values among Caucasians [37,38].

*CYP1A2*1A* and *1B* have normal function and *CYP1A2*1C* has decreased function. Both *CYP1A2*1D* and *CYP1A2*1F* are inducible. For example, both *CYP1A2 *1A* and *1F* express the extensive metabolizer phenotype in the absence of an inducer, but in the presence of tobacco smoke, insulin, modafinil, nafcillin, omeprazole or cruciferous vegetables, the hyper-inducible (HI) phenotype is expressed by *1F* [38]. Among the pharmacogenetic results from the Genelex company, the *1F* haplotype was identified as having the HI phenotype. To achieve consistency across the data set for *CYP1A2* in Table 1, we combined the results of HI into EM.

The gene for *CYP1A2* is located on chromosome 15 (15q24.1) outside the PWS critical region. Therefore, it is possible that in the PWS patient with maternal uniparental disomy 15 (UPD), the *CYP1A2* alleles may be identical. The clinical relevance of this depends upon the phenotypic activity determined by the *CYP1A2* alleles seen in the mother. Almost all people have 2 copies of the *CYP1A2* gene [38]. Among our cohort of patients with UPD, there were 3 duplications of alleles, whereas cohorts with DEL and PWS Unspecified had only one. Also, there were complex genotypes of *CYP1A2*, some with as many as 4 alleles. Clinical implications for treatment with these *CYP1A2* findings in PWS are discussed in Sections 4.1 and 4.2.

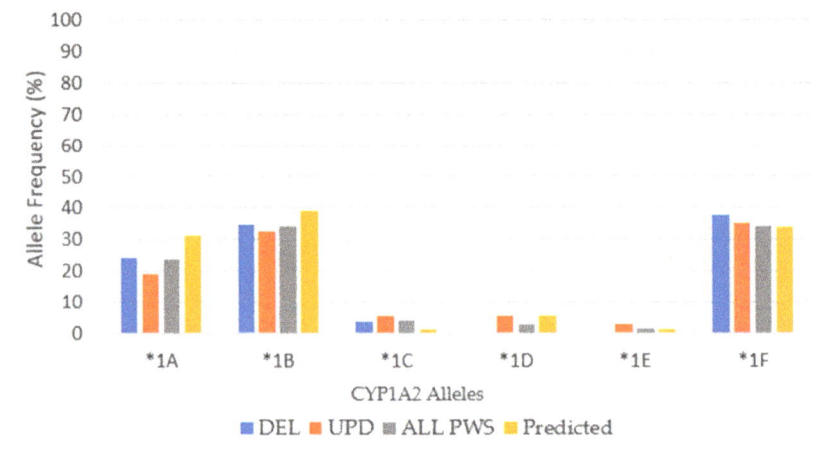

Figure 11. *CYP1A2* allelic frequencies in PWS DEL (*n* = 14), UPD (*n* = 16) and combined cohort (ALL PWS, *n* = 35) compared to normative Caucasian predicted values [37,38].

4. Discussion

The use of pharmacogenomic testing is now commonly obtained, particularly after an untoward result of a medication treatment trial. It provides guidance for medication selection and dosing. There are several studies suggesting that genotypically informed medication selection for treatment of depression increases response and remission rates, decreases adverse effects, and guides the use of adjunctive medications in challenging cases [39,40].

Knowledge of the pharmacogenetic phenotype can inform time parameters of treatment response. Ultra-rapid metabolizers are more likely to have a quicker, positive clinical response to antidepressant medication with several studies suggesting an increased risk of rehospitalization and emergency room visits [41]. In a study performed at the Institute of Living, those patients with the CYP2D6 ultra-rapid metabolizing genotype were more likely to be discharged early and to have at least one readmission within the month after discharge [42]. On the other hand, those patients with intermediate or slow metabolizing genotypes were likely to take a longer time to achieve a clinical treatment response, a longer duration of hospital stay, and a decreased likelihood of readmission in the 30 days after discharge [42]. In another study, intermediate metabolizers were more likely to have adverse effects to medications metabolized by CYP2D6 than extensive metabolizers at comparable doses [43].

Knowledge of the pharmacogenetic phenotype can inform dose response parameters [44]. For example, if a person has the poor metabolizing phenotype of CYP2D6, which metabolizes paroxetine exclusively, a typical starting dose of medication may produce a therapeutic effect, and according to Kirchheiner et al. the dose required for remission may be 65% of the standard dose [30]. If the person is an intermediate metabolizer, they may tolerate low to moderate doses of medication, but as the dose is titrated, their metabolic capacity may be exceeded resulting in side effects [45]. On the other hand, if a person is an ultra-rapid metabolizer, the half-life of the medication will be reduced and the patient may experience unpleasant withdrawal symptoms during the day [29], such as headache and gastrointestinal upset without fever, mood instability, and what is been described as the perception of a lightning bolts radiating down the arms. With this ultra-rapid genotype, these symptoms can be addressed by increasing the schedule of administration of medication across the day. As a result, and following the standard of care, the patient may require a higher total daily dose, e.g., for paroxetine, 135% of the standard dose, than typically recommended by the FDA for that medication and condition as discussed in Kirchheiner et al. [30].

Knowledge of the pharmacogenetic phenotypes can inform other parameters of medication response, including potential adverse effects. If a medication requires conversion to an active metabolite by the cytochrome enzyme system, the phenotype will determine the rate of activation. The best example of this is codeine, which requires CYP2D6 for conversion to the active metabolite morphine. Poor metabolizers of CYP2D6 are at risk for a poor analgesic response, as ultra-rapid metabolizers are at risk for toxicity [29]. Another example is risperidone, one of the most widely prescribed second generation antipsychotic medications among children and adolescents, including with PWS, with known efficacy and adverse effects, especially among those with autism spectrum disorder (ASD) and intellectual and developmental disabilities (IDD) [46]. Risperidone is primarily metabolized by CYP2D6 into another active metabolite, paliperidone, which is linearly related to serum prolactin level. Individuals with the ultra-rapid metabolizing phenotype of CYP2D6 may be more likely to display hyperprolactinemia [47]. In a study of 257 children and adolescents who received risperidone, 76 experienced a variety of adverse effects, and these were more commonly seen in the poor or intermediate metabolizing phenotype of CYP2D6 [48].

Knowledge of potential drug interactions can inform treatment and minimize adverse effects. Drug interactions can occur when using prescribed medications as well as over the counter (OTC) agents and nutraceuticals (herbs, supplements, or vitamins) [14].

4.1. Drug–Drug Interactions

Drug-drug interactions are a common cause of adverse events or failed treatment efficacy. Checking for potential drug interactions can be accomplished by examining the pharmacokinetic pathways for medication metabolism at https://www.pharmgkb.org/pathways and https://drug-interactions.medicine.iu.edu [32]. The Flockhart table is updated frequently and delineates the pharmacogenetic action of specific drugs that use the cytochrome P450 enzyme system. Drugs are delineated as substrates, inhibitors, or inducers for one or more cytochrome P450 enzymes. Medications administered concurrently that are substrates for the same cytochrome enzyme overwhelm the metabolic capacity of the cytochrome and interfere with efficacy or may result in toxicity [45]. If two drugs have the same affinity for an enzyme, they become competitive inhibitors in a dose related way [49]. If one of the drugs is a substrate for another cytochrome P450 enzyme with less affinity, metabolism may be shunted toward those less preferred pathways. An inducer is a drug or agent (e.g., cigarette smoking) that causes an increase in the production of the cytochrome enzyme by action at the promoter site on the gene and usually takes 1–2 weeks to occur [39,40]. An inhibitor is a drug or agent (e.g., cruciferous vegetables) that binds to the cytochrome enzyme and blocks its use; its effect is immediate and persistent for as long as the inhibitor remains in the system. Some medications act as both substrate and inhibitor (e.g., fluoxetine with CYP2D6), or substrate and inducer (e.g., carbamazepine with CYP3A4) [35].

Phenoconversion describes the process whereby a given CYP phenotype, inferred from genotype, is functionally converted to a higher or lower metabolic status on the basis of drug-drug interactions or the influence of non-genetic factors [50]. The resulting phenotype carries the designation of phenocopy because it imitates a different metabolic status. Phenoconversion is more likely to occur in drug-drug interactions when a substrate has a high affinity for a single CYP. For example, clozapine and olanzapine are selectively metabolized by CYP1A2; in the presence of cigarette smoking, phenoconversion to a higher metabolizing phenotype results in the reduction of serum drug levels by 20% [43]. In the case of aripiprazole, concurrent administration of a CYP2D6 inhibitor, such as bupropion or sertraline, can convert the 2D6 extensive metabolizing status downward, driving serum drug levels upward by 20–50%, precipitating adverse effects [51]. In another example, ratios of metabolic phenotypes that were inferred from genotype across cytochromes 2C9, 2C19, 2D6 and 3A4 were converted to a lower status in the presence of inflammation, as reviewed by Klomp et al. [50].

Table 2 itemizes psychotropic and other prescribed medications, OTC agents, nutraceuticals, and dietary/lifestyle factors that are substrates, inhibitors, or inducers of cytochrome P450 enzymes. Most of the items in this table were generated from clinical experience with persons who have PWS and by referencing Flockhart [32]. This table does not constitute a complete list of medications, nor is it a compendium of recommended therapeutic agents for patients with PWS.

Drug–drug interactions may occur with prescribed medications as well as OTC agents and nutraceuticals. OTC antihistamines, such as loratadine (substrate of CYP3A4), may interfere with metabolism of some antidepressants and antibiotics [52]. Chlorpheniramine and dextromethorphan, OTC agents used for common cold symptoms, are substrates for CYP2D6 [32]. Competition at the site of the enzyme receptor can displace risperidone and potentiate its efficacy producing increased sedation or extrapyramidal side effects such as akathisia. The anti-acid medication ranitidine, which was recently removed from the market, is a substrate for CYP2D6 and competes with several atypical antipsychotic medications, including risperidone [18]. Toxic side effects have been reported, including incapacitating sedation that was misdiagnosed as dementia in a patient with PWS. Similarly, omeprazole is a substrate for CYP2C19 and CYP2C9 and inhibits metabolism of many antidepressants contributing to the potential toxicity. Acetaminophen, a substrate for CYP1A2, and ibuprofen, a substrate for CYP2C9, may affect efficacy of psychotropic medications administered concurrently [38]. Melatonin, a substrate of CYP1A2, is commonly used for treatment of insomnia, and treatment with fluvoxamine results in increased serum melatonin [53].

Herbal or plant-based agents may also interact with psychotropic medications. Ginkgo biloba, used to treat memory and dyskinesias, has been associated with increased risk of hemorrhage in combination with SSRIs or SNRIs [54]. Ginseng, used to increase energy, stamina and well-being, has been associated with serotonin syndrome in combination with SSRIs or SNRIs, and ventricular arrythmias in combination with haloperidol [54]. Goldenseal, used for upper respiratory and gastrointestinal tract symptoms, is a potent inhibitor of CYP3A and CYP2D6 [53]. Milk thistle, used for diabetes or liver disease, has resulted in pancreatitis when co-administered with haloperidol or risperidone, and hepatotoxicity may occur with aripiprazole [54]. St. John's Wort, a natural occurring antidepressant, interferes with the efficacy of many pharmaceuticals due to induction of cytochromes 1A2, 2C9 and 3A4 [55]. Both cannabis and cannabidiol are substrates for CYP2C19 and CYP3A4 and inhibitors of CYP2D6 and CYPC9; also, cannabis is a substrate for CYP2C9, and cannabidiol is an inhibitor of CYP2C19 [56]. Their concurrent use with fluoxetine, a substrate for CYP2D6, CYP2C9, and CYP2C19 and an inhibitor of CYP2C9 and CYP2C19, can be expected to produce a complex drug interaction that may result in mood activation. Because each of these agents has a relatively long half-life, the onset of any clinically relevant interaction may be delayed, and once it is identified, the discontinuation of one of the medications will take a while to clear the body, so unpleasant symptoms may linger. The persistence of mood and behavioral symptoms may lead to the diagnosis of a co-morbid psychiatric condition or may require management with yet another psychotropic medication.

Table 2. Psychotropic medications, nutraceuticals, agents, and related cytochrome P450 enzymes.

Cytochrome	CYP1A2	CYP2B6	CYP2C19	CYP2C9	CYP2D6	CYP3A4-5
Substrate	Acetaminophen Amitriptyline, 3 Benztropine, 2 Caffeine Cannabidiol, 3 Chlorpromazine, 2 Clomipramine, 2 Clozapine, 1 Duloxetine, 1 Estradiol Fluvoxamine, 1 Haloperidol, 3 Imipramine, 2 Melatonin Mirtazapine, 3 Olanzapine, 1 Pimozide Propranolol, 1 Tacrine Thioridazine, 2	Bupropion, 1 Selegiline Sertraline, 1 Sibutramine	Amitriptyline, 1 Benztropine, 3 Cannabis, 1 Cannabidiol, 2 Citalopram, 1 Clomipramine, 1 Clozapine, 2 Diazepam Doxepin, 2 Escitalopram, 1 Estradiol Fluoxetine,3 Imipramine, 1 Nortriptyline, 2 Omeprazole Phenytoin Progesterone, 1 Sertraline, 2 Testosterone, 1 Venlafaxine, 2	Amitriptyline, 2 Benztropine, 4 Cannabidiol, 3 Cannabis, 3 Celecoxib Fluoxetine, 2 Ibuprofen, 1 Progesterone, 2 Sertraline, 3 Valproate Warfarin	Amitriptyline, 2 Amphetamine Aripiprazole, 2 Asenapine Atomoxetine Bupropion, 2 Cannabidiol, 3 Chlorpromazine, 1 Citalopram, 4 Clomipramine, 4 Clonidine Clozapine, 3 Desipramine, 4 Dextromethorphan Diphenhydramine Doxepin, 1 Escitalopram, 3 Fluoxetine, 1 Fluvoxamine, 2 Haloperidol, 1 Hydroxyzine Imipramine, 2 Mirtazapine, 2 Nortriptyline, 1 Olanzapine, 2 Paroxetine, 1 Perphenazine Propranolol, 2 Quetiapine, 2 Ranitidine Risperidone, 1 Sertraline, 2 Thioridazine, 1 Trazadone, 2 Venlafaxine, 1 Ziprasidone, 3	Alprazolam Aripiprazole, 1 Benztropine, 1 Bupropion, 2 Buspirone Cannabis, 2 Cannabidiol, 1 Cisapride Citalopram, 2 Clomipramine, 3 Clonazepam Carbamazepine Desvenlafaxine Dextromethorphan Duloxetine, 3 Escitalopram, 2 Estradiol Erythromycin Fexofenadine Guanfacine Haloperidol, 2 Loratadine Lurasidone Mirtazapine, 1 Modafinil Pimozide Progesterone, 3 Quetiapine, 1 Risperidone, 2 Sertraline, 3 Testosterone Trazadone, 1 Tiagabine Ziprasidone, 1 Zolpidem
Inhibitor	Cannabidiol Cannabis Celecoxib Cimetidine Citalopram Ciprofloxacin Clarithromycin Erythromycin Estradiol Fluvoxamine Isoniazid Ketoconazole Modafinil	Cannabidiol Cannabis	Cannabidiol Cannabis Cimetidine Contraceptives Fluconazole Fluoxetine Fluvoxamine Indomethacin Isoniazid Ketoconazole Lansoprazole Modafinil Omeprazole Oxcarbazepine Probenecid Topiramate	Cannabidiol Cannabis Cimetidine Contraceptives Fluconazole Fluoxetine Fluvoxamine Isoniazid Ketoconazole Methylphenidate Modafinil Omeprazole Paroxetine Sertraline Sulfonamides Tacrine	Asenapine Bupropion Cannabis Cannabidiol Diphenhydramine Fluoxetine Goldenseal Haloperidol Hydroxyzine Methylphenidate Paroxetine Propranolol Quinidine Ranitidine	Cannabidiol Cimetidine Ciprofloxacin Clarithromycin Cyclosporine Erythromycin Goldenseal Grapefruit juice Isoniazid Ketoconazole Prednisone Sertraline Verapamil
Inducer	Carbamazepine Cruciferous vegetables Cannabis (smoke) Char-grilling Omeprazole Phenytoin St. John's wort Tobacco (smoke)	Carbamazepine Modafinil Phenytoin Phenobarbital Rifampin	Rifampin	Carbamazepine Phenobarbital Rifampin St. John's wort		Carbamazepine Cruciferous vegetables Ginseng Modafinil Phenytoin Rifampin St. John's wort

Note: Pertinent information about medications and cytochrome selectivity in Table 2 was obtained from multiple sources including literature review, [http://www.pharmgkb.org/pathways] and the Flockhart website [32]. Substrates metabolized by more than one cytochrome are numbered 1, 2, or 3 to indicate binding affinity and to delineate primary, secondary, or tertiary pathways. Inhibition in one pathway has the potential to shunt metabolism through another pathway.

Another common drug-drug interaction is seen with SSRIs (citalopram, escitalopram and sometimes sertraline) and estradiol and/or progesterone (taken for hormone therapy, oral contraception, or occurring naturally with monthly menstrual cycles), which are substrates for CYP2C19. A woman receiving sertraline for depression who experiences premenstrual dysphoria may benefit from a transient dose increase during the luteal phase as progesterone levels increase [57,58]. Because puberty is often delayed or absent in PWS, hormone therapy is usually initiated during the age of typical adolescence. If SSRIs had been started previously, the addition of estradiol or a combination pill may compete with CYP2C19 metabolism altering serum levels and potentially precipitating mood and behavioral difficulties requiring a dose adjustment. Hormone therapy is likely to continue into adulthood in PWS to address lifelong osteopenia and osteoporosis.

The frequency of polypharmacy use identified in the NIH PWS Registry suggests that drug interactions, like the ones identified above, may be commonplace. Knowledge of pharmacogenetics may inform dose parameters as well as potential drug interactions. For patients with PWS, like others with intellectual and developmental disabilities, it is always advisable to try one medication at a time, or to add another medication after a new behavioral baseline has been established. This applies for hormone therapies and use of nutraceuticals as well.

4.2. Specific Relevance of Cytochrome P450 Enzyme System to PWS

There are factors that can change the phenotypic expression of the cytochrome P450 genes that are particularly relevant to PWS. *CYP3A4,5* is sexually dimorphic due to gonadal steroid effects on gene activity. There is evidence to suggest that growth hormone is a modulator of this gender specificity of function. Sinues and colleagues [59] examined CYP3A enzyme activity in 35 unrelated growth hormone deficient children (ages 2.9–13.1 years) both at baseline and after growth hormone replacement. At baseline, the level of activity of CYP3A was elevated compared to controls in a non-sex dependent manner. Then, after growth hormone replacement for 30 days, CYP3A activity was reduced to normal range in males but was unchanged in females. This typical sexual dimorphic level of activity for the CYP3A enzyme impacts serum levels of testosterone, gonadal steroids, as well as psychotropic drugs. This has special relevance for individuals with PWS who are likely to be growth hormone deficient and require growth hormone replacement as well as gonadal steroid therapy [1].

The activity of CYP1A2 has gender specificity also, with lower metabolic function in women than in men. [60,61]. The primary function of CYP1A2 is to purge potential environmental toxins, e.g., heterocyclic amines, and polycyclic hydrocarbons, that may act as carcinogens from the body. Pharmacogenetic studies have explored polymorphisms of these alleles as predisposing factors to the incidence of cancers of the urinary tract, colon, and rectum [37]. CYP1A2 is inhibited by estradiol, oral contraceptives, some antibiotics (ciprofloxacin and levofloxacin), and other drugs (fluvoxamine, celecoxib, and amiodarone). Polymorphisms of *CYP1A2* have been explored as predisposing factors for psychiatric illness [62]. Yenilmez et al. found that the allelic frequency of *CYP1A2*1F* among those with bipolar disorder was 25.5% and among those with schizophrenia, it was 69.4%, which is twice that predicted for normative population frequencies [62]. Because many psychotropic medications used for treating these conditions are also substrates for CYP1A2 (e.g., olanzapine, clozapine, haloperidol, fluvoxamine, duloxetine, tricyclic antidepressants, and clomipramine) [18], their metabolism is subject to the effects of induction, which reduces serum concentration and can interfere with treatment efficacy. Because of hypogonadism and delayed puberty in PWS, females are often prescribed estradiol or estrogen/progesterone combinations found in oral contraceptives, both of which inhibit gene expression and activity of CYP1A2. This inhibition may result in increased drug levels of substrates of CYP1A2 with potential toxicity [32,63].

CYP1A2 is highly inducible by dietary factors and lifestyle considerations [18]. Caffeine is a well-recognized substrate of CYP1A2, and it is used to determine enzyme activity [37]. The CYP1A2*1D and CYP1A2*1F alleles predict the ultra-rapid metabolizing phenotype when the enzymes are induced. Common inducers are tobacco and cannabis smoke, chargrilled meats, cruciferous vegetables (e.g., brussels sprout, broccoli, cauliflower, cabbage, radish, rocket, watercress, and wasabi), insulin, modafinil, nafcillin, omeprazole, and carbamazepine [14,38]. Xie at al. reviewed the magnitude of induction effects, with 3.5-fold increase in smokers vs. non-smokers and 25% increase with broccoli containing diets [63]. The inducibility of CYP1A2 by diet is particularly important to persons with PWS, many of whom follow the Red Yellow Green Diet that contains a high percentage of cruciferous vegetables that are low in calories and high in fiber [64]. Further, many persons with PWS are prescribed modafinil (CYP1A2 inhibitor) for excessive daytime sleepiness. Cigarette smoking and overuse of caffeinated beverages (CYP1A2 inducers) are not uncommon among adults with PWS. Severe skin picking may result in cellulitis that requires systemic antibiotic treatment (CYP1A2 inhibitors) [65]. Gastroesophageal reflux is common in PWS and often treated with proton pump inhibitors such as omeprazole (CYP1A2 inducer) [65,66].

4.3. Non-Genetic Factors Affecting Drug Pharmacokinetics in PWS

There are non-genetic pharmacokinetic factors determining dose response efficacy, and these factors are especially important in the pediatric population. In this report, the cytochrome system pertains to those enzymes in the liver responsible for metabolizing medications. Overall, the metabolic activity of the liver is increased during the developmental years before puberty such that metabolic clearance in children is twice as fast as in adolescence [29]. Therapeutic doses of medications metabolized by CYP1A2, CYP2C9 and CYP3A4 are much higher in children than compared to adults, and the bioavailability of medications that require first pass metabolism for activation is decreased [56]. Increased metabolism suggests a shorter half-life and indicates that the medication should be dosed more frequently through the day. These developmental changes are not seen with CYP2D6 or CYP2C19 [61].

Diseases or nutritional status that affect the liver function will impair metabolism at any age, such as steatohepatitis. In a study by Li et al., CYP2C19 activity was decreased by as much as 80% in adolescents with steatohepatitis (not steatosis) while activity of CYP1A2, CYP2C9 and CYP3A4 was unaltered, unlike the pattern of change in adults resulting in decreased activity of CYP2C19, CYP1A2 and CYP3A4, and increased activity of CYP2C9 [67].

There are other factors affecting drug metabolism such as body weight or body surface area that determine the daily dosage of medication before puberty. As reviewed by Li et al., obesity is associated with an increase in CYP1A2, CYP2C9, CYP2C19, and CYP2D6 activity in children, and a decrease in CYP1A2 and CYP3A4 activity in adults [67]. Body composition is also important, because lipophilic drugs accumulate in adipose tissue and prolong rate of excretion. The mode of delivery of medication (intramuscular, subcutaneous, or intravenous injection; intranasal, sublingual, or rectal administration; or topical application) can affect speed of onset of action, effectiveness on the target symptom, and extent of systemic side effects. Lifestyle factors can also affect cytochrome function, e.g., consumption of chargrilled foods and cruciferous vegetables induces CYP1A2 and CYP3A4 activity; grapefruit juice inhibits CYP3A4; caffeinated beverages inhibit CYP1A2, and smoking cigarettes or cannabis will induce CYP1A2 [60]. Stomach acidity can also affect absorption, and urine pH can affect excretion, especially with amphetamines [68].

Finally, compliance is the most important variable in determining medication efficacy. In general, the more frequently a medication must be administered, the higher the likelihood that doses will be missed. In the experience of PWS experts who administer care to patients with PWS, it is always preferable to start a regular acting medication first to ascertain dose and side effects before converting to a sustained release form (J.F, personal communication; [69]).

4.4. Limitations and Future Directions

The data presented in this clinical case series were obtained from approved commercial laboratories. Not all commercial pharmacogenomic platforms test the same cytochrome P450 genes and polymorphisms. Companies select the polymorphisms to test based on the patient population, the frequency of polymorphisms, and the clinical relevance for a particular field of medicine, e.g., oncology or psychiatry. Also, the clinical interpretation of testing results may differ. The genetic data obtained may be the same, e.g., both the number and type of alleles, but the designated phenotype is determined by combining results from several genes. The algorithm for this combinatorial approach is proprietary [19].

The idea for reporting this clinical case series was conceptualized after the initial collection of data within our respective clinical practices. The patients who received pharmacogenomic testing met medical necessity criteria set forth by the companies based on insurance coverage, including failure of at least one psychiatric medication. Therefore, our cohort represented a biased population of PWS patients who might be expected to have some alterations of cytochrome P450 function. In this case report, there is no PWS control group for comparison. In addition, the information available for each patient came from three different clinical centers, was subject to record availability (age, gender, ethnicity), and was deidentified prior to data collation and analysis. A history of psychotropic medication use as well as family history of psychiatric conditions and medication response was not discoverable. Also, non-genetic, environmental factors that may influence how these patients metabolize psychotropic medications were not known. Our data was limited to the genetic polymorphisms of selected cytochrome P450 enzymes, our interpretation of these findings, and the PWS genetic subtype of the patient. We have provided a descriptive analysis of these results.

This data set was limited in number and did not reach sufficient power for PWS-subtype analysis in all cases. In particular, the numbers were too small to undertake analysis of gene allele frequencies via Hardy-Weinberg equilibrium studies. None the less, we found statistically significant differences in the metabolizing status of cytochromes 2D6, 2C9, 2C19, 3A4 and 1A2. The results from our cohort may not reflect the general PWS patient population, as the patients referred to our specialty centers are often those who have complicated health/behavior/psychiatric concerns and have failed previous medication management. Further, our PWS cohort consisted of more patients with UPD (46%), which is higher than predicted based on studies showing that 35% of PWS individuals have this genetic subtype [1–3]. This may reflect that those with UPD may have more behavioral/psychiatric problems and are more likely to seek mental health intervention. In the future, a larger study of at least 100 subjects from the general population of persons with PWS would provide sufficient statistical power to correlate pharmacogenetic data with factors of age, gender, ethnicity, and family psychiatric history. Also, a larger study would offer greater insight and guidance into medication management in this rare population often presenting with significant psychiatric needs. Until a larger study is performed, the authors realize that the interpretation and generalization of these results is limited to our cohort of referred patients.

Except for *CYP1A2*, which is located on Ch 15, we cannot explain the frequency of phenotypic differences in the cytochrome P450 system noted in this case series. UPD status due to maternal isodisomy 15 may have altered *CYP1A2* allele frequencies in our referred cohort [2]. The most common etiology for CYP polymorphism is familial, which includes variations associated with ethnicity. The ethnicity of our 35 patients was deidentified, and we did not have access to familial psychiatric history. However, the NIH PWS Registry enrolled patients from PWS clinics at 4 sites in the USA, and the racial/ethnic diversity of these 355 patients was minimal with 93% Caucasian. As such, our phenotypic comparisons and statistical correlations were all based on normative Caucasian populations. It is highly unlikely that our pharmacogenetic findings in this PWS cohort were due to ethnic variability.

Finally, one of the criteria for obtaining pharmacogenetic testing includes failure to respond to current treatment with psychotropic medications. The PWS phenotype is a complicated mix of anxiety, stress sensitivity, mood lability, and disruptive behavior. Clinicians assume that these symptoms will respond to psychotropic medication. But it is possible that these symptoms require environmental, psychological, or behavioral management strategies for optimal response. Therefore, treatment failure with psychotropic medications alone cannot necessarily be attributed to polymorphisms of the cytochrome enzyme system.

5. Conclusions

This clinical case series of patients with known PWS subtype is the largest reported cohort to receive commercial pharmacogenomic testing. At first glance, the results from our combined cohort suggest that our patients with PWS had a wide array of alleles that were distributed in a manner consistent with natural variation. However, these patients were referred for evaluation and treatment, and not surprisingly, group differences were noted when comparing the results of PWS testing with normative population data. For example, 48.6% of the combined PWS cohort ($n = 35$) were extensive metabolizers of CYP2D6 compared to the typical population frequency of 63.6% among Americans. There were 36% intermediate metabolizers and 17.1% poor metabolizers compared to 23.6% and 2.2% respectively among Americans, which means that more than half of our PWS cohort had reduced function of CYP2D6. Further, there were differences between the molecular classes of PWS with the deletion subtype having fewer extensive metabolizers and more intermediate metabolizers; both DEL and UPD subtypes had more poor metabolizers compared to the normative American population. These results suggest that increased vigilance is required by clinicians for dose selection and speed of titration of psychotropic medications used in patients with PWS that are substrates for CYP2D6, such as aripiprazole, bupropion, chlorpromazine, citalopram, clonidine, doxepin, escitalopram, fluoxetine, haloperidol, imipramine, mirtazapine, olanzapine, quetiapine, risperidone, sertraline, trazodone, venlafaxine and ziprasidone. The clinical mantra of *start low and go slow* is recognized and indicated in the treatment of clinical symptoms among patients with PWS as well as other intellectual and developmental disabilities [45]. The increased frequency of ultra-rapid metabolizing status of CYP1A2 in PWS, especially among those with UPD, suggests that careful selection of drug dose is indicated for agents that are substrates, such as acetaminophen, benztropine, chlorpromazine, clomipramine, clozapine, duloxetine, estradiol, fluvoxamine, haloperidol, imipramine, mirtazapine, and olanzapine [32]. Further, growth hormone status and gender may play a role in pharmacokinetic parameters of patients receiving medications that are substrates for CYP3A4 primarily, such as aripiprazole, guanfacine, mirtazapine, modafinil, quetiapine, trazodone, and ziprasidone [32,69]. Also, both estradiol and testosterone are substrates for CYP3A4. Increased expression of the *CYP3A4*1B* allele was seen only among UPD in this case series. This allele has been associated with risk of prostate cancer, leukemia, early puberty and major depressive illness [64]. Gender may play a role in the dose selection for persons receiving bupropion or sertraline, as the number of CYP2B6 extensive metabolizers may be higher in PWS as a whole and among females with deletion subtype specifically [70]. A larger cohort of non-referred persons with PWS is needed to substantiate these preliminary pharmacogenetic findings and their applications to the clinical setting where patients with this rare disorder are treated.

In conclusion, like any medical test, pharmacogenetics testing requires that medical necessity criteria be met. These criteria include symptom severity, co-morbid illnesses, and number of failed medication treatment responses. These factors increase the likelihood that more than one medication will be used, as is often seen in PWS. Polypharmacy increases the potential for drug interactions. The pharmacogenetic data from this case series of referred PWS patients underscores the benefit of knowing the phenotypic function of the cytochrome P450 enzyme system to inform selection of psychotropic medication and dose to improve the care and treatment of those with this rare genetic condition. Although our cohort was too small to discover a unique pharmacogenetic phenotype among our patients, we did identify some statistically significant differences in phenotypic function compared to population norms and also between PWS genetic subtypes. Going forward, a larger cohort of non-referred persons with PWS must be studied to confirm these observations for widespread clinical application. Nonetheless, this data supports the use of pharmacogenetics testing in Prader-Willi syndrome.

Author Contributions: Conceptualization—J.F. and J.D.; Data collection—J.F., J.D., M.G.B.; Writing—original draft, J.F.; Writing, review, editing—J.F., J.D., M.G.B. All authors have read and agreed to the published version of the manuscript.

Funding: This case report received no external funding.

Institutional Review Board Statement: Ethical oversight and IRB approval were not required because the clinical care described in this article was not part of a research project. The results presented in this paper have been deidentified, will not affect the patient's clinical care, nor will they have the potential to cause the patient any harm. This article is a scholarly report of a clinical cohort of patients with PWS who received pharmacogenetic testing as part of their medical care at one of three specialty programs across the USA. This report will both inform and hopefully improve the quality of care of patients with PWS.

Informed Consent Statement: Patient consent for this case report was waived because all pertinent private and protected health information about each patient was eliminated prior to collation and analysis of data, except for the genetic subtype of PWS and the pharmacogenetic genotype.

Data Availability Statement: The data presented in this paper were obtained through public websites including literature review using PUBMED, public access websites, such as https://www.pharmgkb.org and http://drug-interactions.medicine.iu.edu [32], and standard reference books by Mrazek [38] and the PWS management book edited by Butler, Lee and Whitman [1]. The pharmacogenetic data obtained from the testing of our patients can be found in the Tables A2–A4. All the tables and figures contained in this article are derived from these data.

Acknowledgments: We thank Grace Graham for her expert preparation of this manuscript. We also acknowledge Linda Gourash, who is a Pittsburgh Partnership collaborator, Waheeda Hossain for statistical analysis, the patients with PWS and their families along with the Prader-Willi Syndrome Association (USA) for their support.

Conflicts of Interest: The authors declare no conflict of interest.

Appendix A

Table A1. Chromosome location for genes producing cytochrome P450 (CYP) enzymes, their common polymorphisms and phenotypic activity [38]; https://www.pharmgkb.org.

Cytochrome P450	Chromosome Location	Common Alleles and Phenotypic Action
CYP2D6	22q13.1	*1 (wildtype); *2 (normal); *2A (increased action); *9, *10, *17, *41 (decreased action); *4, *3,* 5, *6 (inactive).
CYP2B6	19q13.2	*1 (wildtype); *2, *5, *17 (normal); *4, *22 (increased action); *6, *7, *9, *16, *19, *20 (decreased action); *8, *12, *13, *18,*24 (inactive).
CYP2C19	10q24.1–q24.3	*1 (wildtype); *11, *13, *15, *18,*28 (normal); *17 (increased action); *9, *10, *16, *19, *25, *26 (decreased action); *2-*8, *22, *24, *35-*37 (inactive).
CYP2C9	10q23.33	*1 (wildtype); *9 (normal); *2, *3 (decreased action); *6, *15, *25 (inactive).
CYP3A4	7q22.1	*1 (wildtype); *7, *9, *10 (normal); *1B, *2-*6, *8, *11-*13, *15-*18, *22 (decreased action); *20, *26 (inactive).
CYP1A2	15q24.1	*1, *1A, *1B (wildtype); *1D (T-delT), *1F(C/A) increased action when induced; *1C(G/A); *1K(C/A); *3(T/C), *4(A/T), *7(G/A) (decreased action).

Table A2. Pharmacogenetic data for cytochrome P450 enzymes in PWS cohort with Deletion: Testing laboratory, CYP genotype, and CYP phenotype.

	CYP2D6		*CYP2B6*		*CYP2C19*		*CYP2C9*		*CYP3A4*		*CYP1A2*	
Lab	**Alleles**	**PT**	**Alleles**	**PT**	**Alleles**	**PT**	**Alleles**	**PT**	**Alleles**	**PT**	**Alleles**	**PT**
GS	*1/*1	EM	*1/*6	IM	*1/*1	EM	*1/*1	EM	*1/*1	EM	*1F/*1B	UM
GS	*4/*41	PM	*1/*6	IM	*1/*17	EM	*1/*1	EM	*1/*1	EM	*1A/*1B	EM
GS	*2/*17 DUP	EM	*1/*6	IM	*1/*17	EM	*1/*1	EM	*1/*1	EM	*1A/*1B	EM
GS	*2/*4	IM	*1/*1	EM	*1/*17	EM	*1/*1	EM	*1/*22	IM	*1A/*1B	EM
GS	*1/*10	IM	*1/*6	IM	*17/*17	UM	*1/*1	EM	*1/*1	EM	*1F/*1B	UM
GL	*2A/*5	IM	*1/*5	EM	*1/*1	EM	NA	NA	*1/*22	IM	*1A/*1A	EM
GS	*4/*4	PM	*1/*1	EM	*1/*1	EM	*1/*1	EM	*1/*1	EM	*1F/*1B	UM
GS	*1/*41	EM	*1/*1	EM	*1/*2	IM	*1/*1	EM	*1/*1	EM	*1F/*1B	UM
GS	*1/*9	IM	*1/*6	IM	*1/*17	EM	*1/*1	EM	*1/*1	EM	*1F/*1B	UM
GS	*1/*9	IM	*1/*1	EM	*1/*17	EM	*1/*2	IM	*1/*1	EM	*1A/*1B	EM
GL	*1/*4	IM	*1/*5	EM	*1/*1	EM	*1/*2	IM	*1/*1	EM	*1A/*1F	HI
GL	*1/*4	IM	*1/*6	IM	*1/*1	EM	*1/*1	EM	*1/*1	EM	*1C*1F/*1F	HI
GS	*1/*4	IM	*1/*1	EM	*1/*1	EM	*1/*2	IM	*1/*1	EM	*1F/*1B	UM
GL	*1/*1	EM	*5/*6	IM	*1/*17	UM	*1/*1	EM	*1/*1	EM	*1F/*1F	HI

Key: Genesight (GS), Genelex (GL); PT—Phenotype; PM—poor metabolizer; IM—intermediate metabolizer; EM—extensive (normal) metabolizer; UM—ultra-rapid metabolizer; NA—result not available; HI—hyperinducer.

Table A3. Pharmacogenetic data for cytochrome P450 enzymes in PWS cohort with UPD: Testing laboratory, CYP genotype, and CYP phenotype.

	CYP2D6		*CYP2B6*		*CYP2C19*		*CYP2C9*		*CYP3A4*		*CYP1A2*	
Lab	**Alleles**	**PT**	**Alleles**	**PT**	**Alleles**	**PT**	**Alleles**	**PT**	**Alleles**	**PT**	**Alleles**	**PT**
GS	*1/*1	EM	*1/*6	IM	*1/*1	EM	*1/*1	EM	*1/*1	EM	*1C*1D/ *1F*1B	UM
GS	*1/*4	IM	*1/*6	IM	*1/*1	EM	*1/*3	IM	*1/*1	EM	*1F/*1B	UM
GS	*1/*2A	EM	*1/*6	IM	*1/*1	EM	*1/*1	EM	*1/*1	EM	*1F/*1B	UM
GS	*1/*41	EM	*1/*6	IM	*1/*17	EM	*1/*1	EM	*1/*1	EM	*1A*1C/ *1B	IM
GS	*1/*4	EM	*1/*6	IM	*1/*1	EM	*1/*2	IM	*1/*1	EM	*1D*1E/ *1F*1B	UM
GS	*2A/*4	EM	*1/*1	EM	*2/*17	EM	*1/*1	EM	*1/*1	EM	*1F/*1B	UM
GS	*1/*2A	EM	*1/*6	IM	*1/*17	EM	*1/*1	EM	*1/*1	EM	*1F/*1B	UM
GS	*10/*41	PM	*1/*1	EM	*1/*17	EM	*1/*1	EM	*1/*1	EM	*1A/*1B	EM
GS	*1/*5	IM	*1/*1	EM	*1/*1	EM	*1/*2	IM	*1/*1	EM	*1F/*1B	UM
GS	*1/*3	IM	NA	NA	*1/*1	EM	*1/*3	IM	*NA*	NA	*1F/*1B	UM
GS	*1/*41	EM	*1/*6	IM	*2/*17	EM	*1/*1	EM	*1/*1	EM	*1A/*1A	EM
GS	*4/*41	PM	*1/*1	EM	*1/*17	EM	*1/*1	EM	*1/*1	EM	*1A/*1A	EM
GS	*4/*41	PM	*1/*6	IM	*1/*1	EM	*2/*2	PM	*1/*1	EM	*1F/*1B	UM
GM	*2/*41 Dup	EM	*1/*6	IM	*1/*1	EM	*1/*1	EM	*1/*22	IM	*1A/*1F	EM
GS	*1/*4	IM	*1/*1	EM	*1/*1	EM	*1/*2	IM	*1/*22	IM	*1F/*1B	UM
GL	*1/*2A	EM	*2/*5	IM	*1/*1	EM	*1/*2	IM	*1/*1B	IM	*1F/*1F	HI

Key: Genesight (GS), Genelex (GL), and Genomind (GM); PT—Phenotype; PM—poor metabolizer; IM—intermediate metabolizer; EM—extensive (normal) metabolizer; UM—ultra-rapid metabolizer; HI—hyperinducer; NA—result not available.

Table A4. Pharmacogenetic data for cytochrome P450 enzymes in PWS Unspecified cohort (DNA methylation positive, subtype unspecified): Testing laboratory, CYP genotype, and CYP phenotype.

	CYP2D6		CYP2B6		CYP2C19		CYP2C9		CYP3A4		CYP1A2	
Lab	Alleles	PT	Alleles	PT	Alleles	PT	Alleles	PT	Alleles	PT	Alleles	PT
GS	*2A/*4	EM	*1/*1	EM	*1/*1	EM	*1/*3	IM	*1/*1	EM	*1A/*1B	EM
GS	*1/*1	EM	*1/*1	EM	*1/*8	IM	*1/*2	IM	*1/*1	EM	*1F/*1B	UM
GS	*1/*1	EM	*1/*1	EM	*1/*1	EM	*1/*2	IM	*1/*1	EM	*1A/*1B	EM
GS	*6/*41	PM	*1/*1	EM	*1/*17	EM	*1/*1	EM	*1/*1	EM	*1F/*1B	UM
GS	*1/*1	EM	*1/*1	EM	*1/*2	IM	*1/*1	EM	*1/*1	EM	*1A/*1A	EM

Key: Genesight (GS); PT—Phenotype; PM—poor metabolizer; IM—intermediate metabolizer; EM—extensive (normal) metabolizer; UM—ultra-rapid metabolizer.

Table A5. Ratios of Cytochrome P450 phenotypes among PWS genetic subtypes.

PWS	CYP2D6	CYP2B6	CYP2C19	CYP2C9	CYP3A4	CYP1A2
DEL	4EM:8IM:2PM	7EM:7IM	2UM:11EM:1IM	10EM:3IM	12EM:2IM	6UM:3HI:5EM
UPD	9EM:4IM:3PM	6EM:9IM	16EM	9EM:6IM:1PM	12EM:3IM	10UM:1HI:4EM:1IM
UnSpec	4EM:1PM	5EM	3EM:2IM	2EM:3IM	5EM	2UM:3EM

Key: UM—ultra-rapid metabolizer; EM—extensive (normal) metabolizer; IM—intermediate metabolizer; PM—poor metabolizer; HI—hyperinducer; DEL—deletion; UPD—uniparental disomy; UnSpec—unspecified genetic subtype.

References

1. Butler, M.G.; Lee, P.D.K.; Whitman, B.Y. *Management of Prader-Willi Syndrome*; Springer: New York, NY, USA, 2006.
2. Butler, M.G.; Hartin, S.N.; Hossain, W.A.; Manzardo, A.M.; Kimonis, V.; Dykens, E.; Gold, J.A.; Kim, S.J.; Weisensel, N.; Tamura, R.; et al. Molecular genetic classification in Prader-Willi syndrome: A multisite cohort study. *J. Med. Genet.* **2019**, *56*, 149–153. [CrossRef] [PubMed]
3. Butler, M.G.; Manzardo, A.M.; Forster, J.L. Prader-Willi syndrome: Clinical genetics and diagnostic aspects with treatment approaches. *Curr. Pediatr. Rev.* **2016**, *12*, 136–166. [CrossRef] [PubMed]
4. Miller, J.L.; Lynn, C.H.; Driscoll, D.C.; Goldstone, A.P.; Gold, J.A.; Kimonis, V.; Dykens, E.; Butler, M.G.; Shuster, J.J.; Dris-coll, D.J. Nutritional phases in Prader-Willi syndrome. *Am. J. Med. Genet. A* **2011**, *155*, 1040–1049. [CrossRef] [PubMed]
5. Crinò, A.; Fintini, D.; Bocchini, S.; Grugni, G. Obesity management in Prader-Willi syndrome: Current perspectives. *Diabetes Metab. Syndr. Obes.* **2018**, *11*, 579–593. [CrossRef]
6. Skokauskas, N.; Sweeny, E.; Meehan, J.; Gallagher, L. Mental health problems in children with Prader-Willi syndrome. *J. Can. Acad. Child. Adolesc. Psychiatry* **2012**, *21*, 194–203. [CrossRef] [PubMed]
7. Zarcone, J.; Napolitano, D.; Peterson, C.; Breidbord, J.; Ferraioli, S.; Caruso-Anderson, M.; Holsen, L.; Butler, M.G.; Thomp-son, T. The relationship between compulsive behaviour and academic achievement across the three genetic subtypes of Prader-Willi syndrome. *J. Intellect. Disabil. Res.* **2007**, *51 Pt 6*, 478–487. [CrossRef]
8. Novell-Alsina, R.; Esteba-Castillo, S.; Caixàs, A.; Gabau, E.; Giménez-Palop, O.; Pujol, J.; Deus, J.; Torrents-Rodas, D. Compulsions in Prader-Willi syndrome: Occurrence and severity as a function of genetic subtype. *Actas Esp. Psiquiatr.* **2019**, *47*, 79–87. [PubMed]
9. Bennett, J.A.; Germani, T.; Haqq, A.M.; Zwaigenbaum, L. Autism spectrum disorder in Prader-Willi syndrome: A systematic review. *Am. J. Med. Gen. A* **2015**, *167*, 2936–2944. [CrossRef]
10. Sinnema, M.; Boer, H.; Collin, P.; Maaskant, M.A.; van Roozendaal, K.E.; Schrander-Stumpel, C.T.; Curfs, L.M. Psychiatric illness in a cohort of adults with Prader-Willi syndrome. *Res. Dev. Disabil.* **2011**, *32*, 1729–1735. [CrossRef]
11. Manzardo, A.M.; Weisensel, N.; Ayala, S.; Hossain, W.; Butler, M.G. Prader-Willi syndrome genetic subtypes and clinical neuropsychiatric diagnoses in residential care adults. *Clin. Genet.* **2018**, *93*, 622–631. [CrossRef]
12. Butler, M.G.; Kimonis, V.; Dykens, E.; Gold, J.A.; Miller, J.; Tamura, R.; Driscoll, D.J. Prader-Willi syndrome and early-onset morbid obesity NIH rare disease consortium: A review of natural history study. *Am. J. Med. Genet. A* **2018**, *176*, 368–375. [CrossRef] [PubMed]
13. Forster, J.L. Pearls: Use of psychotropic medication in PWS. In Proceedings of the Scientific Conference of the Prader-Willi Syndrome Association-USA Conference, Orlando, FL, USA, 23–24 October 2019.
14. Samer, C.F.; Lorenzini, K.I.; Rollason, V.; Daali, Y.; Desmeules, J.A. Applications of CYP450 testing in the clinical setting. *Mol. Diag.* **2013**, *17*, 165–184. [CrossRef] [PubMed]
15. Miksys, S.L.; Tyndale, R.F. Drug-metabolizing cytochrome P450s in the brain. *J. Psychiatry Neurosci.* **2002**, *27*, 406–415. [PubMed]
16. Nebert, D.W.; Wikvall, K.; Miller, W.L. Human cytochromes P450 in health and disease. *Philos. Trans. R. Soc. Lond. B Biol. Sci.* **2013**, *368*, 20120431. [CrossRef] [PubMed]

17. Zanger, U.M.; Schwab, M. Cytochrome P450 enzymes in drug metabolism: Regulation of gene expression, enzyme activities, and impact of genetic variation. *Pharmacol. Ther.* **2013**, *138*, 103–141. [CrossRef]
18. Butler, M.G. Pharmacogenetics and psychiatric care: A review and commentary. *J. Ment. Health Clin. Psychol.* **2018**, *2*, 17–24. [CrossRef] [PubMed]
19. Gross, T.; Daniel, J. Overview of pharmacogenomic testing in clinical practice. *Ment. Health Clin.* **2018**, *8*, 235–241. [CrossRef]
20. Zhou, Y.; Ingelman-Sundberg, M.; Lauschke, V.M. Worldwide distribution of cytochrome P450 alleles: A meta-analysis of population-scale sequencing projects. *Clin. Pharm.* **2017**, *102*, 688–700. [CrossRef]
21. Roof, E.; Dykens, E. The use of psychotropic medications in Prader-Willi syndrome. *Gathered View* **2006**, *31*, 3.
22. Durette, J.R.; Gourash, L.G.; Forster, J.L. Risks and benefits of SSRI medication in young people with PWS. In Proceedings of the PWSA Scientific Conference, Baton Rouge, LA, USA, 17–20 October 2012.
23. Gourash, L.M.; Durette, J.R.; Forster, J.L. SSRI medication in children, adolescents and young adults with PWS: A cautionary report. In Proceedings of the PWS Mental Health Research Strategy Workshop, Bethesda, ML, USA, 1–3 March 2015.
24. Martis, S.; Peter, I.; Hulot, J.S.; Kornreich, R.; Desnick, R.J.; Scott, S.A. Multi-ethnic distribution of clinically relevant CYP2C genotypes and haplotypes. *Pharm. J.* **2013**, *13*, 369–377. [CrossRef]
25. Li-Wan-Po, A.; Girard, T.; Farndon, P.; Cooley, C.; Lithgow, J. Pharmacogenetics of CYP2C19: Functional and clinical im-plications of a new variant CYP2C19*17. *Br. J. Clin. Pharmacol.* **2010**, *69*, 222–230. [CrossRef] [PubMed]
26. Butler, M.A.; Lang, N.P.; Young, J.F.; Caporaso, N.E.; Vineis, P.; Hayes, R.B.; Teitel, C.H.; Massengill, J.P.; Lawsen, M.F.; Kadlubar, F.F. Determination of CYP1A2 and NAT2 phenotypes in human populations by analysis of caffeine urinary me-tabolites. *Pharmacogenetics* **1992**, *2*, 116–127. [CrossRef] [PubMed]
27. Muscat, J.E.; Pittman, B.; Kleinman, W.; Lazarus, P.; Stellman, S.D.; Richie, J.P., Jr. Comparison of CYP1A2 and NAT2 pheno-types between black and white smokers. *Biochem. Pharmacol.* **2008**, *76*, 929–937. [CrossRef]
28. Al-Ahmad, M.M.; Amir, N.; Dhanasekaran, S.; John, A.; Abdulrazzaq, Y.M.; Ali, B.R.; Bastaki, S. Genetic polymorphisms of cytochrome P450-1A (CYP1A2) among Emiratis. *PLoS ONE* **2017**, *12*, e0183424. [CrossRef] [PubMed]
29. Wehry, A.M.; Ramsey, L.; Dulemba, S.E.; Mossman, S.A.; Strawn, J.R. Pharmacogenomic Testing in Child and Adolescent Psychiatry: An Evidence-Based Review. *Curr. Probl. Pediatr. Adol. Health Care* **2018**, *48*, 40–49. [CrossRef] [PubMed]
30. Kirchheiner, J.; Nickchen, K.; Bauer, M.; Wong, M.L.; Licinio, J.; Roots, I.; Brockmöller, J. Pharmacogenetics of antidepres-sants and antipsychotics: The contribution of allelic variations to the phenotype of drug response. *Mol. Psychiatry* **2004**, *9*, 442–473. [CrossRef] [PubMed]
31. Flockhart, D.A.; Oesterheld, J.R. Cytochrome P450-mediated drug interactions. *Child. Adolesc. Psychiatr. Clin. N. Am.* **2000**, *9*, 43–76. [CrossRef] [PubMed]
32. Flockhart, D.A. Drug Interactions: Cytochrome P450 Drug Interaction Table. Indiana University School of Medicine. 2007. Available online: https://drug-interactions.medicine.iu.edu (accessed on 12 July 2020).
33. Zeigler-Johnson, C.M.; Walker, A.H.; Mancke, B.; Spangler, E.; Jalloh, M.; McBride, S.; Deitz, A.; Malkowicz, S.B.; Ofori-Adjei, D.; Gueye, S.M.; et al. Ethnic differences in the frequency of prostate cancer susceptibility alleles at SRD5A32 and CYP3A4. *Hum. Hered.* **2002**, *54*, 13–21. [CrossRef]
34. Saiz-Rodríguez, M.; Almenara, S.; Navares-Gómez, M.; Ochoa, D.; Román, M.; Zubiaur, P.; Koller, D.; Santos, M.; Mejía, G.; Borobia, A.M.; et al. Effect of the Most Relevant CYP3A4 and CYP3A5 Polymorphisms on the Pharmacokinetic Parameters of 10 CYP3A Substrates. *Biomedicines* **2020**, *8*, 94. [CrossRef]
35. Elens, L.; van Gelder, T.; Hesselink, D.A.; Haufroid, V.; van Schaik, R.H. CYP3A4*22: Promising newly identified CYP3A4 variant allele for personalizing pharmacotherapy. *Pharmacogenomics* **2013**, *14*, 47–62. [CrossRef]
36. Świechowski, R.; Jeleń, A.; Mirowski, M.; Talarowska, M.; Gałecki, P.; Pietrzak, J.; Wodziński, D.; Balcerczak, E. Estimation of CYP3A4*1B single nucleotide polymorphism in patients with recurrent Major Depressive Disorder. *Mol. Genet. Genom. Med.* **2019**, *7*, e669. [CrossRef] [PubMed]
37. Sachse, C.; Bhambra, U.; Smith, G.; Lightfoot, T.J.; Barrett, J.H.; Scollay, J.; Garner, R.C.; Boobis, A.R.; Wolf, C.R.; Gooderham, N.J. Colorectal Cancer Study Group Polymorphisms in the cytochrome P450 CYP1A2 gene (CYP1A2) in colorectal cancer patients and controls: Allele frequencies, linkage disequilibrium and influence on caffeine metabolism. *Br. J. Clin. Pharm.* **2003**, *55*, 68–76. [CrossRef] [PubMed]
38. Mrazek, D. *Psychiatric Pharmacogenomics*; Guilford Press: New York, NY, USA, 2010.
39. Bradley, P.; Shiekh, M.; Mehra, V.; Vrbicky, K.; Layle, S.; Olson, M.C.; Maciel, A.; Cullors, A.; Garces, J.A.; Lukowiak, A.A. Improved efficacy with targeted pharmacogenetic-guided treatment of patients with depression and anxiety: A randomized clinical trial demonstrating clinical utility. *J. Psychiatr. Res.* **2018**, *96*, 100–107. [CrossRef] [PubMed]
40. Greden, J.F.; Parikh, S.V.; Rothschild, A.J.; Thase, M.E.; Dunlop, B.W.; DeBattista, C.; Conway, C.R.; Forester, B.P.; Mondimore, F.M.; Shelton, R.C.; et al. Impact of pharmacogenomics on clinical outcomes in major depressive disorder in the GUIDED trial: A large, patient- and rater-blinded, randomized, controlled study. *J. Psychiatr. Res.* **2019**, *111*, 59–67. [CrossRef]
41. Takahashi, P.Y.; Ryu, E.; Pathak, J.; Jenkins, G.D.; Batzler, A.; Hathcock, M.A.; Black, J.L.; Olson, J.E.; Cerhan, J.R.; Bielinski, S.J. Increased risk of hospitalization for ultra-rapid metabolizers of cytochrome P450 2D6. *Pharm. Pers. Med.* **2017**, *10*, 39–47. [CrossRef]

42. Ruaño, G.; Szarek, B.L.; Villagra, D.; Gorowski, K.; Kocherla, M.; Seip, R.L.; Goethe, J.W.; Schwartz, H.I. Length of psychiatric hospitalization is correlated with CYP2D6 functional status in inpatients with major depressive disorder. *Biomark. Med.* **2013**, *7*, 429–439. [CrossRef]
43. Laika, B.; Leucht, S.; Heres, S.; Steimer, W. Intermediate metabolizer: Increased side effects in psychoactive drug therapy. The key to cost-effectiveness of pretreatment CYP2D6 screening? *Pharm. J.* **2009**, *9*, 395–403. [CrossRef]
44. Seeringer, A.; Kirchheiner, J. Pharmacogenetics-guided dose modifications of antidepressants. *Clin. Lab. Med.* **2008**, *28*, 619–626. [CrossRef]
45. Mrazek, D.A. Psychiatric pharmacogenomic testing in clinical practice. *Dialogues Clin. Neurosci.* **2010**, *12*, 69–76, PM-CID:PMC3181940. [PubMed]
46. Fallah, M.S.; Shaikh, M.R.; Neupane, B.; Rusiecki, D.; Bennett, T.A.; Beyene, J. Atypical Antipsychotics for Irritability in Pe-diatric Autism: A Systematic Review and Network Meta-Analysis. *J. Child. Adolesc. Psychopharmacol.* **2019**, *29*, 168–180. [CrossRef]
47. Troost, P.W.; Lahuis, B.E.; Hermans, M.H.; Buitelaar, J.K.; van Engeland, H.; Scahill, L.; Minderaa, R.B.; Hoekstra, P.J. Prolac-tin release in children treated with risperidone: Impact and role of CYP2D6 metabolism. *J. Clin. Psychopharmacol.* **2007**, *27*, 52–57. [CrossRef] [PubMed]
48. Oshikoya, K.A.; Neely, K.M.; Carroll, R.J.; Aka, I.T.; Maxwell-Horn, A.C.; Roden, D.M.; Van Driest, S.L. CYP2D6 genotype and adverse events to risperidone in children and adolescents. *Pediatr. Res.* **2019**, *85*, 602–606. [CrossRef] [PubMed]
49. Guengerich, F.P. A history of the roles of cytochrome P450 enzymes in the toxicity of drugs. *Toxicol. Res.* **2020**, 1–23. [CrossRef] [PubMed]
50. Klomp, S.D.; Manson, M.L.; Guchelaar, H.J.; Swen, J.J. Phenoconversion of Cytochrome P450 Metabolism: A Systematic Re-view. *J. Clin. Med.* **2020**, *9*, 2890. [CrossRef] [PubMed]
51. Kiss, Á.; Menus, Á.; Tóth, K.; Déri, M.; Sirok, D.; Gabri, E.; Belic, A.; Csukly, G.; Bitter, I.; Monostory, K. Phenoconversion of CYP2D6 by inhibitors modifies aripiprazole exposure. *Eur. Arch. Psychiatry Clin. Neurosci.* **2020**, *270*, 71–82. [CrossRef] [PubMed]
52. Kloosterboer, S.M.; McGuire, T.; Deckx, L.; Moses, G.; Verheij, T.; van Driel, M.L. Self-medication for cough and the common cold: Information needs of consumers. *Aust. Fam. Physician* **2015**, *44*, 497–501. [PubMed]
53. Härtter, S.; Wang, X.; Weigmann, H.; Friedberg, T.; Arand, M.; Oesch, F.; Hiemke, C. Differential effects of fluvoxamine and other antidepressants on the biotransformation of melatonin. *J. Clin. Psychopharm.* **2001**, *21*, 167–174. [CrossRef]
54. Woroń, J.; Siwek, M. Unwanted effects of psychotropic drug interactions with medicinal products and diet supplements containing plant extracts. *Psychiatry Pol.* **2018**, *52*, 983–996. [CrossRef]
55. Zhang, X.L.; Chen, M.; Zhu, L.L.; Zhou, Q. Therapeutic risk and benefits of concomitantly using herbal medicines and con-ventional medicines: From the perspectives of evidence based on randomized controlled trials and clinical risk manage-ment. *Evid. Based Complement. Altern. Med.* **2017**, *2017*, 9296404. [CrossRef]
56. Lucas, C.J.; Galettis, P.; Schneider, J. The pharmacokinetics and the pharmacodynamics of cannabinoids. *Br. J. Clin Pharmacol.* **2018**, *84*, 2477–2482. [CrossRef]
57. Miller, L.J.; Girgis, C.; Gupta, R. Depression and related disorders during the female reproductive cycle. *Women's Health (Lond.)* **2009**, *5*, 577–587. [CrossRef] [PubMed]
58. Roomruangwong, C.; Carvalho, A.F.; Comhaire, F.; Maes, M. Lowered plasma steady-state levels of progesterone com-bined with declining progesterone levels during the luteal phase predict peri-menstrual syndrome and its major subdo-mains. *Front. Psychol.* **2019**, *10*, 2446. [CrossRef] [PubMed]
59. Sinués, B.; Mayayo, E.; Fanlo, A.; Mayayo, E., Jr.; Bernal, M.L.; Bocos, P.; Bello, E.; Labarta, J.I.; Ferrández-Longás, A. Effects of growth hormone deficiency and rhGH replacement therapy on the 6beta-hydroxycortisol/free cortisol ratio, a marker of CYP3A activity, in growth hormone-deficient children. *Eur. J. Clin. Pharm.* **2004**, *60*, 559–564. [CrossRef]
60. Landi, M.T.; Sinha, R.; Lang, N.P.; Kadlubar, F.F. Human cytochrome P4501A2. *IARC Sci. Publ.* **1999**, *148*, 173–195. [PubMed]
61. Anderson, G.D.; Lynn, A.M. Optimizing pediatric dosing: A developmental pharmacologic approach. *Pharmacotherapy* **2009**, *29*, 680–690. [CrossRef]
62. Yenilmez, E.D.; Tamam, L.; Karaytug, O.; Tuli, A. Characterization of CYP1A2, CYP2C9, CYP2C19 and CYP2D6 polymor-phisms using HRMA in psychiatry patients with schizophrenia and bipolar disease for personalized medicine. *Comb. Chem High Throughput Screen.* **2018**, *21*, 374–380. [CrossRef]
63. Xie, C.; Pogribna, M.; Word, B.; Lyn-Cook, L., Jr.; Lyn-Cook, B.D.; Hammons, G.J. In vitro analysis of factors influencing CYP1A2 expression as potential determinants of interindividual variation. *Pharmacol. Res. Perspect.* **2017**, *5*, e00299. [CrossRef]
64. Gourash, L.M.; Hanchett, J.E.; Forster, J.L. Inpatient Crisis Intervention for Persons with PWS. In *Management of Prader-Willi Syndrome*, 3rd ed.; Butler, L., Whitman, Eds.; Springer: Cham, Switzerland, 2006; p. 418.
65. Butler, M.G.; Miller, J.L.; Forster, J.L. Prader-Willi Syndrome—Clinical Genetics, Diagnosis and Treatment Approaches: An Update. *Curr. Pediatr. Rev.* **2019**, *15*, 207–244. [CrossRef]
66. Saeves, R.; Strøm, F.; Sandvik, L.; Nordgarden, H. Gastro-oesophageal reflux—An important causative factor of severe tooth wear in Prader-Willi syndrome? *Orphanet. J. Rare Dis.* **2018**, *13*, 64. [CrossRef]
67. Li, H.; Canet, M.J.; Clarke, J.D.; Billheimer, D.; Xanthakos, S.A.; Lavine, J.E.; Erickson, R.P.; Cherrington, N.J. Pediatric cyto-chrome P450 activity alterations in nonalcoholic steatohepatitis. *Drug Metab. Dispos.* **2017**, *45*, 1317–1325. [CrossRef]

68. López, F.A.; Leroux, J.R. Long-acting stimulants for treatment of attention-deficit/hyperactivity disorder: A focus on ex-tended-release formulations and the prodrug lisdexamfetamine dimesylate to address continuing clinical challenges. *Atten. Defic. Hyperact. Disord.* **2013**, *5*, 249–265. [CrossRef] [PubMed]
69. Lamba, J.K.; Lin, Y.S.; Schuetz, E.G.; Thummel, K.E. Genetic contribution to variable human CYP3A-mediated metabolism. *Adv. Drug Del. Rev.* **2002**, *54*, 1271–1294. [CrossRef]
70. Anderson, G.D. Gender differences in pharmacological response. *Int. Rev. Neurobiol.* **2008**, *83*, 1–10. [CrossRef] [PubMed]

MDPI

St. Alban-Anlage 66

4052 Basel

Switzerland

Tel. +41 61 683 77 34

Fax +41 61 302 89 18

www.mdpi.com

Genes Editorial Office

E-mail: genes@mdpi.com

www.mdpi.com/journal/genes

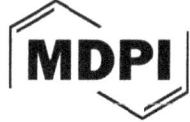

www.ingramcontent.com/pod-product-compliance
Lightning Source LLC
Chambersburg PA
CBHW042022080526
44654CB00092B/222